Blackwell's Five-Minute
Veterinary Consult
Clinical Companion

Small Animal Endocrinology and Reproduction

Edited by

Deborah S. Greco
&
Autumn P. Davidson

WILEY Blackwell

Registered Offices
John Wiley & Sons, Inc., 111 River Street, Hoboken, NJ 07030, USA

Editorial Office
1606 Golden Aspen Drive, Suites 103 and 104, Ames, Iowa 50010, USA

For details of our global editorial offices, customer services, and more information about Wiley products visit us at www.wiley.com.

Wiley also publishes its books in a variety of electronic formats and by print-on-demand. Some content that appears in standard print versions of this book may not be available in other formats.

Library of Congress Cataloging-in-Publication Data applied for

A catalogue record for this book is available from the British Library.

ISBN: 9781118356371

Cover image: Courtesy of the editors

Set in 10.5/13pt Berkeley by Aptara Inc., New Delhi, India

Printed and bound by CPI Group (UK) Ltd, Croydon, CR0 4YY

C9781118356371_241024

Blackwell's Five-Minute
Veterinary Consult

Clinical Companion

Small Animal Endocrinology and Reproduction

Contents

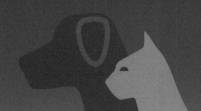

Contributor List

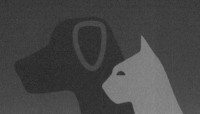

Sarah G. J. Alwen BSc, MSc, DVM

Giovana Bassu DVM, DECAR

Julia Bates DVM, DACVIM

Michela Beccaglia DVM, PhD, DECAR

David Beehan MVB MS DACT

Ellen N. Behrend VMD, PhD, DACVIM

Annika Bergstrom DVM, DECAR

David Bruyette DVM, DACVIM

Janice Cain DVM, DACVIM (Internal Medicine)

Margret L. Casal Dr med vet, MS, PhD, DECAR

Karen Copley RNC BSN

Emily Cross DVM, DABVP (Canine/Feline)

Autumn P. Davidson DVM, MS, DACVIM (Internal Medicine)

Bruce Eilts DVM, DACT

Wenche Farstad DVM, PhD, DECAR

Linda M. Fleeman BVSc, PhD, MANZCVS

Melinda Fleming DVM

Joni L. Freshman DVM, DACVIM (Internal Medicine) CVA

Cathy J. Gartley DVM, DVSc, DACT

J De Gier DVM, DECAR

Virginia Gill DVM, DACVIM (Oncology)

Chen Gilor DVM, PhD, DACVIM

Melissa Goodman DVM

Deborah S. Greco DVM, PhD, DACVIM

Clare Gregory DVM, DACVS

Sophie A. Grundy BVSc, MACVSc, DACVIM (Internal Medicine)

Nili Karmi PhD, DVM

Margaret R. Kern DVM, DACVIM

Peter P. Kintzer DVM, DACVIM

E. Freya Kruger DVM, DACVIM (Internal Medicine)

Jennifer Bones Larsen DVM, MS, PhD, DACVN

James Lavely DVM, DACVIM (Neurology)

Xavier Lévy DVM, DECAR

Cheryl Lopate MS, DVM, DACT

Sarah K. Lyle DVM, PhD, DACT

Elisa M. Mazzaferro MS, DVM, PhD, DACVECC

Rhett Nichols DVM, ACVIM (Internal Medicine)

Stijn J. Niessen DVM, PhD, DECVIM

Danielle O'Brien DVM, DACVIM (Oncology)

Mark E. Peterson DVM, Dip. ACVIM

Carlos Rodriguez DVM, PhD, DACVIM (Oncology)

Michael Schaer DVM, DACVIM, DACVECC

Laura Slater DVM

Aline B. Vieira DVM, MSc, PhD

Benita von Dehn DVM, DACVIM (Internal Medicine)

Foreword

I have had the privilege, following graduation from veterinary school, of completing an internship, a three-year residency, several years in private practice, joining my first veterinary school faculty at the Western College of Veterinary Medicine in Saskatoon and then, for the past 35+ years, on faculty at the University of California, Davis. The absolute high point of my career, of any decade, year, month or day would certainly be having the opportunity to participate in 'rounds.' Sitting around a table or on the floor of a hospital ward, reviewing the presenting complaint and history, physical examination, laboratory and imaging studies … trying to figure out the cause for an abnormality in a cat or dog … these were the greatest of challenges, and they were consistently stressful, exciting and fun! Rounds were always a wonderful complement to my seeing cases, because they offered a place to share observations and thought processes with colleagues, to learn how they may have done or thought differently. Always a learning experience. However, it must be admitted, I always entered rounds with fear, honestly two fears: first, that my ignorance would be revealed; and/or second, that the rounds I was conducting would be boring. So, I always tried to determine ahead of time the case or cases to be presented – whether as a student or an intern – when I was going to be presenting a case and asked questions, or as a faculty member attempting to take advantage of a 'teaching opportunity.' As a person who was often a 'leader' in rounds (usually defined as being the oldest person in the room), it seemed that I was always expected to know the answer to any question asked, while having to shoulder the responsibility for making rounds interesting, logical, and practical. Quickly reviewing a subject prior to rounds or before any case discussion always added to my sense of confidence and competence.

The Blackwell Five-Minute Veterinary Consult's Clinical Companion; Small Animal Endocrinology and Reproduction will serve as a wonderful aid to those who may be preparing for rounds, for those concerned that their differential diagnosis is incomplete, or that their chosen strategy in managing a newly diagnosed condition may not be up-to-date, or for those preparing to meet and discuss one of these conditions with an owner, student, colleague, or teacher.

Among the many students with whom I had the honor and pleasure to share time on my internal medicine service were Deborah Greco and Autumn Davidson. Teachers love to impart their knowledge to their students. A few students absorb that knowledge and then dedicate their careers to build from that foundation while also teaching the next generation of 'students.' This should always be viewed as a wonderful compliment to their teachers. Doctors Greco and Davidson have evolved to become world-renowned and respected small animal endocrine and reproduction experts. As one of their early instructors, I take great pride in their successes. Deb Greco and Autumn Davidson are to be congratulated on assembling a thorough list of topics relative to canine and feline endocrinology and reproduction, with more than 60 chapter titles that encompass a huge number of conditions and biochemical abnormalities encountered in small animal practice. Most importantly, the authors who were assembled to carry out the task of presenting each subject are among the world's best veterinary clinicians and clinical researchers. These individuals bring vast experience and a wealth of knowledge to their assignments. Each subject is succinctly reviewed practically and logically, while being cost-effective. When appropriate, discussions begin with typical client concerns, history and physical examination features, diagnostic approaches, therapeutic strategies, and prognosis.

This *Clinical Companion* should be on the bookshelf of every small animal veterinary hospital. The information it provides can be easily applied to the clinical diagnosis and treatment of endocrine or reproductive disorders for the benefit of the patient, owner, veterinarian and the entire veterinary health team.

Enjoy!

Edward C. Feldman, DVM
Diplomate, ACVIM (SAIM)
Emeritus Professor of Small Animal Internal Medicine
University of California, Davis, USA

Preface

As internal medicine consultants, Dr Davidson and I observed the need for a readily accessible, concise reference on endocrinology and reproduction for the busy veterinary practitioner. This book was developed as an expanded companion book to the *Five-Minute Veterinary Consult*, but also serves as a bridge to more comprehensive texts such as *Canine and Feline Endocrinology and Reproduction* by Feldman and Nelson. We would like to thank our contributors for sharing their expertise. We look forward to providing veterinary practitioners with another tool to manage challenging reproductive and endocrine cases. Thank you Dr Davidson for your friendship, unwavering support and hard work – all of which made this book possible.

Deborah S. Greco DVM, PhD, DACVIM (Internal Medicine)

I credit Dr Greco for first coming up with the idea of a comprehensive but concise reference text covering clinical conditions in small animal endocrinology and reproduction. She did not have to work hard to convince me that this would be a welcome addition to the library of small animal clinicians. Veterinarians in clinical practice – both generalists and specialists – are always pressed for time, but are also committed to providing the best care for their patients and the most current information to their clients. Excellent textbooks of endocrinology and reproduction already exist; their comprehensiveness begat lengthiness, and are difficult to peruse in 10 minutes between cases. Our thought was to create a reference text covering all of the topics we thought were relevant to the practice of endocrinology and reproduction, in a format that could be read in 5 minutes (well, maybe 10 minutes), yet permitted the reader to gain excellent knowledge of the topic (or to confirm their knowledge already in place). The list of topics grew alarmingly, but our list of knowledgeable and willing authors made it all seem possible. Voila! *Blackwell's Five-Minute Veterinary Consult Clinical Companion Small Animal Endocrinology and Reproduction*! Thank you Dr Greco, thank you to all our contributing authors for time spent preparing manuscripts in their already overly busy lives, and finally, thank you Tom (my loving husband) for patiently waiting for me to finish working on the computer every night.

A. P. Davidson DVM, MS, DACVIM (Internal Medicine)

About the Companion Website

This book is accompanied by a companion website:

www.fiveminutevet.com/endocrinology

The website includes:
- Client education handouts

chapter 1

Anthelmentics in Pregnant and Breeding Dogs

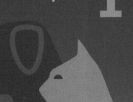

DEFINITION

- Dogs are subject to both external and internal parasites, putting them at risk for communicable diseases, severe anemia, as well as other complications.
- Parasites most commonly indicated include ectoparasites, heartworm and intestinal parasites.
- The Companion Animal Parasite Council (CAPC) recommends administering year-round broad-spectrum parasite control with efficacy against heartworm, intestinal parasites, fleas, and ticks.
- Some parasite preventives are contraindicated for use in pregnant bitches, as they may cause developmental toxicity or prenatal mortality.
- Similar precautions may also exist for breeding studs and neonates.

ETIOLOGY/PATHOPHYSIOLOGY

- Ectoparasites – ticks are small arachnids in the order Ixodida and subclass Acarina, whereas fleas are insects forming the order Siphonaptera. Both are ectoparasites living by hematophagy and are vectors of a number of diseases. Tick and flea prevalence varies by region within North America.
- Ectoparasites generally acquire pathogens when feeding on infected reservoir hosts, transmitting pathogens and toxins during hematophagy.
- Heartworm (*Dirofilaria immitis*) is a parasitic roundworm that is spread from host to host through the bites of mosquitoes.
- The heartworm resides in the pulmonary arterial system causing damage to the lung vessels and tissues.
- Transmission of intestinal parasites may occur through ingestion of paratenic hosts, infective larvae or fleas, transmammary, transplacental transmission, or parasitic vectors.
- Pathophysiology of intestinal parasites varies widely but they live primarily as adults in the dog's intestinal tract.

Blackwell's Five-Minute Veterinary Consult Clinical Companion: Small Animal Endocrinology and Reproduction, First Edition. Edited by Deborah S. Greco and Autumn P. Davidson. © 2017 John Wiley & Sons, Inc. Published 2017 by John Wiley & Sons, Inc. Companion Website: www.fiveminutevet.com/endocrinology

- *Giardia*, the most common non-helminthic intestinal parasite, is a flagellated protozoan parasite that colonizes and reproduces in the small intestine, causing giardiasis.
- *Giardia* infection can occur through the ingestion of dormant microbial cysts in contaminated water, food, or feces.
- Neonates may have an increased risk of infection through physical interaction with (transmammary), or the ingestion of infective eggs disseminated by dams with postgestational infection or infected breeding studs still on premises.
- Transplacental transmission to the fetus can occur in some intestinal parasites; e.g., roundworms.

 ## SIGNALMENT/HISTORY

- Ectoparasites can affect any breed and any age, though are most commonly found in dogs averaging 3–6 years and atopic breeds.
- Species-specific prevalence related to geographic distribution exists for ticks, intestinal parasites and heartworm.
- Heartworm is prevalent among medium to large breeds aged 3–8 years (outdoor dogs).
- Hookworm infection causes acute disease in neonates and young puppies, and chronic blood-loss anemia in mature dogs.
- Roundworm clinical disease is most severe in young puppies.
- Tapeworm and whipworms show no sex, breed, or age predilection.
- *Giardia* is seen primarily in young dogs.

Historic Findings

- Ectoparasites cause symptoms such as scratching or rubbing, licking, chewing or biting, skin abrasions, or pyoderma (caused by secondary bacterial infection).
- Heartworm-infected dogs are primarily asymptomatic until late in the course of disease.

 ## CLINICAL FEATURES

- Clinical features of parasitic infection vary based on species and severity (parasite load).
- Visualization of parasite evidence (fleas, flea dirt, attached ticks, tick-feeding cavities, vomit, diarrhea, or perianal coat containing eggs or worms).
- Lesions or abrasions are primarily caused by self-trauma.
- Wide variation of gastrointestinal signs, including vomit, diarrhea, abdominal distention, weight loss, obstruction.
- Wide variation of associated parasitic-borne diseases.
- Heartworm infection can result in varying severity of cardiac and pulmonary abnormalities.
- Neonates are often at higher risk for increased severity of symptoms.

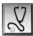 ## DIFFERENTIAL DIAGNOSIS

- Skin irritation can be caused by:
  - Food allergy
  - Atopy
  - Sarcoptic mange
  - Cheyletiellosis.
  - Primary keratinization defects
  - Drug reaction
- Diarrhea and vomiting can be caused by:
  - Diet change
  - Food intolerance or sensitivity
  - Bacterial infection
  - Viral infection
  - Toxins
  - Idiopathic hemorrhagic gastroenteritis
  - Small intestinal bacterial overgrowth (SIBO); also called antibiotic-resistant diarrhea
  - Lymphangiectasia
  - Infiltrative disease
  - Exocrine pancreatic insufficiency
  - Idiopathic inflammatory bowel disease
  - Histoplasmosis
  - Intestinal obstruction
  - Histiocytic ulcerative colitis
- Cardiopulmonary dysfunction
  - Pulmonary hypertension
  - Pulmonary bacterial, viral, or mycotic infection
  - Inflammatory lung disease
  - Acquired or congenital cardiac disease

 ## DIAGNOSTICS

- Physical examination of skin, perianal coat, or feces for parasites, parasite dirt or resulting abrasions/lesions.
- Blood + fecal testing (large variation).

 ## THERAPEUTICS

- Refer to *The 5-Minute Veterinary Consult Clinical Companion Canine and Feline Infectious Diseases and Parasitology* for specific therapies by parasite species.

Prevention

- Therapeutic precautions in pregnant/lactating bitches, breeding studs and puppies are indicated below.

TABLE 1.1. Parasite Preventive Charts

Commercial name	Active ingredient(s)	Indicated use	Dosage	Route	Pregnant and lactating bitch	Breeding stud	Puppy
Comfortis	Spinosad	Fleas	Spinosad (30 mg/kg PO)	Oral	Unsafe	NPA	14 Weeks
Program Tablets	Lufenuron	Fleas	Lufeneron 10mg/kg monthly PO	Oral	Safe	Safe	4 Weeks
Program Flavor Tabs	Lufenuron	Fleas	Lufeneron 10mg/kg monthly PO	Oral	Safe	Safe	4 Weeks
Vectra for Dogs and Puppies	Dinotefuran + Pyriproxyfen	Fleas	Available in 1.3, 2.0, 4.0 and 6.0ml sizes. Apply every month.	Topical	Unsafe	NPA	8 Weeks
NexGard	Afoxolaner	Fleas + Ticks	2.5 mg/kg monthly	Oral	NE	NE	8 Weeks
Activyl	Indoxacarb	Fleas	Available in 0.51 ml, 0.77 ml, 1.54 ml, 3.08 ml, and 4.62 ml sizes. The topical solution should be applied monthly as a single spot between the dog's shoulder blades.	Topical	Unsafe	NE	8 Weeks
Scalibor Protector Band	Deltamethrin	Ticks	Deltamethrin (4%); one colar every 6 months	Collar	Safe	Safe	12 Weeks
Preventic	Amitraz	Ticks		Collar	Safe	NPA	12 Weeks
Sentry Natural Defense	Peppermint + Cinnamon + Lemongrass + Clove + Thyme	Fleas + Ticks	Available in 1.5 ml, 3.0 ml, and 4.5 ml sizes. Apply the entire contents in a single spot to the animal's skin.	Topical	NPA	NPA	12 Weeks
Sentry Pro XFT	Etofenprox + Pyriproxyfen	Fleas + Ticks	The topical solution should be applied monthly as a single spot between the dog's shoulder blades.	Topical	Unsafe	NPA	12 Weeks
Bio Spot Flea & Tick Collar with IGR For Dogs	Propoxur + (S)-Methoprene	Fleas + Ticks	One collar every 5 months	Collar	Unsafe	NPA	12 Weeks

Seresto	Flumethrin + Imidacloprid	Fleas + Ticks	One collar every 8 months	Collar	NE	NE	7 Weeks
Bravecto	Fluralaner	Fleas + Ticks	25 mg/kg q 8-12 weeks	Oral	Safe	Safe	24 Weeks
Advantage II	Imidacloprid + Pyriproxyfen	Fleas + Chewing lice	Imidacloprid (10 mg/kg) and Pyriproxyfen (0.5 mg/kg) minimum	Topical	NPA	NPA	7 Weeks
Fiproguard	Fipronil	Fleas + Ticks + Chewing lice	Available in 0.67 ml, 1.34 ml, 2.68 ml, and 4.02 ml sizes. Apply the entire contents in a single spot to the animal's skin.	Topical	Safe	Safe	12 Weeks
Fiproguard Max	Fipronil + Cyphenothrin	Fleas + Ticks + Chewing lice	The topical solution should be applied monthly as a single spot between the dog's shoulder blades.	Topical	Unsafe	NPA	12 Weeks
PetArmor	Fipronil	Fleas + Ticks + Chewing lice	Available in 0.67 ml, 1.34 ml, 2.68 ml, and 4.02 ml sizes. Apply the entire contents in a single spot to the animal's skin.	Topical	Safe	Safe	8 Weeks
Certifect for Dogs	Fipronil + (S)-Methoprene + Amitraz	Fleas + Ticks + Chewing lice	Available in 1.70 ml, 2.14 ml, 4.28 ml, and 6.42 ml sizes. Apply the entire contents in a single spot to the animal's skin.	Topical	Safe	Safe	8 Weeks
Frontline Plus	Fipronil + (S)-methoprene	Fleas + Ticks + Chewing lice	Available in 0.67 ml, 1.34 ml, 2.68 ml, and 4.02 ml sizes. Apply the entire contents in a single spot to the animal's skin.	Topical	Safe	Safe	8 Weeks
Frontline Top Spot	Fipronil	Fleas + Ticks + Chewing lice	Available in 0.67 ml, 1.34 ml, 2.68 ml, and 4.02 ml sizes. Apply the entire contents in a single spot to the animal's skin.	Topical	Safe	Safe	8 Weeks

(Continued)

TABLE 1.1. (*Continued*)

Commercial name	Active ingredient(s)	Indicated use	Dosage	Route	Pregnant and lactating bitch	Breeding stud	Puppy
Parastar	Fipronil	Fleas + Ticks + Chewing lice	The topical solution should be applied monthly as a single spot between the dog's shoulder blades.	Topical	Safe	Safe	8 Weeks
Parastar Plus	Fipronil + Cyphenothrin	Fleas + Ticks + Chewing lice	The topical solution should be applied monthly as a single spot between the dog's shoulder blades.	Topical	Unsafe	Unsafe	Unsafe
Flea4X	Fibronil	Fleas + Ticks + Chewing lice	Available in 0.67 ml, 1.34 ml, 2.68 ml, and 4.02 ml sizes. Apply the entire contents in a single spot to the animal's skin.	Topical	Safe	Safe	8 Weeks
Bio Spot Defense Flea & Tick Control For Dogs	Etofenprox + (S)-Methoprene	Fleas + Ticks + Mosquitoes	The topical solution should be applied monthly as a single spot between the dog's shoulder blades.	Topical	Unsafe	NPA	10 Weeks
Heartgard Chewables	Ivermectin	Heartworm	Ivermectin (0.006 mg/kg) monthly PO	Oral	Safe	Safe	6 Weeks
ProHeart6	Moxidectin	Heartworm + Hookworms	0.05 ml of the constituted suspension/kg body weight (0.0227 ml.lb) every six months subcutaneously.	Injection	Safe	Safe	6 Months
Tri-Heart Plus Chewable Tablets	Ivermectin + Pyrantel	Heartworm + Roundworms + Hookworms	Ivermectin (0.006 mg/kg) and Pyrantel (5 mg/kg) monthly PO	Oral	Safe	Safe	6 Weeks
Heartgard Plus Chewable Tablets	Ivermectin + Pyrantel	Heartworm + Roundworms + Hookworms	Ivermectin (0.006 mg/kg) monthly PO	Oral	Safe	Safe	6 Weeks

Product	Ingredients	Parasites	Dosage	Route			Interval
IverhartPlus Flavored Chewables	Ivermectin + Pyrantel	Heartworm + Roundworms + Hookworms	Ivermectin (0.006 mg/kg) and Pyrantel (5 mg/kg) monthly PO	Oral	Safe	NPA	6 Weeks
Iverhart Max Chewable tablets	Ivermectin + Pyrantel pamoate + Praziquantel	Heartworm + Roundworms + Hookworms + Tapeworms	Ivermectin (0.006 mg/kg) and Pyrantel pamoate (5 mg/kg) and Praziquantel (5 mg/kg) monthly PO	Oral	Unsafe	NPA	8 Weeks
Trifexis	Spinosad + Milbemycin Oxime	Heartworm + Roundworms + Hookworms + Whipworms	Milbemycin oxime (0.5 mg/kg) and Spinosad (30 mg/kg) monthly PO	Oral	Safe	Safe	8 Weeks
Interceptor Flavor Tabs	Milbemycin Oxime	Heartworm + Roundworms + Hookworms + Whipworms	Milbemycin (0.5 mg/kg) monthly PO	Oral	Safe	Safe	2 Weeks
Droncit	Praziquantel	Tapeworm	Praziquantel (5.0 mg/kg) PO, SC, or IM minimum	Oral	Safe	Safe	4 Weeks
Cestex	Epsiprantel	Tapeworm	Epsiprantel (5.5 mg/kg PO)	Oral	Unsafe	NPA	7 Weeks
Nemex Tabs	Pyrantel Pamoat	Roundworms + Hookworms	Pyrantel pamoate (5 mg/kg PO)	Oral	Safe	Safe	6 Weeks
Virbantel	Pyrantel Pamoate + Praziquantel	Tapeworms + Roundworms + Hookworms	Pyrantel pamoate (5 mg/kg) and Praziquantel (5 mg/kg) PO	Oral	Safe	Safe	12 Weeks
Drontal Plus	Praziquantel + Pyrantel Pamoate + Febantel	Tapeworm + Roundworms + Hookworms + Whipworms	Praziquantel (5 mg/kg) and Pyrantel pamoate (5 mg/kg) and Febantel (25 mg/kg) minimum PO	Oral	Unsafe	NPA	4 Weeks
Safe-Guard Canine	Fenbendazole	Tapeworm + Roundworms + Hookworms + Whipworms	Fenbendazole (50 mg/kg x 3 days PO)	Oral	Safe	Safe	6 Weeks

(Continued)

TABLE 1.1. (Continued)

Commercial name	Active ingredient(s)	Indicated use	Dosage	Route	Pregnant and lactating bitch	Breeding stud	Puppy
Dog Worms 3	Pyrantel pamoate + Praziquantel	Tapeworm + Roundworms + Hookworms + Whipworms	Small dogs (30mg tablets) - 6.0-12.0 lbs: 1 tablet, 12.1-25 lbs: 2 tablets Medium-Large dogs (114mg tablets) - 25.1-50 lbs: 1 tablet, 50.1-100lbs: 2 tablets, 100.1-150 lbs: 3 tablets, 150.1-200 lbs: 4 tablets		NE	NE	12 Weeks
Panacur C Canine Dewormer	Fenbendazole	Tapeworm + Roundworms + Hookworms + Whipworms	Fenbendazole (50 mg/kg x 3 days PO)	Oral	Safe	Safe	6 Weeks
Revolution	Selamectin	Fleas + Ticks + Heartworm + Roundworms + Hookworms	Selamectin (6 mg/kg) monthly TOPICAL	Topical	Safe	Safe	6 Weeks
Advantage Multi for Dogs	Imidacloprid + Moxidectin	Fleas + Heartworm + Roundworms + Hookworms + Whipworms	10% Imidacloprid and 2.5% Moxidectin topical spot-on	Topical	NPA	NPA	7 Weeks
Sentinel Flavor Tabs	Lufenuron + Milbemycin oxime	Fleas + Heartworm + Roundworms + Hookworms + Whipworms	Milbemycin (0.5 mg/kg) and lufenuron (10 mg/kg) monthly PO	Oral	NPA	NPA	4 Weeks

Trifexis	Spinosad + Milbemycin Oxime	Fleas, Heartworm, Roundworm, Whipworm, Hookworm	30 mg/kg Spinosad; 0.5 mg/kg Milbemycin oxime monthly	Oral	Safe	NE	8 Weeks
K9 Advantix	Imidacloprid + Permethrin	Fleas + Ticks + Mosquitoes + Chewing lice + Biting flies	Imidacloprid (10 mg/kg) and Permethrin (50 mg/kg) and Pyriproxyfen (0.5 mg/kg) minimum	Topical	NPA	NPA	7 Weeks
Vectra 3D	Dinotefuran + Pyriproxyfen + Permethrin	Fleas + Ticks + Mosquitoes + Lice + Sand flies + Mites	Available in 1.6ml, 3.6ml, 4.7ml, 8.0ml sizes	Topical	Unsafe	NPA	7 Weeks

NPA = No Problems Anticipated
NE = Not Evaluated

COMMENTS

- Companion Animal Parasite Council recommends year-round flea and tick control.
- Veterinarians are encouraged to evaluate new products not included in this chapter by reading the package insert or direct manufacturer consultation.

See Also

Canine Breeding Management.
Feline Pre-Breeding Examination and Breeding Husbandry.

Suggested Reading

Bowman, D.D., Barr, S.C. (eds) (2006) *Refer to The 5-Minute Veterinary Consult Clinical Companion Canine and Feline Infectious Diseases and Parasitology.* 1st edn. John Wiley & Sons.
http://www.capcvet.org/resource-library/parasite-product-applications-for-dogs.

Author: Sarah G. J. Alwen BSc, MSc, DVM

Antimicrobial Stewardship in Small Animal Reproduction

chapter 2

DEFINITION

- Veterinarians recognize the need to maintain the usefulness of antimicrobial drugs in animals as well as humans, and that indiscriminant use of antimicrobial drugs contributes to the development of pathogen resistance. It is the responsibility of the veterinarian to prescribe antimicrobial drugs only when indicated to treat infection.

ETIOLOGY/PATHOPHYSIOLOGY

- Bacteria can be resistant to the action of antimicrobial drugs because of their inherent structure or physiology, or they can develop mechanisms to circumvent the action of the drugs through spontaneous genetic mutation. Antimicrobial use then applies a selective pressure to bacteria favoring resistant populations.

Systems Affected

- Cardiovascular
- Endocrine/metabolic
- Gastrointestinal
- Hemic/lymphatic/immune
- Hepatobiliary
- Musculoskeletal
- Nervous
- Neuromuscular
- Ophthalmic
- Renal/urologic
- Reproductive
- Respiratory
- Skin/exocrine

Blackwell's Five-Minute Veterinary Consult Clinical Companion: Small Animal Endocrinology and Reproduction, First Edition. Edited by Deborah S. Greco and Autumn P. Davidson. © 2017 John Wiley & Sons, Inc. Published 2017 by John Wiley & Sons, Inc. Companion Website: www.fiveminutevet.com/endocrinology

CLINICAL FEATURES

- Breeders commonly express concern that infertility or subfertility in bitches is related to vaginal and uterine flora, requesting pre-breeding vaginal cultures and antimicrobial therapy based on the results. Stud dog owners specifically fear that a bitch will expose their male to pathologic bacteria and damage his fertility. It has been shown that normal flora is exchanged during natural breedings without any detriment to either the bitch or the stud dog, or to their fertility or fecundity.

- The normal female reproductive tract harbors a variety of aerobic bacterial (including *Mycoplasma*) populations in the vaginal vault and uterus. Mixed vaginal cultures can be present in healthy, fertile bitches; the most common isolates include *Pasteurella multocida*, β-hemolytic streptococci, *Escherichia coli*, and *Mycoplasma* spp. The only bacterial species that is proven to be a specific cause of infertility in the bitch is *Brucella canis*. Recent development of transcervical uterine cannulation has enabled intrauterine cultures and biopsies to be collected noninvasively, and these may provide more accurate evaluation of actual infectious problems in the uterus than cranial vaginal cultures acquired with guarded swabs. During normal canine estrus, bacteria ascend the reproductive tract and are present within the uterus, subsequently regressing spontaneously. Vaginal and intrauterine cultures must both be interpreted with caution as many bacterial populations represent normal bacterial flora and do not indicate disease or explain infertility.

- The indiscriminant use of antibiotics before and during pregnancy is counterproductive and associated with the development of resistant organisms; it is not contributory to improved fertility or fecundity. It is unjustified to treat all positive vaginal cultures with antimicrobials, or to assume that all positive vaginal or uterine bacterial cultures are associated with infertility. As a general rule, growth of bacteria from the vagina or uterus in conjunction with clinical signs of excessive, malodorous or abnormal vaginal discharge, vaginal mucosal inflammation, peripheral leukocytosis and systemic illness, is significant and warrants treatment with antimicrobial agents. If possible, uterine cytology or biopsy should be examined for evidence of inflammation or infection.

- Breeders are less likely to request pre-breeding semen cultures of normal stud dogs, as commonly occurs with normal bitches. Previously fertile stud dogs currently failing to impregnate normal bitches with good husbandry and normal breeding behavior should have a semen evaluation performed; if the semen is abnormal and inflammatory in character, it should be submitted for aerobic, anaerobic and *Mycoplasma* spp. culture, and *B. canis* testing should be performed.

- If the semen contains excessive numbers of other cells such as white blood cells, macrophages, or red blood cells (pyospermia, hemospermia), an infectious/inflammatory disease should be considered.

- Bacterial infection of the testes (orchitis), epididymides (epididymitis), or scrotum can cause alterations in spermatogenesis as a result of the destructive properties of the organisms themselves, and as a result of local swelling and hyperthermia. Focal lesions can become generalized. Prostatic disorders can cause abnormal semen due to the prostatic fluid component.

■ The normal bacterial flora of the prepuce and distal urethra are the same organisms most frequently isolated from normal canine semen, and also from dogs with bacterial orchitis, epididymitis, or prostatitis. The normal flora of the distal urethra and prepuce consist predominantly of aerobic organisms, but anaerobic organisms are also found. *Pasteurella multocida*, β-hemolytic streptococci and *E. coli* are the organisms most commonly isolated from dogs. Because of this, collecting semen for culture can be misleading, as the normal urethral flora will contaminate the sample. The number of colony-forming units (CFUs) per milliliter of semen attributable to urethral contamination (normal urethral flora) reportedly varies from 100 to 10,000. A separate culture of the material from a urethral swab, obtained just before ejaculation, could be used to identify urethral organisms. Quantitative culture of the urethra can then be compared to quantitative culture of the semen. Gentle cleansing of the prepuce should precede semen collection; semen should be collected with sterile equipment (artificial vagina and collection tubes). Semen evaluation should not be performed on these samples because of the spermicidal effects of cleansing and sterilizing agents. A greater than 3 logs increase in the number of an organism identified in both the semen and the urethral cultures could be considered significant.

■ Quantitative aerobic, anaerobic and mycoplasma cultures of both the urethra and semen are often prohibitively expensive. Specific sampling of the urine (cystocentesis), prostate, epididymides and testes can be more efficient and meaningful, and is facilitated by ultrasound-guided technique. Cytologic samples of these areas can also be acquired; suppurative inflammation of the prostate, epididymides and testes is characterized by infiltration of neutrophils and macrophages.

■ Concluding that an infertile or subfertile dog has infectious etiology on the basis of a positive semen culture is unjustified without supportive data. Dogs with infectious orchitis, epididymitis and/or prostatitis tend to have clinical signs supporting the etiology (heat, pain, redness and swelling of the affected organ) readily apparent on the physical examination as well as abnormal semen. Semen collection may be difficult due to pain associated with ejaculation.

■ Documented infectious diseases in breeding dogs and bitches include:
  • Pyometra
  • Abortion (*Brucella canis*)
  • Post-partum metritis
  • Mastitis
  • Orchitis/epididymitis
  • Prostatitis
  • Balanoposthitis
  • Cystourethritis/pyelonephritis
  • Neonatal bacterial sepsis
  • Neonatal herpes

DIAGNOSTICS

- Perform *Brucella* screening.
- Consider canine herpesvirus-1 (CHV1) serology (I find this of little value and it is not routinely recommended).
- Intrauterine sampling compared to vaginal flora in *infertility work-ups* in the bitch where inflammatory/infectious disease is a concern (interpretation of normal flora in the vagina versus disease-causing flora).
- Quantitative semen and urethral cultures in subfertility work-ups in the dog where inflammatory/infectious disease is a concern (very high cost).
- Ultrasound-guided sampling in cases of prostatitis, orchitis, epididymitis, cystitis.
- Vaginal sampling in cases of open pyometra, post-partum metritis.
- Routine vaginal cultures prior to breeding, in an otherwise healthy bitch are *not* recommended.

THERAPEUTICS

- Therapeutic antimicrobial use should be confined to appropriate clinical indications.
- Therapeutic alternatives should be considered prior to antimicrobial therapy.
- Culture and susceptibility results aid in the appropriate selection of antimicrobials.
- Use narrow-spectrum antimicrobials whenever appropriate, for the minimum time needed to eradicate true infection.
- Antimicrobials considered important in treating refractory infections in human or veterinary medicine should be used in animals only after careful review and reasonable justification. In particular, veterinarians should avoid prescribing extra-label use of fluoroquinolones and extended-spectrum beta-lactam antimicrobials (e.g., third- or fourth-generation cephalosporins) or recommending drugs such as carbapenems, glycopeptides, and oxazolidinones used for treatment of multidrug-resistant pathogens in humans.
- Judicious use of antimicrobials in animals requires the oversight of a veterinarian. Antibiotics should not be provided to breeders for indiscriminant use.
- The routine prophylactic use of antimicrobials should never be used as a substitute for good animal health management.
- Treatment with an antimicrobial prior to breeding, in an attempt to improve fertility, is absolutely not recommended and is contraindicated.

See Also

Infectious causes of pregnancy loss – canine.
Infectious causes of pregnancy loss – feline.
Canine Prostate Disease: Benign Prostatic Hyperplasia, Cystic Benign Prostatic Hyperplasia, Prostatitis.
Pyometra, Cystic endometrial hyperplasia (Hydrometra, Mucometra, Hematometra).
Canine Semen Abnormalities Orchitis/Epididymitis.

Suggested Reading

Morley, P.S., Apley, M.D., Besser, T.E., Burney, D.P., Fedorka-Cray, P.J., Papich, M.G., Traub-Dargatz, J.L., Weese, J.S. (2005) Antimicrobial Drug Use in Veterinary Medicine. ACVIM Consensus Statement. *J. Vet. Intern. Med.*, **19**, 617–629.

Prescott JF, Baggot JD. American Veterinary Medical Association. *AVMA Guidelines for Judicious Therapeutic Use of Antimicrobial Drugs.* Available at: http:// www.avma.org/scienact/jtua/default.asp. Accessed May **30**, 2004. 6.

Doig, P. A., Ruhnke, H.L., Bosu, W.T. (1981) The genital *Mycoplasma* and *Ureaplasma* flora of healthy and diseased dogs. PMCID: PMC1320213.

Bjurström, L., Linde-Forsberg, C. (1992) Long-term study of aerobic bacteria of the genital tract in stud dogs. *Am. J. Vet. Res.*, **53** (5), 670–673.

Bjurström, L., Linde-Forsberg, C. (1992) Long-term study of aerobic bacteria of the genital tract in bitches. *Am. J. Vet. Res.*, **53** (5), 665–669.

Ström, B., Linde-Forsberg, C. (1993) Effects of ampicillin and trimethoprim-sulfamethoxazole on the vaginal bacterial flora of bitches. *Am. J. Vet. Res.*, **54** (6), 891–896 (PMID:8323058).

Weese, J.S., Blondeau, J.M., Boothe, D., Breitschwerdt, E.B., Guardabassi, L., Hillier, A., Lloyd, D.H., Papich, M.G., Rankin, S.C., Turnidge, J.D., Sykes, J.E. (2011) Antimicrobial Use Guidelines for Treatment of Urinary Tract Disease in Dogs and Cats: Antimicrobial Guidelines. SAGE-Hindawi Access to Research Veterinary Medicine International, Volume 2011, Article ID 263768, 9 pages doi:10.4061/2011/263768.

Marques, C., *et al.* (2016) Emergence of CMY-2-producing *Proteus mirabilis* in companion animals with UTI: 16 years study. ASM Microbe 2016, Boston, June 20, 2016.

Marques, C. (2016) European Multicenter Study on Antimicrobial Resistance in Companion Animal Urinary Tract Infection. ASM Microbe 2016, Boston, June 20, 2016.

Marques, C., *et al.* (2016) Ctx-M-15-Producing Multidrug Resistant *Klebsiella pneumoniae* High-risk Lineages Cause Urinary Tract Infection in Companion Animals. ASM Microbe 2016, Boston, June 20, 2016.

Abraham, S., *et al.* (2014) Carbapenemase-producing bacteria in companion animals: a public health concern on the horizon. *J. Antimicrob. Chemother.*, **69**, 1155. doi: 10.1093/jac/dkt518.

Rosen, M. (2016) Bacteria resistant to last-resort antibiotic appears in U.S. Science News Online, May 27.

Authors: Autumn P. Davidson DVM, MS, DACVIM (Internal Medicine); Janice Cain DVM, DACVIM (Internal Medicine)

chapter 3

Autoimmune Polyglandular Syndrome

DEFINITION

- Autoimmune polyglandular syndromes (APSs) include: APS Type 1 (diabetes, ectodermal mucositis, etc.), APS Type 2 (hypoadrenocorticism, hypothyroidism, type 1 diabetes mellitus, premature ovarian failure), and APS Type 3 (liver cirrhosis plus endocrinopathies).
- Autoimmune polyglandular syndrome type II is defined as the occurrence of two or more of the following disorders in the same individual: adrenal insufficiency; primary hypothyroidism; insulin-dependent diabetes mellitus (IDDM); primary hypogonadism (premature ovarian failure, immune-mediated orchitis); myasthenia gravis; immune-mediated hemolytic anemia (IMHA); immune-mediated thrombocytopenia (ITP); hypoparathyroidism; hypopituitarism; and celiac disease.

ETIOLOGY/PATHOPHYSIOLOGY

- Circulating organ-specific autoantibodies are commonly present in APS type 2. Environmental factors combined with an HLA-associated genetic predisposition are thought to trigger the process. Cell-mediated immune abnormalities in the Type II syndrome include defects and alterations of cell-surface markers, but the most consistent abnormality is a functional defect leading to a decrease in suppressor T-cell activity.
- Approximately 45% of all patients with idiopathic (autoimmune) adrenal insufficiency will develop one or more additional endocrinopathies (usually hypothyroidism). APS II is inherited as an autosomal dominant trait in humans associated with the presence of human leukocyte antigens (HLAs).
- Hypothyroidism is the most common initial endocrinopathy in the dog.
- Hypoadrenocorticism is usually followed by the development of hypothyroidism, but some dogs will develop hypothyroidism first. All three endocrinopathies in a single dog is rare.
- Type 1 diabetes combined with immune-mediated thyroid disease (Hashimoto's thyroiditis) is the most common initial endocrinopathy in humans and dogs.

Blackwell's Five-Minute Veterinary Consult Clinical Companion: Small Animal Endocrinology and Reproduction, First Edition. Edited by Deborah S. Greco and Autumn P. Davidson. © 2017 John Wiley & Sons, Inc. Published 2017 by John Wiley & Sons, Inc.
Companion Website: www.fiveminutevet.com/endocrinology

- In a retrospective of 225 cases of canine hypoadrenocorticism, 4% of the dogs also suffered from hypothyroidism, two dogs had concurrent IDDM and hypoadrenocorticism, and one dog had concurrent hypoadrenocorticism, hypothyroidism, IDDM, and hypoparathyroidism.
- Another retrospective study of 45 dogs with adrenal insufficiency reported four dogs with concurrent hypothyroidism, one dog with concurrent IDDM, and one dog with concurrent primary gonadal hypoplasia.
- A single case of Type II APS has been described in a middle-aged female dog presenting in a hypothyroid crisis; treatment of the hypothyroid state resulted in precipitation of the hypoadrenocorticism. The presence of serum autoantibodies to thyroid and adrenal tissue was observed in this dog as evidence of autoimmune polyglandular syndrome Type II.

 ## SIGNALMENT/HISTORY

- Hypoadrenocorticism and hypothyroidism – mean age of onset of the disease was in young adulthood (5.4 years).
- Second endocrinopathy less than one year (hypoadrenal and hypothyroidism) or 18 months (IDDM and hypothyroidism) after the first endocrinopathy.
- Slight female predilection.

 ## CLINICAL FEATURES

- Dogs diagnosed with hypoadrenocorticism, most common clinical signs include:
  - Lethargy
  - Collapse
  - Vomiting
  - Weight loss
  - Weakness
  - Ataxia
  - Anorexia
  - Bradycardia
  - Megaesophagus
  - Diarrhea
- A decreasing insulin requirement is often the earliest sign of adrenal insufficiency.
- Concurrent hypothyroidism and IDDM often have increasing insulin requirements as hypothyroidism may cause insulin resistance.
- In dogs diagnosed with hypopadrenocorticism as the initial endocrinopathy, thyroid evaluation was performed because of:
  - Continued lethargy despite adequate mineralocorticoid replacement therapy.
  - Persistent hyponatremia and/or hypercholesterolemia.
  - Dermatologic disease.
  - Bradycardia.

- Obesity.
- Heat-seeking behavior.

DIFFERENTIAL DIAGNOSIS

- Inadequate glucocorticoid or mineralocorticoid supplementation in dogs with hypoadrenocorticism.
- In dogs with diabetes mellitus, rule out other causes of insulin resistance.
- In dogs with hypothyroidism, rule out other causes of weakness or electrolyte disturbances (e.g., hyperkalemia).

DIAGNOSTICS

- Complete blood count (CBC)/Chemistry profile/Urinalysis abnormalities.
  - Hyponatremia
  - Hypercholesterolemia
  - Hyperkalemia
  - Hypochloremia
  - Azotemia
  - Hypocalcemia
  - Hypercalcemia
- ACTH response test.
- Serum TT4 and endogenous canine TSH.
- Acetycholine receptor antibody titer.

THERAPEUTICS

Drug(s) of Choice

- Levothyroxine 22–44 µg/kg/day.
- Deoxycorticosterone pivilate 1 mg/kg IM q. 25–30 days.

Precautions/Interactions

- Avoid generic levothyroxine.

Alternative Drugs

- Florinef (0.1 mg/10 lb PO q. 24 h).

Appropriate Health Care

- Not applicable.

Nursing Care

- Not applicable.

Diet

- Not applicable.

Activity

- Not applicable.

Surgical Considerations

- Not applicable.

 COMMENTS

Patient Monitoring

- Serum potassium and sodium.
- Post pill total thyroxine (TT4) or canine endogenous TSH (cTSH) levels.

Prevention/Avoidance

- Not applicable.

Possible Complications

- Precipitation of Addisonian crises in dogs with concurrent hypothyroidism and hypoadrenocorticism. Cautious thyroid supplementation with monitoring of serum potassium.

Expected Course and Prognosis

- Excellent with thyroid hormone/corticosteroid and mineralocorticoid replacement.

Synonyms

- Polyendocrine gland failure.

Abbreviations

APS = Autoimmune polyglandular syndrome.

See Also

Hypothyroidism
Hypoadrenocorticism
Diabetes mellitus (canine)

Suggested Reading

Peterson, M.E., Kintzer, P. (1996) Review of 225 cases of canine hypoadrenocorticism. *J. Am. Vet. Med. Assoc.*, **208** (1), 85–91.

Feldman, E.C., Nelson, R.W. (1996) *Canine and Feline Endocrinology and Reproduction*, 2nd edition. WB Saunders, Philadelphia, pp. 55–57.

Bowen, D., Schaer, M., Riley, W. (1986) Autoimmune polyglandular syndrome in a dog: A case report. *J. Am. Anim. Hosp. Assoc.*, **22**, 649–654.

Nuefeld, M., Maclaren, N.K., Blizzard, R.M. (1981) Two types of autoimmune Addison's disease associated with different polyglandular autoimmune syndromes. *Medicine*, **60**, 355–362.

Eisenbarth, G.S., Jackson, R.A. (1981) Immunogenetics of polyglandular failure and related diseases in HLA, in *Endocrine and Metabolic Disorders* (ed. N.Farid). Academic Press, New York, pp. 235–264.

Volpe, R. (1977) The role of autoimmunity in hypoendocrine and hyperendocrine function. *Ann. Intern. Med.*, **87**, 86–99.

Author: Deborah S. Greco DVM, PhD, DACVIM

Breeding Management of the Bitch and Ovulation Timing for Optimal Reproductive Efficiency

INDICATIONS

- Optimal reproductive success.
- Breed healthy bitches in an ethical manner.
- Use ovulation timing (OT) to determine when to breed and predict due date.

EQUIPMENT

- Standard equipment needed for a complete health examination (stethoscope).
- Cotton-tipped swabs and other materials needed for routine in-house cytology.
- Scope for vaginoscopy: Pediatric proctoscope for all but toy breeds (Welch Allyn USA model 32020; Fig. 4.1); otoscope for toy breeds.
- Routine materials to draw and submit blood to reference laboratory including plain red-topped blood collection tubes for progesterone submission. Alternatively: in-house progesterone measurement by an automated analyzer. In-house progesterone semi-quantitative kits are not reliable, and laboratory testing for actual concentration is recommended.
- In-house LH assay kit (Witness LH, Zoetis, Kansas City, MO, USA).
- Semen collection materials (see chapter on semen collection).
- Vaginal insemination pipettes (Infusion pipette, 0.2 OD × 22" long, K1-2250, Kalayjian Industries, Signal Hill, CA; can be cut to shorter length as needed).
- Scope for transcervical insemination (TCI; Karl Storz model 27027 KL and NL with a 30° telescope model 28325BA; Fig. 4.1).
- Polypropylene catheters, for insemination via the TCI scope (Argyle polypropylene 8 Fr and 5 Fr, Coridien, Mansfield, MA).
- Syringes for insemination (latex free, Norm-Ject 1×100, Henke Sasswolf, Germany, CE0535).
- Materials, facility, pharmaceuticals (including proper anesthesia, monitoring and patient support) as needed for standard aseptic abdominal surgery.

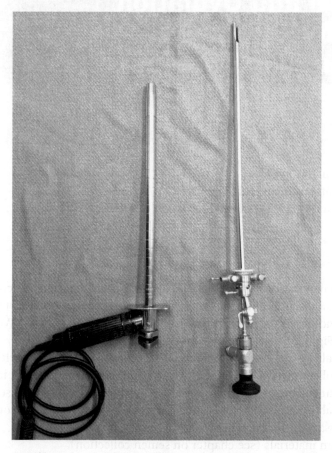

■ **Fig. 4.1.** Rigid scopes used in canine reproduction. Right: Storz cystourethrascope used for TCI. Left: Welch Allyn pediatric proctoscope used for vaginoscopy.

PROCEDURES

Breeding Management

Medical History

- Determine if bitch is in good health for breeding: current significant medical disease, chronic medication, advanced age might all indicate bitch is not appropriate for breeding.
- Question owner as regards commitment to ethical breeding.
- Assess whether breeding consecutive estrous cycles is advisable (may be considered appropriate for some breeds that historically have early onset of endometrial disease), but must be weighed in view of ethical concerns (adequate pup placement and responsibility of breeder for all pups produced).
- Determine that bitch has passed all appropriate pre-breeding genetic/orthopedic/ocular testing as deemed appropriate for the breed. If the owner refuses to obtain such

pre-breeding clearances, the veterinarian is encouraged not to provide reproductive services, other than that needed to protect health of the bitch.

Examination
- General health: a complete examination is imperative prior to each breeding.
- Vaginal examination for a maiden bitch: need to assess vulvar/vestibular/vaginal anatomy and to determine if annular strictures or vagino-vestibular septa or other anomalies are present (see Chapter on Vulvovaginal malformations).
- Vaginoscopy can be performed to further assess normal vaginal anatomy and determine presence of vaginal neoplasia in older bitches.

Breeding Plan
- Determine plan to obtain semen: natural breeding, fresh artificial insemination (AI), chilled (shipped) semen, or frozen semen.
- Fresh semen (natural breeding or side-by-side AI) if from a male with a normal semen analysis and history of producing offspring, will typically yield the highest conception rate. This choice must be weighed in consideration of pedigree analysis and gene pool available locally.
- Chilled-shipped semen (semen is collected and processed for overnight shipment) is an excellent alternative to a local male. If semen quality is good and is processed for shipping correctly, and OT is performed properly, the conception rate is similar to that with fresh semen breedings (natural or side-by-side AI). Costs are higher, but there is an advantage to increase the available gene pool without shipping the bitch.
- Frozen semen is often more convenient as it can be shipped in advance of the breeding. It can allow breeding to a sire that is no longer living, but for which excellent longevity and health information is known. Disadvantages include increase cost to obtain and ship semen, slight decrease in conception rate as compared to fresh or chilled semen, and the expertise needed to properly handle frozen semen.
- Dual-sire breedings can be considered. DNA analysis of all pups, dam and both sires are required to determine paternity. This can be an excellent choice when using semen of questionable viability. Often, the second choice male, with more viable semen, is used after (up to 24 hours later) breeding with the first choice male that has lower-quality or frozen semen. This method will increase success in obtaining pregnancy when attempting to use semen of questionable quality.

Ovulation Timing

Physiology
- Vaginal epithelial cells cornify (superficial cells) in response to estrogen produced from developing ova. The degree of cornification will not determine the time of ovulation. The end of estrus is typically associated with a 'shift' in cytology to more than 20% parabasal cells.

- Luteinizing hormone (LH) released from the pituitary, triggers ovulation to occur approximately 48 hours later. Ova then require an additional 48 hours to complete meiosis.
- The peak period of fertility is approximately 4–6 days after the LH peak.
- Progesterone, produced from pre-ovulatory luteinization of follicles, starts to increase at approximately the time of the LH peak. Progesterone continues to rise throughout ovulation and the fertile period. Serum progesterone concentration will stay elevated throughout diestrus/pregnancy.
- Expected whelping date will be 65 days (±1 day) after the LH peak. This information is helpful for management during gestation and for planning an elective Cesarean section prior to the onset of labor.

Vaginal Cytology
- Evaluation is helpful to determine onset of proestrus and differentiate from other causes of vaginal discharge.
- Can be used to confirm estrus at the time of breeding, but will not determine if pre- or post-ovulation.
- Can be used to determine the onset of diestrus.

Vaginoscopy
- The appearance of the vaginal mucosa changes due to the influence of estrogen. Evaluation of these changes can correlate to pre- or post-ovulation status.
- During proestrus, when estrogen levels are highest, the vaginal mucosa is edematous.
- After ovulation, as estrogen levels wane, the vaginal mucosa starts to shrink and becomes crenulated: angular and wrinkled.
- At the onset of diestrus, the vaginal mucosa becomes thin and flattened.

Serum Progesterone Concentration
- Sequential measurement is used to determine the time of ovulation (Table 4.1).
- Laboratory reference ranges can vary, but typically baseline pre-ovulatory levels are less than 1.5 ng/ml.
- When at the baseline range (prior to ovulation), the levels can fluctuate within that range.
- The initial progesterone rise (1.5–2.5 ng/ml) correlates with the LH peak. Typically, ovulation will occur 2 days later and peak fertility will be 4–6 days later.

TABLE 4.1. Progesterone testing protocol for ovulation timing.

- Owner to determine onset of proestrus by observation of bloody vaginal discharge. This day is assigned day 1 of the cycle.
- Start progesterone testing by day 5–7 of the cycle.
- Continue progesterone testing every other day until determination of ovulation and onset of the fertile period.
- Typically: LH peak occurs when progesterone level is 1.5–2.5 ng/ml; ovulation two days later with progesterone range of 4–10 ng/ml; peak fertile period four days after LH peak with progesterone range of 6–20 ng/ml.
- Typically breed 4–6 days after the LH peak (2–4 days after ovulation).

- Progesterone levels at the time of ovulation vary, but range from 4 to 10 ng/ml.
- After ovulation, during peak fertility and also during diestrus, progesterone levels range from 6 to 20 ng/ml.
- Evaluation of sequential progesterone levels, every 24–28 hours, is the best method currently available to determine the time of ovulation. Each bitch is unique and looking for a specific progesterone level (e.g., 5 ng/ml) can lead to errors in interpretation.

LH Testing

- The LH rise can occur in 24 hours or less.
- LH testing is best accomplished with concurrent progesterone testing, and can be used to confirm the LH peak (Table 4.2).
- Typically, serum is analyzed every 24–48 hours for progesterone concentration, and 0.5 ml is saved and frozen *daily* for later LH analysis.
- If serum is not obtained daily, the LH peak can be missed.
- Once the progesterone rise is detected, serum samples can be thawed and then analyzed for LH.
- LH testing is helpful to confirm the fertile window for bitches with atypical progesterone curves. It is also helpful for increasing accuracy when using frozen semen, which is extremely dependent on correct timing for success. It is not necessary, and is costly and time-consuming, when breeding with fresh semen.
- Some bitches have a LH peak that is not detected with daily sampling (peak is less than 24 hours in duration); therefore, LH testing alone (without progesterone analysis) is not recommended.

Insemination Technique and Semen Handling

Indications and Considerations

- *Natural breeding*: excellent choice when breeding pair is available and semen is of good quality. For some breeds, natural breeding is not practical (e.g., English Bulldogs, French Bulldogs, some giant-sized breeds). Relatively high conception rate expected with proper

---

Table 4.2. Progesterone and LH testing protocol for ovulation timing.

- Follow same protocol as in Table 4.1 for progesterone testing.
- In addition: save serum every day. This will require removing and saving some serum from days for progesterone blood draws, and also to obtain serum on the in-between, non-progesterone testing days.
- As serum is obtained: save in individually date-labeled tubes.
- Once the first rise of progesterone is detected (1.5–2.5 ng/ml), obtain frozen serum from the date of this progesterone rise, and one day prior. Both of these samples are then sampled for presence of LH (follow directions included in test kit).
- Determination of LH will more accurately determine the day of the LH rise. Continue to assess progesterone concentrations to confirm ovulation and the fertile period.
- Since there can be several fertile days within the fertile period, determination of the day of the LH peak can help with selection of the absolute peak fertile day when using frozen semen (day 5–6 after the LH peak in most cases).

OT and viable semen. Breeding plan: two to three natural breedings within the fertile window (4–6 days after LH peak). Can also start one day prior to fertile window as semen is expected to survive several days within oviducts. Breeding more than once per day is not necessary, but breeding on consecutive days is acceptable.

- *Fresh semen (side-by-side) AI*: vaginal insemination: commonly performed when natural breeding is not possible, but breeding pair available. Semen is collected, evaluated and immediately inseminated into the cranial segment of the vaginal canal. Conception rate similar to natural breeding when proper OT is conducted and semen is viable.
- *Transcervical (intrauterine) insemination (TCI)*: Semen is deposited into the uterine lumen. The main advantage with TCI is to bypass the cervix, thereby providing a potentially greater amount of sperm into the uterus; however, sperm must still travel to oviduct for fertilization. The technique is difficult to learn and master, and specialized equipment is necessary.
  - *Advantages*: no requirement for tranquilization or anesthesia, very low risk of injury when properly performed, achieves same location of semen deposition as does a surgical procedure, can be very rapid to perform: 5 minutes in some cases (Fig. 4.2a,b).
  - *Indications*: chilled or frozen semen; semen of substandard quality; bitch with a history of subfertility. Semen must be properly prepared: only sperm-rich fraction of the ejaculate is used. Adding a semen extender (commercially available) containing an antibiotic is recommended due to placement directly into the uterus and therefore, bypassing the natural barrier (cervix).
- *Surgical intrauterine insemination*: Standard anesthesia, preparation for surgical laparotomy, and routine ventral mid-line approach to abdomen to exteriorize the uterus. Semen

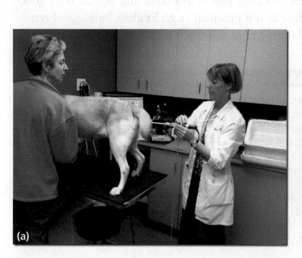
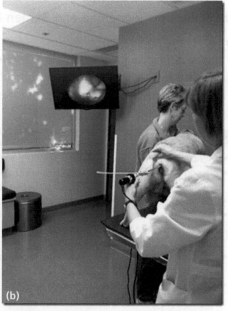

■ **Fig. 4.2.** (a,b) The TCI procedure: Note that the dog is standing with minimal restraint and is not sedated.

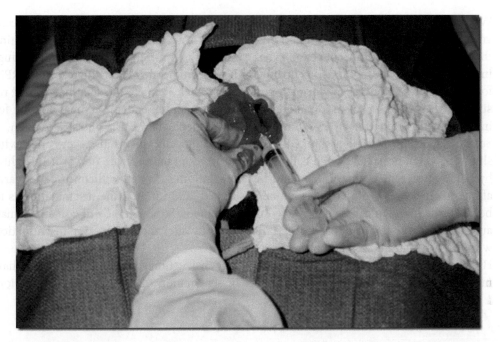

■ **Fig. 4.3.** Surgical insemination. Standard ventral midline surgical approach to exteriorize the uterus. Use a standard hypodermic needle, attached to a semen-filled syringe, to puncture through the uterine wall to inject semen into the uterine lumen; repeat into the other uterine horn.

is inseminated into both uterine horns (lumen) via trans-uterine puncture with standard hypodermic needle attached to semen-filled syringe (Fig. 4.3). Routine surgical closure and postoperative care, avoiding medications contraindicated in pregnancy. Indications and semen preparation: similar to TCI procedure. Care must be taken to avoid spillage of semen into the abdomen because semen-induced peritonitis can be a serious complication.

Semen Handling Considerations

- Canine semen is relatively hardy: exposure to light and mild temperature changes are not significant. If an extender is added, it should be the same temperature as the semen or at room temperature.
- When thawing frozen semen or warming chilled-shipped semen, care must be taken to avoid contact with water. Water is spermicidal.
- Do not use any type of lubricant on the insemination pipette or scope; natural lubrication from vaginal secretions is typically sufficient. If a lubricant is necessary, ensure it is a non-spermicidal type.
- Semen collection materials must be non-spermicidal and aseptic (clean and dry or disposable).
- All equipment/materials must be clean and dry. Specific syringes are used for insemination: the rubber stopper of most syringes might contain spermicidal residues. Either purchase syringes without a rubber stopper or prepare syringes (take apart, wash or soak in a dilute chlorhexidine solution for 5 minutes, rinse thoroughly and allow to completely dry).

- When preparing semen for chilled shipment or intrauterine insemination (TCI or surgical), very little to no prostatic fluid should be used. This is accomplished either by separating the semen fractions during collection (saving only the sperm-rich fraction) or by centrifuging the semen: round-bottomed centrifuge tubes recommended, centrifuge at 3000 RPM for 3–5 minutes, avoiding the formation of a firm pellet. Remove the supernatant and re-suspend the semen pellet in a commercial chilled-semen extender. Maximal volume for intrauterine insemination is 1.5–2.5 ml; volume will depend on parity and size of bitch.
- Semen handling for chilled-shipped semen: follow specific instructions provided with shipment when possible. Semen can be brought to room temperature or warmed slightly by holding the semen tube in the hand for a few minutes. Semen will continue to warm after insemination. If too large a volume is shipped, and intrauterine insemination is to be performed, semen can be centrifuged post-shipment. Supernatant will contain a small amount of sperm and can be deposited intravaginally after the intrauterine insemination with the concentrated semen portion.
- Handling/thawing of frozen semen: follow specific instructions provided. Proprietary thaw media may be provided with the shipment. Thaw semen immediately prior to insemination.

 ## COMMENTS

- Pitfalls of spot progesterone checking: The progesterone concentration increase is not typically linear and cannot be predicted. It is not unusual for relatively large increases to occur within 24–48 hours. Alternate-day evaluation is strongly recommended for accuracy, in some cases daily sampling is beneficial.
- Pitfalls of waiting for the progesterone concentration to reach a certain number (i.e., 5 ng/ml): Each bitch is rather unique and there is a considerable range of progesterone concentration-associated ovulation and the peak fertile period. Detecting the initial progesterone rise from baseline and confirming the rise by subsequent testing will improve the accuracy of OT and success.
- Pitfalls of predicting ovulation based on previously evaluated cycles: there can be considerable variation from cycle to cycle. It is highly recommend to perform OT for each cycle in which the bitch will be bred.

(Layout: box):

- Presentation of a bitch for AI without prior OT: It is not unusual for clients to seek veterinary assistance for an AI after an unsuccessful attempt at natural breeding.

RECOMMENDATIONS

- Perform complete physical examinations of both the male and female (including vaginal palpation to rule out a vaginal anomaly as a cause for the unsuccessful breeding attempt).
- Evaluate vaginal cytology: if fully cornified (90% or more superficial cells), the bitch is in estrus but it cannot be determined if this is pre- or post-ovulatory.

- Evaluate using vaginoscopy if possible to determine if vaginal edema (pre-ovulation) or crenulation (post-ovulation) is present.
- If unsure if pre- or post-ovulation, perform AI and collect serum for progesterone assay. If progesterone is 5–20 ng/ml and the vaginal cytology is fully cornified, very possibly timing was appropriate. If progesterone is less than 4 ng/ml, the bitch is unlikely to be in her fertile period and further progesterone testing and breeding are recommended.
- If vaginal cytology is compatible with diestrus (>50% of the cells are not superficial cells) and progesterone is elevated (usually >20 ng/ml), advise the client that the fertile window has likely been missed and to start timing earlier during the next cycle.

Abbreviations

OT = Ovulation timing: the methods evaluated to determine when ovulation occurs.
AI   = Artificial insemination: usually this term refers to a side-by-side breeding involving semen collection immediately prior to vaginal insemination.
LH = Luteinizing hormone: an ovulatory hormone released spontaneously from the pituitary that causes ovulation to occur about 2 days later.
TCI = Trans-cervical insemination: a procedure utilizing a specific scope (Storz) that will allow visualization and catheterization of the cervix during the fertile period. This method of insemination is used most frequently when breeding with chilled or frozen semen, or in situations of less than optimal fresh semen quality. It is also an augmented procedure when breeding a bitch that has apparently failed to conceive with prior breeding attempts.

See Also

Estrous Cycle Abnormalities
Medical Manipulation of the Estrous Cycle
Evaluation of Ovulation with Ultrasound

Suggested Reading

Goodman, M. (2001) in *Clinical Theriogenology. Veterinary Clinics of North America: Small Animal Practice*, Vol. 31 (2) (ed. A. Davidson), WB Saunders. Philadelphia PA.
Concannon, P.W., Hanse, I.W., McEntee, K. (1977) Changes in LH, progesterone and sexual behavior associated with preovulatory luteinization in the bitch. *Biol. Reprod.*, **17**, 604–613.
de Gier, J., Kooistra, H.S., Djajadiningrat-Laanen, S.C., *et al.* (2006) Temporal relations between plasma concentrations of luteinizing hormone, follicle-stimulating hormone, estradiol-17[beta], progesterone, prolactin, and [alpha]-melanocyte stimulating hormone during the follicular, ovulatory, and early luteal phase in the bitch. *Theriogenology*, **65**, 1346–1359.
Feldman, E.C., Nelson, R.W. (2004) Ovarian cycle and vaginal cytology, in *Canine and Feline Endocrinology and Reproduction,* 3rd edition. Saunders-Elsevier Science, St Louis, pp. 752–774.
Johnston, S.D., Root Kustritz, M.V., Olson, P.N. (2001) Breeding management and artificial insemination of the bitch, in *Canine and Feline Theriogenology.* Saunders, Philadelphia, pp. 49–63.

Author: Janice Cain DVM, DACVIM (Internal Medicine)

chapter 5

Breeding Management of the Queen: Pre-Breeding Examination and Breeding Husbandry

DEFINITION

- Maintaining a well-run breeding colony or a cattery relies on proper environmental conditions, including a photoperiod of ≥12 hours, high-quality nutrition, proper control of infectious diseases, and healthy breeding stock. The most common complaints include infertility, ovulation without conception, fetal losses, small litter sizes, and fading kittens.

ETIOLOGY/PATHOPHYSIOLOGY

- Sex determination: chromosomal sex, normal karyotype: 38, XX (queen) and 38, XY (tom); gonadal sex (ovaries or testes), and phenotypic sex (female or male).
- Normal puberty occurs on average at 9–10 months of age (range 4 months to 2 years); puberty may set in later in large breeds, Manx, and some longhaired cats; onset is also seasonal and weight (2.3– 2.5 kg) -dependent; males mature a little later than females.
- Queens (Fig. 5.1)
  - Seasonally polyestrous; estrus dependent on natural light; no cycles in winter months.
  - Induced ovulators.
  - Proestrus: short if seen (1–2 days); behaviors similar to estrus but queen will not allow mating by tom.
  - Estrus: range 3–16 days; average 4.4 days if bred and 7.4 days if not bred, signs of receptivity include lordosis, loud and frequent vocalization, increased affection, positive stimulation and allowing the male to mount; phase of estrogen dominance.
  - Postestrus (Interestrus): in queens that did not ovulate; 13–18 days' length (average 9 days); queen will return to estrus; cycle every 2–3 weeks.
  - Diestrus: progesterone dominance; in queens induced to ovulate; in a fertile mating, diestrus length 65 days (range 63–71 days); non-fertile mating but ovulation, 40–50 days length.
  - Seasonal anestrus: hormonal quiescence.
  - Reproductive life: 8–10 years; max. litter sizes at 2 years of age.

Blackwell's Five-Minute Veterinary Consult Clinical Companion: Small Animal Endocrinology and Reproduction, First Edition. Edited by Deborah S. Greco and Autumn P. Davidson. © 2017 John Wiley & Sons, Inc. Published 2017 by John Wiley & Sons, Inc.
Companion Website: www.fiveminutevet.com/endocrinology

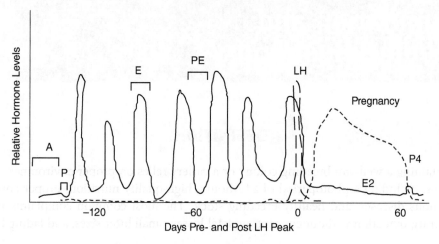

■ **Fig. 5.1.** Example of a typical estrous cycle in a cat. Mating results in induced ovulation and the LH peak. A fertile breeding results in diestrus (pregnancy) of 65 days. A, Anestrus; P, Proestrus; E, Estrus; PE, Postestrus; E2, Estradiol; P4, Progesterone; LH, Luteinizing hormone.

- ■ Toms
  - • Spines on penis: testosterone production (Fig. 5.2).
- ■ Breeding systems:
  - • Healthy parents with no genetic diseases or illnesses.
  - • Parents should be from healthy, good-sized litter.
  - • Indoor only cats; FeLV, FIV, FIP, *Toxoplasma*-negative.
  - • Quarantine new cats.

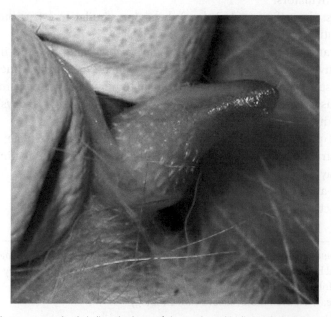

■ **Fig. 5.2.** Penile spines are organized circling the base of the penis and indicate the presence of testosterone.

- One to three queens per tom in a breeding room or run.
- Long-day, year-round breeders: at least 12–14 hours of artificial light/day.
- Average litter size four to six kittens, depending on the breed.
- Any disruption of the aforementioned processes will lead to infertility, small litter sizes, or neonatal death.

Systems Affected

- Reproductive

 ## SIGNALMENT/HISTORY

Risk Factors/Problems

- Overcrowding.
- Incorrect lighting (<14 hours daily).
- Poor environmental conditions; malnutrition.
- Congenital defects including chromosomal abnormalities (36 autosomes plus XXX, XXY or XX/XY).
- Systemic viral infections (FIP, FeLV, FIV).
- Bacterial infections.
- Parasitic infections (*Toxoplasma* ssp.).
- Loner.
- Hormonal disorders; false pregnancy.

Historic Findings

- Failure to cycle.
- Failure to conceive.
- Small litter sizes.
- Neonatal deaths, fading kittens.
- Endemic infectious diseases within the cattery (FIP, FHV, FIV, FeLV, ringworm, etc.).
- Medications and/or supplements given during pregnancy.
- Inadequate nutrition.
- Incorrect lighting (e.g., cattery in basement).

 ## CLINICAL FEATURES

- Absent breeding behavior.
- Breeding behavior that does not result in pregnancy.
- Queen cycles every 3 weeks despite being bred.
- Queen shows signs of estrus 25–50 days after being bred – infertile breeding.
- Queen palpates pregnant at 21 days but no kittens are born at term.
- Aged queen and/or tom.

- Congenital malformations of external genitalia; intersex conditions.
- Purulent or bloody vaginal discharge.
- Acute abdomen (queen).
- Spontaneous abortion.
- Small litter sizes.
- Neonatal deaths, fading kittens.

 ## DIFFERENTIAL DIAGNOSIS

- Endemic infectious diseases:
  - Viral: FIP, FeLV, FIV, FHV, FCV.
  - Bacterial: *Mycoplasma*, *Campylobacter*, (contributing to URTIs and chronic diarrhea, respectively and thus to overall poor health in cattery).
  - Parasitic: Toxoplasmosis, tritrichomoniasis, fleas and other parasites that are a sign of poor environmental conditions.
- Infertility
  - Incorrect environment (daily light cycles too short).
  - Congenital defects.
- Chromosomal abnormalities: 39, XXX; 38, XX/XY, 39, XXY.
- Rectovaginal fistula.
- Aplastic/hypoplastic ovaries/testes.
- Persistent penile frenulum.
- Hypoplastic prepuce.
- Cryptorchidism:
  - Insufficient stimulation for ovulation.
  - Hormonal imbalances (ovarian cysts, hormone-producing adrenal tumors).
  - Pyometra.
  - Loner (cats that do not interact with others, even when in season).
  - Concurrent disease.
  - Ovulation without fertilization (false pregnancy).
- Problems during pregnancy, abortion, still births, and small litter sizes:
  - Pyometra (fetuses in one horn and pyometra in the other).
  - Uterine torsion.
  - Medications and/or supplements given during pregnancy.
  - Poor environmental conditions (endemic disease – see above, toxins, overcrowding).
  - Geriatric queen.

 ## DIAGNOSTICS (including pre-breeding examination)

- Historical information:
  - Light cycles?
  - What are the environmental conditions? Sometimes, it is worth going to look at the cattery to get a good impression.

- Signalment of the animals.
- Breeding set-up? (i.e., how many queens per tom?).
- Breeding behavior?
- Is the queen cycling?
- Has she ever cycled before?
- Has she litters before?
- Does she breed readily but not get pregnant?
- Have any pregnancy diagnostics been performed?
- Litter sizes?

■ Thorough physical examination: anatomical abnormalities, concurrent disease; check for the presence of spines on the penis to ensure testosterone production; check for testicular descent.

■ Vaginoscopy: an otoscope can be used carefully to examine the vestibule and vaginal canal for strictures and other malformations.

■ Vaginal cytology: often not recommended in cycling queens, as it may induce ovulation. Cytology dependent on estradiol concentrations and shows changes similar to those found in dogs (Fig. 5.3). Check for inflammatory cells and bacteria. Bacteria are only of concern if intracellular and accompanied by large numbers of neutrophils.

■ Complete blood count, biochemistry screen and UA if systemic disease is suspected.

■ FeLV, FIV, and toxoplasmosis testing.

■ Hormone testing:
  - Queen: estradiol levels during estrus, progesterone several days after mating to assess induction of ovulation and presence of functional corpora lutea (>2 ng/ml).
  - Tom: testosterone: check for penile spines *or* draw baseline testosterone sample (serum), administer 250–500 IU hCG IM and draw two post samples at 1 hour and 2 hours after hCG.

■ Vaginal cultures using guarded swabs or from the uterus directly (hysterotomy).

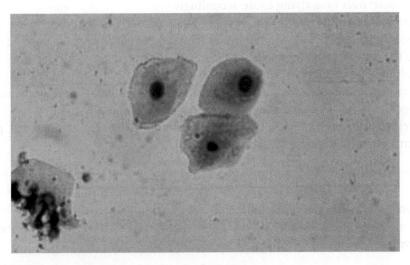

■ **Fig. 5.3.** Feline estrual vaginal cytology showing superficial cells.

- Semen evaluation including cultures: semen collection via artificial vagina (trained tom), electroejaculation or 100 µg/kg medetomidine IM and inserting a tomcat catheter into the urethra but not all the way in to the bladder – the collection will be in the catheter. Normal cat semen shows an average of about 50% motility, 30% forward progressive motility, and 40% normal morphology
- Imaging:
  - Radiography: Generally not helpful other than after day 42 of gestation to assess number of fetuses or retention of fetus or fetal parts after parturition.
  - Ultrasound: Normal ovaries and non-pregnant uterus may not be seen easily; Look for cystic structures on ovaries or on uterine serosa; enlarged uterus may indicate pyometra, pregnancy, or uterine torsion (during pregnancy).
  - Check for fetal viability; fetal heartbeats seen after 21/22 days gestation. Retained placentas, fetuses or fetal parts after parturition.
  - In male cats, check for cryptorchidism (retained testicle not easily visible).
  - Enlarged adrenal gland may indicate hormone-producing neoplasia in both tom and queen.

 ## THERAPEUTICS

- Failure to cycle: increase photoperiod, treat underlying disease. If queen has cycled before, induce estrus.
- Queen cycles but does not ovulate: induce ovulation.
- Queens cycle but male seems uninterested: change male or pair with different females.
- Ovarian cysts: surgical removal or medical treatment with GnRH.
- Pyometra: medical treatment using prostaglandins if breeder is to be retained, otherwise ovariohysterectomy (OHE). To assess medical treatment, ultrasonographic assessment of the uterus should be performed every few days until it is completely evacuated.
- Queens abort: treat underlying cause accordingly.
- Small litter sizes, fading kittens: increase photoperiod; decrease numbers of cats in cattery or in the room; improve hygiene; remove or treat infectious diseases; quarantine new additions to the cattery; provide excellent nutritional support.
- Use healthier and younger breeding stock.
- Repair anatomic abnormalities but other than the persistent penile frenulum, most defects have a genetic basis, and thus may not be suitable for breeding.
- Toms reluctant to breed: check for hair rings around penis and remove; cut persistent frenulum; pair with different females.

Drugs

- Estrus induction or synchronization:
  - 2 mg FSH/cat/day IM for 4–5 days (3–7 days) until estrus is apparent, then induce ovulation with 150–250 IU hCG IM or 25 µg GnRH IM.

- Alternatively, 150 IU PMSG or eCG per cat IM, followed by 100 IU hCG per cat IM 84 hours later.
- Induce ovulation:
  - 5–25 µg GnRH per cat.
  - 50–250 IU hCG per cat IM; ovulation 24–36 hours later.
- Ovarian cysts; both options will cause ovulation and/or luteinization:
  - 25 µg GnRH per cat IM.
  - 250 IU hCG per cat IM.
- Pyometra: Day 1: 100 µg PG-F2alpha (Lutalyse®)/kg SC or IM once, from day 2 on until uterus has been evacuated: 200–250 µg PG-F2 alpha/kg once daily or divided into two- to three-times daily for less side effects.
- Antibiotics for the treatment of genital infections: depends on microbial culture results; in the absence of culture results, marbofloxacin provides good tissue levels of a broad-spectrum antibiotic with less side effects in cats than enrofloxacin.

Procedures

- OHE for pyometra.
- Surgical resection of persistent frenulum.
- Laparotomy or laparoscopy to drain/remove ovarian cysts.

 COMMENTS

Expected Course and Prognosis

- Improving environmental conditions, increasing the photoperiod, and providing high-quality nutrition result in overall increases in litter sizes and improved health of the neonates.
- If other systemic illness is present, fertility may improve after successful treatment of the underlying illness, however, there may be a genetic predisposition or basis for the systemic illness, which may not make the animal a good candidate for breeding.
- Medical treatment of pyometra may result in return of fertility but is not always successful.

Abbreviations

FeLV   = Feline leukemia virus
FIV   = Feline immunodeficiency virus
FIP   = feline infectious peritonitis
FHV   = Feline herpesvirus
FCV   = Feline calicivirus
URTI   = Upper respiratory tract infection
CL   = Corpus luteum
FSH   = Follicle-stimulating hormone

hCG   = Human chorionic gonadotropin
eCG   = Equine chorionic gonadotropin
PMSG = pregnant mare serum gonadotropin
GnRH = Gonadotropin-releasing hormone
OHE   = Ovariohysterectomy

See Also

Infectious Causes of Pregnancy Loss- Feline
Evaluation of Ovulation with Ultrasound
Ultrasonographic Gestational Aging in the Dog and Cat
Nutrition of the Breeding Dog and Cat
Neonatal Resuscitation and Post Partum Neonatology

Suggested Reading

Johnston, S.D., Root Kustritz, M.V., Olson, P.N.S. (2001) *Canine and Feline Theriogenology*. WB Saunders, Philadelphia, PA.
Wiebe, V.J., Howard, J.P. (2009) Pharmacologic advances in canine and feline reproduction. *Top. Companion Animal Med.*, 24, 71–99.
Greene, C.E., Schultz, R.D. (2006) Immunoprophylaxis, in *Infectious Diseases of the Dog and Cat* (eds C.E.Greene, et al.). WB Saunders, Philadelphia, PA.
England, G., von Heimendahl, A. (2011) *Manual of Canine and Feline Reproduction and Neonatology, 2nd edition*. BSAVA Press, London, UK.
Lopate, C. (2012) *Management of Pregnant and Neonatal Dogs, Cats, and Exotic Pets*. Wiley Blackwell, Ames, IA.

Author: Margret L. Casal Dr med vet, MS, PhD, DECAR

chapter 6

Carcinoid and Carcinoid Syndrome

DEFINITION

- Carcinoid tumors are neuroendocrine tumors that arise from amine precursor uptake and decarboxylation (APUD) cells. The APUDoma family of tumors also includes pheochromocytomas, insulinomas, gastrinomas, glucagonomas, medullary thyroid tumors and parathyroid tumors.
- The origins of carcinoids are most commonly the enterochromaffin and enterochromaffin-like cells of the gastrointestinal tract, but they can occur in a variety of locations due to the embryologic nature of these cells.
- Carcinoids may secrete a variety of amines such as histamine, serotonin, and peptides such as bradykinins and tachykinins. In humans, these secretory substances can cause a well-recognized 'carcinoid syndrome' and/or 'carcinoid crisis' in approximately 5–10% of carcinoid patients. The human carcinoid syndrome is most commonly characterized by flushing, abdominal pain, diarrhea, bronchospasm and cyanosis. Domestic small animals have not been reported to date to show these clinical signs, although a dog has been reported to have episodic collapse and melena in association with an ileocecal carcinoid. Morbidity and mortality are more often a function of tumor size and gastrointestinal blockage in dogs and cats with carcinoid. Clinical signs may vary with the location of the primary tumor and whether metastasis is present.
- Primary carcinoid tumors have been reported in the stomach, small intestine, colon, lung, gallbladder and liver in dogs. In cats, carcinoids have been found in the stomach, small intestine, liver, and heart.

ETIOLOGY/PATHOPHYSIOLOGY

- In humans, carcinoids are frequently associated with carcinoid syndrome. This syndrome occurs due to a release of substances from the carcinoid tumors, most frequently serotonin. Serotonin metabolites can be measured in urine in humans. This syndrome has not been demonstrated in veterinary medicine. In dogs and cats, clinical signs are most frequently related to gastrointestinal signs associated with a mass-lesion or signs associated with the presence of metastatic disease.

Blackwell's Five-Minute Veterinary Consult Clinical Companion: Small Animal Endocrinology and Reproduction, First Edition. Edited by Deborah S. Greco and Autumn P. Davidson. © 2017 John Wiley & Sons, Inc. Published 2017 by John Wiley & Sons, Inc. Companion Website: www.fiveminutevet.com/endocrinology

Systems Affected

- Gastrointestinal – weight loss, anorexia, diarrhea, vomiting.
- Hepatobiliary – jaundice, ascites.
- Endocrine/urologic – polyuria/polydipsia.

SIGNALMENT/HISTORY

- Dog: rare, older, >9 years of age.
- Cat: rare, middle-aged to older, >7 years of age.

CLINICAL FEATURES

- Clinical signs generally depend on the location of the primary tumor and/or metastases. Signs range from weight loss, anorexia, diarrhea, polyuria/polydipsia, vomiting, melena, ascites, to jaundice. Carcinoid syndrome in humans is characterized by paroxysmal flushing of the head/neck, diarrhea, abdominal cramping and bronchospasms. Carcinoid heart disease is a known syndrome in humans with advanced carcinoid syndrome, which develops due to the creation of fibrotic endocardial plaques and secondary valvular dysfunction in response to excess secretion of serotonin. Cardiac signs (ventricular tachycardia) have been reported in one dog with an intestinal carcinoid and are thought to possibly be related to tumor-associated vasoactive amines.

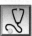

DIFFERENTIAL DIAGNOSIS

- Differentials vary depending on the presenting complaint. They include primary gastrointestinal diseases such as other neoplasia, infection, inflammation, parasites, foreign body ingestion, dietary indiscretion, or other liver/biliary disease.

DIAGNOSTICS

CBC/ Biochemistry/Urinalysis

- Results can appear normal except for a mild anemia that is generally non-regenerative.
- Electrolyte abnormalities and elevated liver enzymes can be present depending on tumor location and clinical presentation.

Other Laboratory Tests

- Serum serotonin levels, serum chromogranin A, and urinary 5-hydroxyindoleacetic acid are measured in humans suspected of carcinoid tumors. This appears more accurate than direct measurement of serum amine and peptide levels. Serum serotonin levels were found to be increased 10-fold in one dog with an intestinal carcinoid with multiple metastases. Other serum and urinary testing has not been documented in animals with carcinoid tumors.

Imaging

- Ultrasound has been used to identify both primary tumors and metastasis in the abdomen and the thorax of dogs and cats.
- CT scans and MRI have been used with mild-moderate success for localization of carcinoids in humans.
- Newer and more sensitive molecular-imaging modalities in humans include the use of: (i) radiolabeled somatostatin receptor scintigraphy ('OctreoScan'); (ii) radioiodinated metaiodobenzylguanidine (MIBG) imaging; and (iii) PET scans.
- Three-view thoracic radiographs should be taken for preoperative staging.

Pathologic Findings

- These tumors typically have a fine fibrovascular stroma with minimal to moderate cellular pleomorphism. The cytoplasm is eosinophilic and usually contains secretory granules which often stain argyrophilic and/or argentaffin-positive.
- Biopsy of the affected tissue with histopathologic examination often confirms the diagnosis. In some cases with equivocal histopathologic results, immunohistochemistry (looking for chromogranin A and/or synaptophysin expression) may be used to determine the amines and peptides actively secreted to aid in the confirmation of a carcinoid diagnosis.

 THERAPEUTICS

- In many cases, surgical excision can be curative, especially when there is no evidence of metastasis. Prognosis is guarded, however, as metastasis may be present at the time of diagnosis. Debulking can decrease hormone secretion in humans, and it may relieve gastrointestinal signs in animals that are obstructed because of tumor size.

Drugs

- Octreotide, a somatostatin analog, is often used in humans for palliative therapy when surgery is not an option. Octreotide inhibits hormone secretion from the tumor cells. Octreotide may be of little benefit in veterinary patients with carcinoids as carcinoid syndrome is not widely reported.
- Chemotherapy and radiotherapy has been reported to have minimal efficacy in humans with carcinoid tumors, as carcinoids are believed to be relatively chemoresistant and radioresistant. **The use of adjuvant carboplatin has been recently reported in a dog with a completely excised non-metastatic jejunal carcinoid.

COMMENTS

Patient Monitoring

- Blood work should be serially monitored postoperatively. Elevated liver enzymes may correlate with hepatic metastasis.
- Abdominal ultrasound and three-view thoracic radiographs should be serially performed postoperatively to delineate liver and/or other organ metastasis.

Expected Course and Prognosis

- Limited survival data available in veterinary medicine
- Complete excision likely associated with a good outcome. Metastasis reported in several cases, leading to a guarded prognosis.

Abbreviations

APUD = amine precursor uptake and decarboxylation
PET   = positron emission tomography

Suggested Reading

Choi, U.S., Alleman, A.R., Choi, J.H., et al. (2008) Cytologic and immunohistochemical characterization of a lung carcinoid in a dog. *Vet. Clin. Pathol.*, **37** (2), 249–252.

Feldman, E.C., Nelson, R.W. (2004) Gastrinoma, Glucagonoma and Other APUDomas, in *Canine and Feline Endocrinology and Reproduction* (eds E.D. Feldman, R.W. Nelson), 3rd edition. Saunders, St Louis, pp. 656–657.

Rossmeisl, J.H., Jr, Forrester, S.D., Robertson, J.L., et al. (2002) Chronic vomiting associated with a gastric carcinoid in a cat. *J. Am. Animal Hosp. Assoc.*, **38** (1), 61–66.

Sugnini, E.P., Gargiulo, M., Assin R., et al. (2008) Adjuvant carboplatin for the treatment of intestinal carcinoid in a dog. *In Vivo*, **22** (6), 759–761.

Tappin, S., Brown, P., Ferasin, L. (2008) An intestinal neuroendocrine tumour associated with paroxysmal ventricular tachycardia and melaena in a 10-year old boxer. *J. Small Anim. Pract.*, **49** (1), 33–37.

Author: Virginia Gill DVM, DACVIM (Oncology)

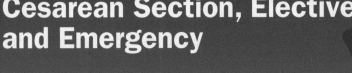

chapter 7

Cesarean Section, Elective and Emergency

DEFINITION

- Cesarean section is defined as the delivery of a fetus by surgical incision through the abdominal wall and uterus; this was derived from the belief that Julius Caesar was born that way. Cesarean sections can be either elective or emergency.

ETIOLOGY/PATHOPHYSIOLOGY

- Indications for acute cesarean section (CS):
  - Primary or secondary uterine inertia nonresponsive to medical therapy (see Dystocia, Chapter 15). If the dystocia is prolonged the risk for fetal death is increased, and early intervention may reduce morbidity and mortality.
  - Uterine rupture secondary to dystocia or inappropriate use of ecbolic drugs, most commonly oxytocin (Fig. 7.1).

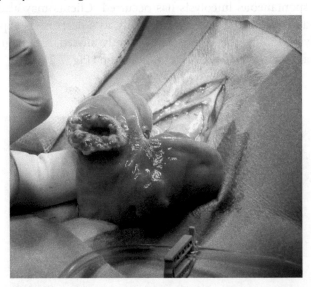

■ Fig. 7.1. Uterine horn rupture secondary to excessive administration of oxytocin in an obstructive dystocia.

Blackwell's Five-Minute Veterinary Consult Clinical Companion: Small Animal Endocrinology and Reproduction, First Edition. Edited by Deborah S. Greco and Autumn P. Davidson. © 2017 John Wiley & Sons, Inc. Published 2017 by John Wiley & Sons, Inc.
Companion Website: www.fiveminutevet.com/endocrinology

- Fetal malposition without success of correction by manipulation vaginally.
- Fetal death (usually includes green vulvar discharge, uteroverdin, in the bitch) with remaining viable but distressed fetuses.
- Fetal distress with decreased heart rate. This is evaluated by ultrasonographic examination or fetal Doppler echocardiograph. If the puppies have a heart rate of 150–170 beats/min, CS should be considered. If the fetal heart rate is <150 beats/min in one or several puppies, CS should be performed without delay. Normal heart rate in at the end of gestation is >200/min in puppies and approximately 230/min in kittens.
- Indications for elective CS:
  - Abnormalities of maternal pelvis (traumatic or congenital).
  - Abnormalities of soft tissues (e.g., vaginal septa).
  - Disease during pregnancy (e.g., Addison's disease or diabetes mellitus).
  - History of earlier dystocia may be an indication for elective CS. However, veterinarians should inform breeders to work proactively to exclude bitches with a history of unexplained dystocia from breeding. Breeders are suggested to primarily use bitches who manage to breed and give birth independently, without medical assistance. This is challenging in bitches with an increased anatomic incidence of dystocia, for example brachycephalic breeds.
- Timing of elective CS is crucial for the survival of puppies. The CS can be safely performed on or after day 62 after the LH surge. Progesterone should ideally be less than 2 ng/ml, indicating that spontaneous luteolysis has occurred. Clients may also be instructed to measure the body temperature several times daily, as a decrease is expected in conjunction with luteolysis, though this can be inadvertantly missed. A radiograph showing fetal dentition mineralization is evidence of term gestation (Fig. 7.2).

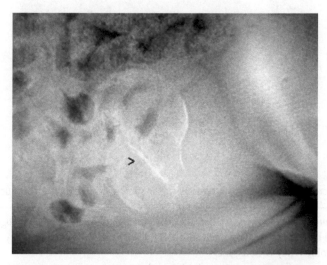

■ **Fig. 7.2.** Mineralization of fetal dentition (arrow) indicating fetal maturation; elective CS can proceed safely.

SIGNALMENT/HISTORY

- Some breeds have been reported to have an increased incidence (or frequency) of dystocia, including brachycephalic breeds, Scottish Terriers, Chihuahuas, and Pomeranians. Some giant breeds have an increased incidence, such as the Irish Wolfhound and Great Dane.

Equipment

- Surgery equipment required for CS is standard, as for most abdominal surgeries.
- Equipment for resuscitation of the puppies includes towels, a warming box, suction devices, supplemental oxygen, and supportive drugs.

Procedure

Preoperative Steps

- Before induction of anesthesia, the bitch or queen should optimally be treated with crystalloid fluids. Pre-anesthetic blood analysis is recommended including, at least packed cell volume (PCV), total solids (TS), ionized calcium, and glucose.
- The dam should be prepped before induction if possible.

Patient Anesthesia and Analgesia

- Many different protocols have been used in the bitch. The goal is both to keep puppy morbidity and mortality minimal while at the same time delivering a safe plane of anesthesia to keep the bitch pain-free and immobile. Premedication with an anticholinergic prevents bradycardia. Glycopyrrolate may be preferable to atropine as it does not cross the placenta. Sedatives and tranquilizers should be avoided due to fetal cardiovascular depression. Pre-oxygenation is very important. Induction of anesthesia with propofol, followed by inhalational anesthesia with isofluorane or sevoflorane, is ideal. A propofol CRI is also an option, but provides less (if any) analgesia. Many bitches will develop respiratory depression from the propofol infusion. Induction with ketamine, thiamylal and thiopental has been reported to reduce puppy vigor and should be avoided. Less has been documented concerning anesthesia for CS in the queen. Propofol induction followed by inhalation is commonly used. However, one retrospective study showed higher survival in kittens when dissociative anesthesia was used in the queen compared to propofol combined with isoflorane. The puppies or kittens should be exposed to isoflorane/sevoflorane for as short a time as possible to reduce apnea after delivery.
- Fetal hypoxia is avoided by ensuring maintenance of airway, blood pressure and circulation in the bitch or queen throughout the procedure. If epidural anesthesia is used the dam cannot be intubated; the bitch or queen can be difficult to restrain when the newborns vocalize.

- When all puppies or kittens have been removed from the uterus, opiates should be administered to the dam (e.g., meperidine, methadone, oxymorphone or morphine could be used). If opiates have been administered before induction the newborns should be treated with an appropriate reversal agent if depressed.
- The additional use of local anesthetic agents (lidocaine, bupivacaine) can complement general anesthesia and facilitate entry into the abdomen and the uterus, as well as providing analgesia postoperatively.

Surgical Procedure

- Celiotomy is the method most commonly performed in the bitch and queen. A flank incision is uncommon in the bitch or queen; its advantage is less pressure on the diaphragm with better oxygenation due to lateral positioning; the uterine horns may be easier to approach. The increased surgical time and the risk for suture complications, as well as possible inexperience with the approach, are disadvantages. The ventral midline incision is started cranial to the umbilicus and ends just cranial to the pubic bone. If the dam carries many puppies/kittens, the incision has to be extended further cranially. The final entry into the abdomen through the thin linea alba must be made carefully as the uterine wall usually is in direct connection with the abdominal wall. The uterus is carefully lifted; the risk of uterine rupture during elevation is high if not supported over large surfaces. When isolated, moist sponges are placed around the area for the uterine incision. The body of the uterus is usually incised; if there are many neonates, more than one incision might be required and this could involve the uterine horns. The puppies or kittens are then milked toward the incision. The puppy or kitten is then elevated from the uterus within the amniotic sac (Fig. 7.3). The amniotic

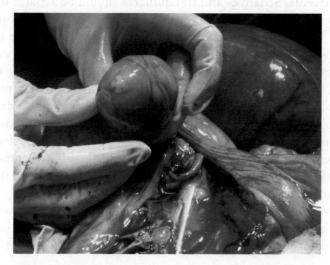

■ **Fig. 7.3.** Neonate head within the amnion.

sac can be opened to allow the puppy/kitten to start to breathe, preferably avoiding amniotic fluid entering the dam's abdomen. The placenta is released from the uterus and the puppy or kitten is handed over to an unsterile assistant. If the placenta is firmly attached to the uterus it should be left in place as the risk for endometrial bleeding is increased; the umbilicus is clamped close (1–3 cm) to the neonate before it is incised. Only careful traction is used when the placentas are removed. When all puppies or kittens have been removed the uterus should be checked again before closure from ovaries to cervix to make sure no neonate has been left behind. The vaginal canal should also be evaluated. Remaining placentas are allowed to pass naturally; ecbolic agents can be used if necessary, but this is unusual. The canine and feline placenta has a zonary configuration (Fig. 7.4).

■ Closure of the uterus is done in one to two layers in an invaginated fashion (Cushing or Lambert). Absorbable monofilament suture 3/0 or 4/0 is used with a taper-point needle. It is important to include the strong submucosa in the suture, the uterine lumen is not perforated or sutured through to reduce risk for complications secondary to scar formation and suture reactions in the endometrial wall. To reduce the amount of adhesions in the peritoneal cavity the suture including the knots may be buried.

■ Oxytocin (0.252 U per dam) can be administered after suturing of the uterus to induce involution; this might be especially important in bitches or queens with uterine inertia. Before closure the abdomen is checked for leakage and debris. The peritoneal cavity is lavaged with warm, sterile fluids. The instruments and gloves may be exchanged if required. The body wall is closed routinely. The cutis may be sutured intradermally to reduce the presence of cutaneous sutures and avoid a need to return for suture removal

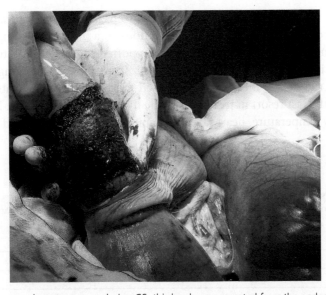

■ **Fig. 7.4.** Canine zonary placenta as seen during CS; this has been separated from the endometrium.

during nursing. Most bitches and queens do not pick on their sutures when caring for their puppies/kittens.

- En-bloc surgery – an ovariohysterectomy in conjunction with CS – is an option in specific cases. Ideally, ovariohysterectomy is only performed when uterine pathology is present, due to the increased anesthetic and surgical time required, inherent blood loss, and concern for lack of estrogen which promotes lactation. The ovarian and uterine arteries are ligated and the entire uterus is handed over to assistants. The recommended time from ligation to delivery of neonates should be less than 1 minute. The survival rate after en-bloc surgery is reported to be 75% in dogs and 42% in cats. Alternatively, ovariohysterectomy can be performed once the neonates have been delivered as described above.

Complications and Follow-Up

- Complications following CS in the bitch and queen are relatively uncommon. Important perioperative complications reported are hypotension, rupture of the uterus, and hemorrhage. Endometritis, peritonitis, wound infection and aspiration pneumonia are complications that may occur after discharge, and owners should be informed to pay attention to signs of these disorders. If the CS was uncomplicated and the dam and also the neonates are healthy before discharge, no new appointment is required. Ideally, discharge should occur once the dam is ambulatory, euthermic, and showing maternal behavior and the neonates have nursed.

 # COMMENTS

- Approximately 60% of dystocias in bitches and queens are treated surgically, most of them on an emergency basis. The risk for complications in a dam undergoing a CS is usually very low as long as she is healthy; survival is reported to be 99% in bitches. The risk of complications is, however, higher for the puppies and kittens. The longer the labor has been ongoing, the higher the risk for increased mortality in the neonates; therefore, CS should not be the last resort in treatment of the dystocia bitch or queen. Normal neonatal values for body temperature, heart rate and respiratory rate are presented in Table 7.1 (see Chapter 46).

TABLE 7.1. Normal values of body temperature, heart rate and respiratory rate in the neonate.

	Puppies	Kittens
Body temperature	35.0–37.2 °C	35.0–37.2°C
Heart rate	200 beats/min	200–250 beats/min
Respiratory rate	10–18/min	10–18/min

Abbreviations

CS = cesarean section

See Also

Canine Breeding Management
Dystocia
Pregnancy Diabetes
Pregnancy Ketosis
Feline Prebreeding Examination and Breeding Husbandry
Evaluation of Ovulation with Ultrasound
Ultrasonographic Evaluation of Gestational Aging in Dogs and Cats
Neonatal Resuscitation and Post-Partum Neonatology

Suggested Reading

Moon-Massat, P.F. (2002) Perioperative factors associated with puppy vigor after delivery by cesarean section. *J. Am. Animal Hosp. Assoc.*, **38**, 90–96.
Robbins, M.A., Mullen, H.S. (2004) En bloc ovariohysterectomy as a treatment for dystocia in dogs and cats. *Vet. Surg.*, **23**, 48–52.
Smith, F.O. (2007) Challenges in small animal parturition – Timing elective and emergency cesarean section. *Theriogenology*, **68**, 348–353.
Smith, F.O. (2012) Guide to emergency interception during parturition in the dog and cat. *Vet. Clin. North Am. Small. Anim. Pract.*, **42**, 489–499.
Traas, A.M. (2008) Surgical management of canine and feline dystocia. *Theriogenology*, **70**, 337–342.

Author: Annika Bergstrom DVM, DECAR

Pyometra, Cystic Endometrial Hyperplasia (Hydrometra, Mucometra, Hematometra)

chapter 8

DEFINITION

- Pyometra – accumulation of purulent material within the uterine lumen. Stump pyometra may occur in spayed bitches. Classified as open or closed based on the presence or absence of vaginal discharge, respectively.
- Hydrometra – accumulation of a watery secretion within the uterine lumen.
- Mucometra – accumulation of a mucoid secretion within the uterine lumen.
- Hematometra – accumulation of blood within the uterine lumen.

ETIOLOGY/PATHOPHYSIOLOGY

- Two possible mechanisms:
  - May occur in association with cystic endometrial hyperplasia (CEH) in middle-aged to older bitches during diestrus. Elevated progesterone concentrations increase glandular secretions, which results in cyst formation and decreased mucosal immunity and myometrial contractility. Bacteria ascend the cervix or colonize hematogenously. Bacterial proliferation occurs in the presence of progesterone. If there are no bacteria present, mucometra, hydrometra or hematometra may develop instead.
  - Subacute endometritis develops without cystic change in the presence of elevated progesterone concentrations in response to bacteria ascending the cervix during estrus. Typically, pseudo-trophoblastic hyperplasia and increased glandular secretions develop during diestrus.
- Pyometra may occur concurrently with pregnancy.
- The most common bacterium is *Escherichia coli*; *Proteus mirabilis*, *Streptococcus* spp., *Staphylococcus* spp., *Pseudomonas* spp. and *Pasteurella* spp. are other common pathogens.

Blackwell's Five-Minute Veterinary Consult Clinical Companion: Small Animal Endocrinology and Reproduction, First Edition. Edited by Deborah S. Greco and Autumn P. Davidson. © 2017 John Wiley & Sons, Inc. Published 2017 by John Wiley & Sons, Inc.
Companion Website: www.fiveminutevet.com/endocrinology

Systems Affected

- Reproductive – may affect future fertility or the viability of a concurrent pregnancy. May cause signs of vaginitis. Peritonitis may result via translocation of bacteria across the uterine wall, from uterine rupture, or leakage or purulent material from the oviductal bursa.
- Renal/Urologic – acute renal failure from sepsis, endotoxemia, dehydration. Antigen/antibody complex-induced glomerulonephritis may result in chronic kidney disease. Cystitis may occur concurrently. May result in multiple organ dysfunction syndrome (MODS). *E. coli*-associated diabetes insipidus can occur.
- Hemic/Immune – may result in endotoxemia, sepsis, septic shock, or systemic inflammatory response syndrome (SIRS).
- Cardiovascular – may result in disseminated intravascular coagulation (DIC), MODS.
- Respiratory – may result in SIRS, MODS.
- Hepatobiliary – hepatic injury from septicemia or endotoxemia, MODS.

 # SIGNALMENT/HISTORY

- Typically occurs between 2 and 8 weeks post-ovulation, but may occur at any stage of the estrous cycle.
- Middle aged to older (>5–8 years), intact, nulliparous bitches are most common, but may occur in multiparous or young bitches. Stump pyometra may occur in spayed bitches or bitches with ovarian remnants.

Risk Factors

- Hormonal treatment with progestagens ± estrogen.
- Increasing age.
- Increased frequency of estrous cycles or other cycle abnormalities (i.e., luteal cyst, neoplasia).
- Subacute, acute or chronic endometritis.
- Prior history of abortion, pregnancy termination.
- Prior history of mucometra, hematometra, hydrometra.

Historic Findings

- Polyuria and polydipsia (PU/PD).
- Lethargy, depression, anorexia.
- Vomiting, diarrhea.
- ± vulvar discharge.
- ± fever.
- Abdominal distension.

CLINICAL FEATURES

- Depression, lethargy.
- ± fever.
- ± vulvar discharge – absence of discharge may indicate closed pyometra or endometritis.
- ± abdominal distension or a palpably enlarged uterus – may be difficult to palpate if uterus is mildly enlarged or the abdomen is tense.
- ± abdominal pain.
- Delayed capillary refill time (CRT) or dark or brick-red mucous membranes if septic or in DIC, SIRS, or MODS.
- Tachypnea and tachycardia if septic, in DIC, SIRS or MODS.
- Mucometra/hematometra/hydrometra typically have no associated clinical signs other than ± vulvar discharge. They are often diagnosed incidentally during ultrasound examination.

 ## DIFFERENTIAL DIAGNSOSIS

- Pregnancy.
- CEH or endometritis.
- Cervicitis or vaginitis.
- Cystitis.
- Vaginal or uterine neoplasia.
- Vaginal or uterine foreign body.
- Post-partum metritis.
- Uterine torsion.
- Other causes of abdominal pain or distension (gastrointestinal, neoplastic, urinary).

 ## DIAGNOSTICS

- Complete blood count (CBC) – leukocytosis with mature neutrophilia ± degenerative left shift; ± toxic neutrophils; monocytosis; ± normochromic, normocytic anemia.
- Serum chemistry – ± elevated renal and hepatic enzymes (pre-renal or renal); electrolyte abnormalities if vomiting or severe diarrhea.
- Urinalysis – cystocentesis is contraindicated if pyometra is suspected or confirmed. Free catch or catheter samples may reveal real changes or be caused by contamination with purulent or hemorrhagic uterine discharge.
- Vaginal cytology – immature epithelial cells most common, presence of metestrual and foam cells increased, increased numbers of degenerate or non-degenerate neutrophils ± intra- and extracellular bacteria.

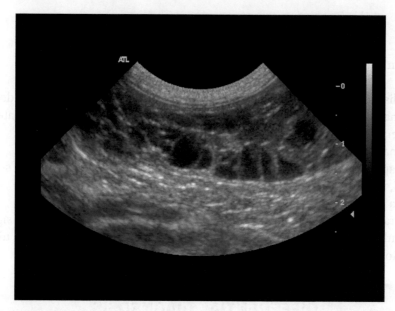

■ **Fig. 8.1.** Sagittal ultrasonographic image of a uterine horn showing marked cystic changes in the endometrium. Image courtesy of T.W. Baker.

- Ultrasonography – required for definitive diagnosis. Ultrasound cannot differentiate the types of fluid present in the uterus, so further diagnostics are required to differentiate the different uterine fluid accumulations. Ultrasound will allow assessment of uterine distention and wall thickness, as well as the presence of cystic changes, bands or septums (Fig. 8.1). The amount of distension or echogenicity of the uterine contents has no reflection of the severity of disease or degree of endotoxemia or sepsis (Fig. 8.2a, b).
- Radiography – may reveal an enlarged ventral abdominal viscus but cannot differentiate early pregnancy from uterine pathology and should never be used as the sole means of diagnosis.
- Progesterone concentration – >2ng/ml if still in diestrus.
- Culture and sensitivity – uterine culture is preferred over vaginal culture, but if not possible, a high guarded vaginal culture should be performed instead. Transcervical endoscopic catheterization technique (TECT) may be used to obtain uterine cultures.

Pathological Findings

- Neutrophilic ± eosinophilic inflammation.
- Lymphoplasmacytic inflammation.
- Cystic endometrial hyperplasia or pseudo-trophoblastic hyperplasia.

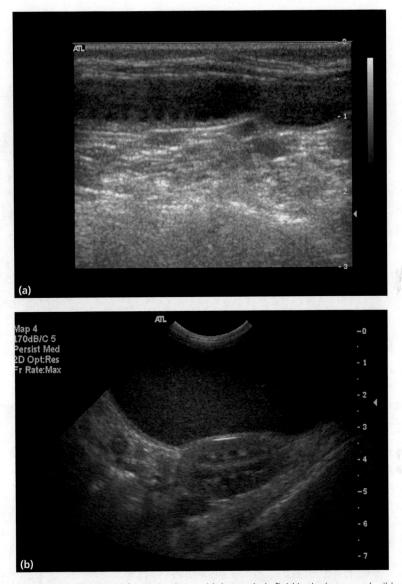

■ **Fig. 8.2.** (a) Ultrasonographic image of a uterine horn with hypoechoic fluid in the lumen and mild endometrial cystic changes. Diagnosis hydrometra. Image courtesy of T.W. Baker. (b) Ultrasonographic image of a close pyometra; marked distension of a uterine horn ventral to the kidney with echogenic fluid. Image courtesy of T.W. Baker.

 THERAPEUTICS

- Stabilization and supportive care followed by ovariohysterectomy is the recommended course of treatment since it is curative. Hysterectomy alone is never recommended for pyometra as any retained uterine tissue will be at risk for development of stump pyometra; thus, ovariectomy should always be performed with hysterectomy (Figs 8.3 and 8.4).

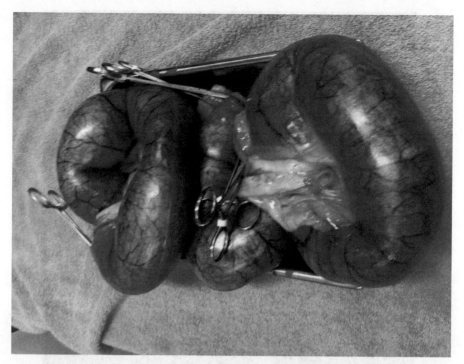

■ **Fig. 8.3.** Markedly distended uterus post ovariohysterectomy performed on an emergency basis for a closed pyometra in a Black Russian Terrier.

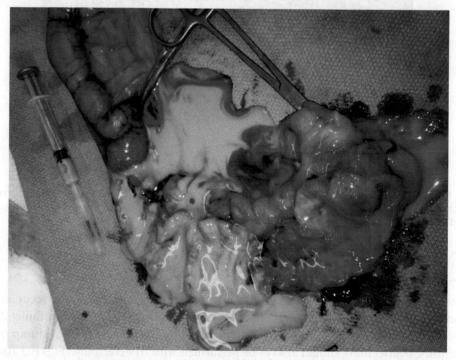

■ **Fig. 8.4.** Typical purulent uterine contents post ovariohysterectomy in a bitch with a closed pyometra associated with *Klebsiella* spp.

■ High-quality broodbitches or poor surgical candidates (heart murmur, coagulopathy, other systemic disease) may be treated medically instead. Luteolysis and uterine emptying are the mainstays to successful treatment. Long-term broad-spectrum antibiotics are necessary until infection is fully resolved. Re-establishment of normal hydration, appetite, attitude are desirable early in the course of treatment.

Supportive Care

■ Intravenous (IV) fluids and electrolyte supplementation with a balanced electrolyte solution should be determined based on bloodwork, degree of dehydration, and severity of vomiting or diarrhea present.
■ Antibiotics – broad-spectrum antibiotics should be initiated immediately.
  • Fluoroquinolones – enrofloxacin 2.5–20 mg/kg PO, IM or IV QD–BID, or ciprofloxacin 5–15 mg/kg PO QD–BID; plus
  • Amoxicillin 10–22 mg/kg PO BID or ampicillin 10–22 mg PO or SQ BID–TID, or 20–40 mg/kg IV TID–QID; or
  • Amoxicillin-clavulanic acid 10–20 mg/kg PO BID (alone or with a fluoroquinolone).
  • Culture and sensitivity results may indicate the need to change antibiotics, and should always be performed before initiating antimicrobial therapy.
  • Antibiotics should be continued for a minimum of 2–4 weeks after uterine evacuation is complete.
■ Mucometra, hydrometra and hematometra do not need to be treated, but the bitch should be monitored carefully for the development of pyometra. Prophylactic antibiotic therapy until conclusion of diestrus may be indicated if CEH is evident or endometritis is suspected based on diagnostics (ultrasound and cytology). Consider abbreviating diestrus with prostaglandin or antiprolactin therapy and breeding on next cycle.

Drugs

■ Prostaglandins
  • PGF2α – Lutalyse (dinoprost tromethamine) or other natural prostaglandins are preferred at a dose of 10–50 µg/kg SQ q 4–6 hours. Synthetic prostaglandins have more potent side effects; dosage must be calculated precisely. Lower doses should be used until cervical opening occurs, and then gradually increased. If side effects (hypersalivation, tachypnea, tachycardia, vomiting, diarrhea, tremors, ataxia, hypovolemic shock) are significant, remain at lower dosages.
■ Prostaglandins should not be used alone to treat a closed pyometra, or uterine rupture may occur. Addition of anti-progestagen or dopamine agonists will facilitate luteolysis and early cervical relaxation.
■ Prostaglandins should be continued until uterine evacuation is complete and luteolysis has been achieved and maintained for at least 72 hours. Corpora lutea are more resistant to luteolysis early in diestrus, and recrudescence of luteal function is common if therapy is not continued long enough, which may result in relapse of pyometra.

- PGF2α may also be used intravaginally to aid in cervical relaxation (25–50 µg total dose diluted in 3–5 ml sterile saline and instilled vaginally with an insemination pipette). Care should be taken to avoid perforation of the vaginal wall during diestrus and anestrus, when it can be quite thin.
  - Misoprostol (prostaglandin E2) – 1–5 µg/kg PO TID–QID or 5–10 µg/kg PO BID until uterine evacuation is complete. It can be used in combination with an anti-progestagen in patients where PGF2α may be contraindicated (i.e., brachycephalics).
- May also be used intravaginally (100 µg tablet dissolved in 3–4 ml sterile water and instilled with an insemination pipette near the cervix) to facilitate cervical relaxation. Care should be taken to avoid perforation of the vaginal wall during diestrus and anestrus, when it can be quite thin.
  - Dopamine agonists hasten luteolysis by blocking production of prolactin, a luteotropic hormone.
  - Cabergoline – 5 µg/kg PO QD or divided Q12 h – has minimal to no gastrointestinal side effects, but is more expensive. This drug is preferable to bromocriptine as it is difficult to differentiate side effects of bromocriptine from those of the disease process; hence, it is harder to determine if therapy may be continued safely. Cabergoline may need to be compounded for small- to medium-sized bitches as it is too difficult to provide the correct dose with the tablet size available.
  - Bromocriptine at 10–50 µg/kg PO BID (dose should be started low and then increased slowly over 4–5 days, stopping when side effects (vomiting, diarrhea, inappetance) become significant. Bromocriptine tablets (2.5 mg) may be mixed with 10 ml distilled water in an amber vial, kept refrigerated, and used for up to 7 days once reconstituted.
  - Anti-progestagens – aglepristone at 10 mg/kg SQ, twice, 24 hours apart and then repeated every 7 days until resolution is complete, or mifepristone 2.5 mg/kg PO QD for 5 days.

Procedures

- TECT may be used to lavage the uterus (lactated Ringer's solution or 0.9% saline) to aid in uterine evacuation. Concurrent use of transabdominal ultrasound to ensure the uterus is not being over-distended is recommended.
- In cases where there is a thick mucoid secretion present and uterine emptying is not occurring, despite complete luteolysis and effective ecbolic therapy, uterine lavage with acetylcysteine solution may facilitate the breakdown of mucoid discharge and allow emptying. For this, 30 ml of acetylcysteine are mixed with 150 ml saline, and small aliquots (5–15 ml) of the dilution are instilled daily until uterine emptying begins.
- Serial daily or alternate-day transabdominal ultrasonography is used to monitor uterine evacuation and uterine wall thickness. Uterine evacuation is typically complete 7–10 days from onset of initiation of cervical drainage.
- Surgical uterine lavage may be performed if TECT is not available, or is ineffective. Uterine biopsy and culture are recommended if surgical lavage is performed.

COMMENTS

- Routine use of prophylactic antibiotics at the time of breeding may predispose bitches to pyometra by promoting resistance to antibiotics and thereby increasing the virulence of the same bacteria.
- Pyometra should be included as a differential for any intact female with non-specific signs of malaise or abdominal pain or distension, particularly in the immediate post estrus period (2–8 weeks).
- Any patient undergoing medical management with prostaglandins should be hospitalized, so that if hypovolemic shock occurs during therapy, rapid fluid replacement can be provided. Inability to provide rapid support may result in patient death.
- Closed and occasionally open pyometras can be life-threatening conditions. The decision to treat medically should not be taken lightly. A complete work-up of the bitch should be performed prior to deciding whether medical management is appropriate. At any point during medical management, if the clinical condition of the bitch begins to deteriorate, medical therapy should be abandoned and ovariohysterectomy should be performed immediately.
- Ovariectomy should always be performed in aged bitches that have possible CEH or endometritis, as pyometra can develop in bitches even if no progesterone is being secreted. Complete ovariohysterectomy is still the recommended course of action for gonadectomy in aged bitches.

Expected Course and Prognosis

- Guarded to good. Depends on type of bacteria, presence of bacteremia, sepsis, other organ system disease. Failure to effect complete uterine emptying within 7 days of cervical opening lowers the prognosis considerably.
- Bitches should be bred on the next heat cycle after treating a pyometra to reduce the risk of recurrence (pregnancy is somewhat protective).
- Some theriogenologists advise that bitches which are not to be bred in the near future should have estrus suppressed with mibolerone or deslorelin (Suprelorin® implant) until the owner is ready to breed. Note: deslorelin may exacerbate CEH in some cases. Long-term studies in breeding bitches are lacking with either of these drugs.
- Approximately 50% of bitches treated medically for pyometra will subsequently conceive and carry to term.

Abbreviations

CEH   = Cystic endometrial hyperplasia
MODS = Multiple organ dysfunction syndrome
SIRS   = Systemic inflammatory response syndrome
DIC   = Disseminated intravascular coagulation

PU/PD = Polyuria and polydipsia
CBC   = Complete blood count
TECT   = Transcervical endoscopic catheterization technique (TECT)
PGF2α = Prostaglandin F2α

See Also

Endometrial Disorders: Post-Partum Metritis/Subinvolution of Placental Sites
Infectious causes of Pregnancy Loss – Canine
Ovarian Remnant Syndrome/Hyperestrogenism
Medical Manipulation of the Estrous Cycle

Suggested Reading

Pretzer, S.D. (2008) Clinical presentation of canine pyometra and mucometra: A review. *Theriogenology*, 70, 359–363.
Schlafer, D.H., Gifford, A.T. (2008) Cystic endometrial hyperplasia, pseudo-placentational endometrial hyperplasia, and other cystic conditions of the canine and feline uterus. *Theriogenology*, 70, 349–358.
Verstegen, J., Dhaliwal, G., Verstegen-Onclin, K. (2008) Mucometra, cystic endometrial hyperplasia, and pyometra in the bitch: advances in treatment and assessment of future reproductive success. *Theriogenology*, 70, 364–374.

Author: Cheryl Lopate MS, DVM, DACT

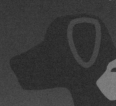

Chapter 9

Cryptorchidism

DEFINITION

- The incomplete descent of one or both testes into the scrotum is a common congenital anomaly of the male reproductive tract with implications on health.
- Cryptorchid dogs are disqualified from conformation competition in the USA; variably in other countries.
- Retained testes can be anywhere caudal to the ipsilateral kidney into the inguinal canal.
- Descent of the testes to the final scrotal position should occur by 6–8 weeks of age and they can often be palpated at 5 weeks of age.
- Ultrasound evaluation of the male abdomen for cryptorchid testes is useful preoperatively (see below).

SIGNALMENT/HISTORY

- Reported in almost all breeds of dogs.
- Unilateral cryptorchidism is threefold more common than bilateral cryptorchidism; the right testis is retained twofold more as often than the left in dogs; the right and left testes are retained at equal frequency in cats.
- Incidence – dogs, ranges of 0.8–10% have been reported; incidence increases with the proportion of purebred dogs in the population, implicating a genetic cause; cats, 1–1.7%.
- Genetics (dogs) – exact mode of inheritance unknown; complex genetic basis; likely polygenic recessive trait; likely heritable; both parents implicated; sex-limited trait.
- Cryptorchidism associated with persistent Müllerian duct syndrome (PMDS; male pseudohermaphroditism) is more common in miniature schnauzer dogs because of inheritance as an autosomal recessive trait. In normal male embryos, Müllerian ducts regress as a result of anti-Mullerian hormone (AMH) secretion by Sertoli cells. In miniature

Blackwell's Five-Minute Veterinary Consult Clinical Companion: Small Animal Endocrinology and Reproduction, First Edition. Edited by Deborah S. Greco and Autumn P. Davidson. © 2017 John Wiley & Sons, Inc. Published 2017 by John Wiley & Sons, Inc.
Companion Website: www.fiveminutevet.com/endocrinology

schnauzers with PMDS, normal amounts of biologically functional AMH are secreted by Sertoli cells during the critical stage of gonadal development; however, the Müllerian ducts fail to regress as a result of mutation in the AMH type II receptor gene. A molecular test for PMDS in miniature schnauzers has been developed based on the identical nature of the *AMHRII* mutation in affected dogs of this breed. Since approximately 50% of PMDS-affected miniature schnauzers have completely normal external genitalia and are fertile, this test could prove to be essential in decreasing and ultimately eliminating this inherited anomaly.

- Genetics (cats) – may be inherited, but no data documents hereditary defect; Persians over-represented in surveys; this suggests a genetic basis.

 ## CLINICAL FEATURES

- Bilaterally cryptorchid animals are infertile due to a lack of spermatogenesis, but virile as testosterone production is normal; unilaterally cryptorchid animals are typically fertile due to the scrotal testis.
- Rarely associated with pain or other signs of disease unless functional malignant transformation occurs or the abdominal testis undergoes torsion; inguinal testes can become strangulated and painful.
- Acute onset of abdominal pain results from torsion of the spermatic cord of retained testes; 36% of retained testes with torsion of the spermatic cord were neoplastic; torsion likely precipitated by increased weight of testis.
- Feminizing paraneoplastic syndrome: estrogen-secreting tumors in retained testes produce feminizing signs: gynecomastia, symmetrical alopecia of trunk and flanks, hyperpigmentation of inguinal skin, pendulous preputial sheath, prostatic squamous metaplasia, hematologic changes.

Causes and Risk Factors

- See Genetics above

DIAGNOSIS

- Intact tomcats have characteristic behaviors (spraying), morphology (prominent cheeks, thickened skin) and urine odor which should raise the index of suspicion for cryptorchidism (normal testosterone production) if no scrotal testes evident.
- Examination of the feline penis may be useful (Figs 9.1 and 9.2).
- Characteristic behaviors in the cryptorchid dog include inter-dog aggression, leg lifting and urine marking, and interest in estrual bitches.

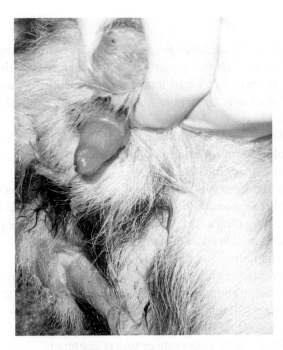

■ **Fig. 9.1.** Smooth penile mucosa in a cheetah under the influence of deslorelin, which reduces testosterone levels to that of a neutered animal.

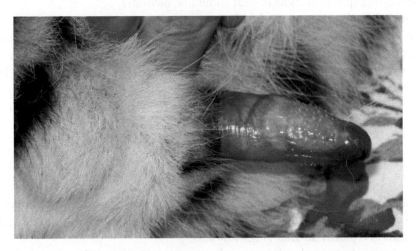

■ **Fig. 9.2.** Same intact male cheetah as in Fig. 9.1, prior to deslorelin implant. Note barbs on penile mucosa. Penile barbs are conserved across feline species.

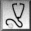 **DIFFERENTIAL DIAGNOSIS**

- Monorchidism is very rare.
- Incomplete castration (most commonly scrotal testis removed).

Laboratory Tests

- An AMH test (commercially available assay (MOFA ®) is useful in the bitch and queen for the identification of ovarian remnant syndrome as it is produced by the ovary post puberty.
- AMH is produced by Sertoli cells in fetal testes in mammals, and inhibits Müllerian (paramesonephric) duct development in males; it is produced until the functional maturation of the testes.
- In one study Sertoli cells from fetuses and neonatal puppies up to 45 days of age expressed AMH, but not in older puppies or adults; thus, the test will not identify post-pubertal cryptorchidism in veterinary medicine.
- Baseline serum testosterone levels vary normally; single levels are not diagnostic.
- Serum testosterone before and 48 hours after hCG injection (250 IU IM) has been used to suggest castration if <20 pg/ml and a twofold increase to suggest the presence of testicular tissue; test results are variable and not always reliable.
- hCG is of human origin; the potential for hypersensitivity exists.
- GnRH IM with blood sample collection pre- and 2–3 hours post-injection: castrated dogs have testosterone concentrations <0.1 ng/ml and should not stimulate with GnRH administration; test results are variable and not always reliable.
- Luteinizing hormone (LH):
  - High LH (>1/liter) suggests the dog or tom is castrated.
  - High LH will only occur in an intact bitch on the day of the LH surge during proestrus/estrus (physical signs of heat should be obvious).
  - Low LH (<1/liter) suggests the dog or tom is intact.
  - Low LH can also occur with exogenous estrogen or progesterone exposure; will not differentiate the presence of a gonad or gonadal remnant from exogenous hormone exposure (i.e., human transdermal hormone replacement therapy in contact with pet).
  - The LH test is not marketed for this purpose in the canine or feline; however, it can be reliable in the author's experience.

Imaging

- Cryptorchid testes can be positioned anywhere between the ipsilateral kidney and the inguinal canal, and can be recognized by the presence of the mediastinum testis; the cryptorchid testis is typically smaller (Figs 9.3–9.5).
- Prostatic hyperplasia in the dog secondary to testosterone influence causes symmetric, mild enlargement of the gland with mildly increased echogenicity which may progress to become patchy. The shape of the gland may change from bi-lobed to circular in the transverse plane. The parenchyma can have a striated appearance. This can be very helpful in diagnosing cryptorchidism as the prostate is easily visualized (Fig. 9.6).
- Visualizing an enlarged neoplastic cryptorchid testis is facilitated by its increased size and abnormal appearance (Figs 9.7 and 9.8).

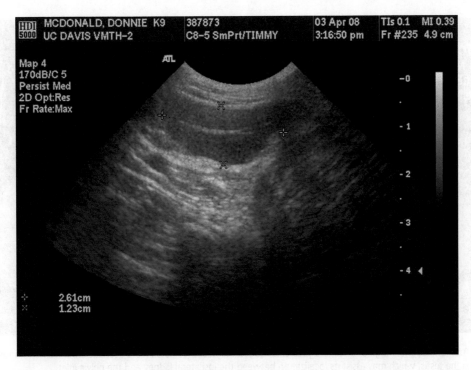

■ **Fig. 9.3.** Sagittal image of a canine cryptorchid, abdominal testis (cursors) measuring 2.61 cm in length. The mediastinum testis is visible.

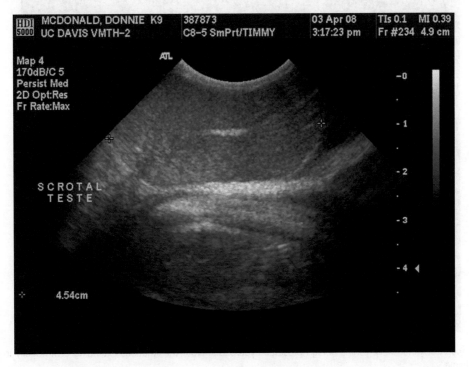

■ **Fig. 9.4.** The scrotal testis from the same dog, measuring 4.54 cm in length.

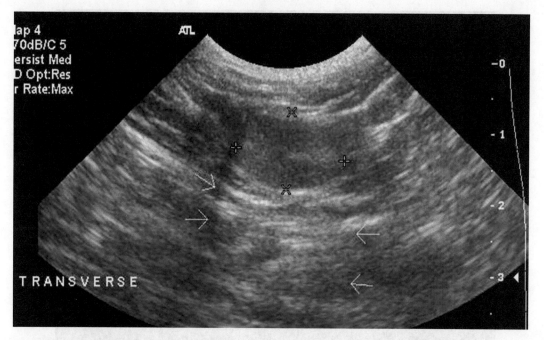

■ **Fig. 9.5.** Ultrasound image of a feline cryptorchid, abdominal testis (cursors). Note acoustic enhancement (arrows) dorsal to the testis, which may assist its localization between the ipsilateral kidney and the pelvic inlet.

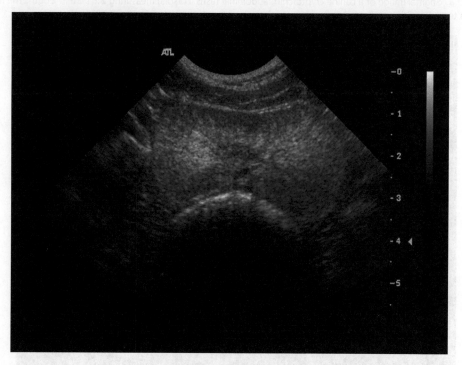

■ **Fig. 9.6.** Transverse view, canine benign prostatic hyperplasia. Note the striations extending centrifugally in the parenchyma.

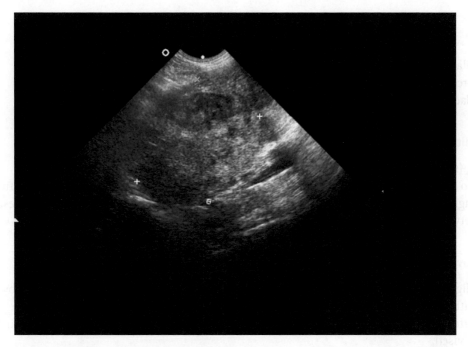

■ **Fig. 9.7.** Canine intra-abdominal testicular torsion. A mid-abdominal mass (cursors) with little recognizable anatomy.

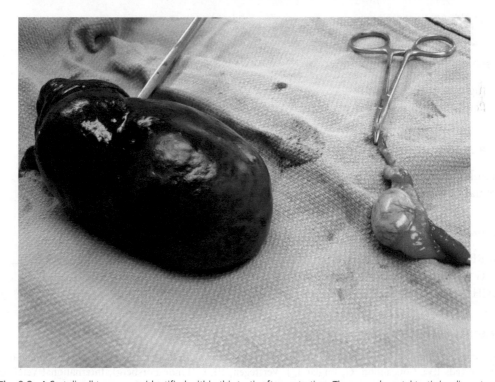

■ **Fig. 9.8.** A Sertoli cell tumor was identified within this testis after castration. The normal scrotal testis is adjacent.

THERAPEUTICS

- Bilateral castration is advised; unilateral if only one testis remains.
- Orchiopexy is unethical.
- Placement of prosthetic testicles in the scrotum is cosmetic.

Medications

Drug(s)

- No effective therapy has been documented in controlled studies; uncontrolled studies suggesting the efficacy of hCG injections in dogs were likely spontaneous late descent between 6 weeks and 4 months of age.

Follow-Up

- Migration of testes into the scrotum at 10 months of age has been documented by the author.
- Late descent is considered a genetic abnormality as is non-descent; neutering is advised.

COMMENTS

Associated Conditions

- Inguinal hernia.
- Penile and preputial defects (e.g., hypospadias).

See Also

Sertoli Cell Tumor
Sexual Development Disorders

Abbreviations

GnRH = Gonadotropin-releasing hormone
hCG = Human chorionic gonadotropin
AMH = Antimullerian hormone

Internet Resources

Memon, M., Tibary, A. (2001) Canine and feline cryptorchidism, in *Recent Advances in Small Animal Reproduction* (eds P.W. Concannon, G. England, J. Verstegen, III, C. Linde-Forsberg), International Veterinary Information Service, Ithaca NY. Available at: www.ivis.org, 2001. A1217.0901.

Suggested Reading

Davidson, A.P., *et al.* (2009) Reproductive ultrasound of the dog and tom. *Top. Companion Anim. Med.*, **24**, 68.

Meyers-Wallen, V.N., Donahoe, P.K., Ueno, S., Manganaro, T.F., Patterson, D.F. (1989) Mullerian inhibiting substance is present in testes of dogs with persistent mullerian duct syndrome. *Biol. Reprod.*, **41**, 881–888.

Felumlee, A.E., Reichle, J.K., Hecht, S., Penninck, D., Zekas, L., Dietze Yeager, A., Goggin, J.M., Lowry, J. (2012) Use of ultrasound to locate retained testes in dogs and cats. *Vet. Radiol. Ultrasound*, **53** (5), 581–585.

Birchard, S.J., Nappier, M. (2008) Cryptorchidism. *Compend. Contin. Educ. Pract. Vet.*, **30** (6), 325–337.

Johnston, S.D., Root Kustritz, M.V., Olson, P.N.S. (2001) Disorders of the canine testes and epididymes, in *Canine and Feline Theriogenology*. Saunders, Philadelphia, pp. 312–332.

Author: Autumn P. Davidson DVM, MS, DACVIM (Internal Medicine)

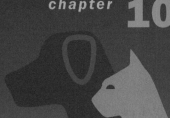

chapter 10

Diabetes Insipidus

DEFINITION

- Diabetes insipidus (DI) is a disorder of water metabolism characterized by polyuria, urine of low specific gravity or osmolality (so-called insipid, or tasteless, urine), and polydipsia.

ETILOGY/PATHOPHYSIOLOGY

- Central DI (CDI) – deficiency in the secretion of antidiuretic hormone (ADH).
- Nephrogenic DI (NDI) – renal insensitivity to ADH.

Systems Affected

- Endocrine.
- Metabolic.
- Renal.
- Urologic.

Incidence/Prevalence

- CDI – Rare.
- NDI – Rare.

SIGNALMENT/HISTORY

- Species/breed – dogs and cats.
- Mean age and range – any age, but usually young.

Blackwell's Five-Minute Veterinary Consult Clinical Companion: Small Animal Endocrinology and Reproduction,
First Edition. Edited by Deborah S. Greco and Autumn P. Davidson. © 2017 John Wiley & Sons, Inc.
Published 2017 by John Wiley & Sons, Inc.
Companion Website: www.fiveminutevet.com/endocrinology

CLINICAL FEATURES

- Polyuria.
- Polydipsia.
- Incontinence – occasional.

Causes

Inadequate Secretion of ADH
- Congenital defect.
- Idiopathic.
- Trauma.
- Neoplasia.

Renal Insensitivity to ADH
- Congenital.
- Secondary to drugs (e.g., lithium, demeclocycline, and methoxyflurane).
- Secondary to endocrine and metabolic disorders (e.g., hyperadrenocorticism, hypokalemia, pyometra, and hypercalcemia).
- Secondary to renal disease or infection (e.g., pyelonephritis, chronic renal failure, pyometra).

 DIFFERENTIAL DIAGNOSIS

- Hyperadrenocorticism.
- Diabetes mellitus.
- Liver disease – portosystemic shunt.
- Hyperadrenocorticism.
- Pyometra.
- Pyelonephritis.
- Hyperthyroidism – cats.
- Hypercalcemia.
- Psychogenic polydipsia.
- Renal failure.

CBC/Biochemistry/Urinalysis

- Usually normal, hypernatremia in some patients.
- Urinary specific gravity low (usually <1.012, often <1.008).

Other Laboratory Tests

- Plasma ADH.

Imaging

- MRI or CT scan if a pituitary tumor is suspected.

 # DIAGNOSTICS

- Modified water-deprivation test (see Table 10.1 for protocol).
- ADH supplementation trial – therapeutic trial with synthetic ADH (DDAVP); a positive response (water intake decreases by 50% in 3–5 days).
- Rule out all other causes of polyuria/polydipsia before conducting an ADH trial.

Pathologic Findings

- Degeneration and death of neurosecretory neurons in the neurohypophysis (CDI).

TABLE 10.1. Procedures for the Modified Water Deprivation test and the ADH supplementation test.

MODIFIED WATER DEPRIVATION TEST

- The animal is confined to a cage with no food or water and is weighed at 1- to 2-hour intervals after emptying the urinary bladder and getting an initial body weight.
- When >5% of body weight has been lost, the urinary bladder should be completely emptied and the urine checked for specific gravity or osmolality.
- A urine specific gravity >1.025 or urine osmolality >900 mOsm/l is generally considered an adequate response to water deprivation.
- Failure to concentrate urine to this degree in the absence of renal disease indicates either central or nephrogenic DI, and/or medullary washout.
- Immediately following water deprivation, if the animal fails to concentrate urine adequately after losing 5% or more of its body weight, an ADH response test is performed.
- A synthetic form of ADH (desmopressin acetate [DDAVP®]) may be given subcutaneously or intravenously, or 20 µg of DDAVP (about 4 drops of the 100 µg/ml intranasal preparation) can be administered as intranasal or conjunctival drops.
- Urine-concentrating ability is then monitored every 2 hours for 6 to 10 hours.
- Increases in urine specific gravity >1.025 or urine osmolality >900 mOsm/l after administration of aqueous vasopressin or DDAVP is suggestive of central DI.
- An inability to concentrate urine after ADH administration indicates nephrogenic DI or severe medullary washout.

DDAVP therapeutic trial

- The owner should measure the animal's 24-hour water intake 2–3 days before the therapeutic trial with DDAVP is initiated, allowing free-choice water intake.
- The intranasal preparation of DDAVP is administered in the conjunctival sac (1–4 drops every 12 hours) for 3–5 days.
- A dramatic reduction in water intake (>50%) during the first few treatment days would strongly suggest an ADH deficiency.
- When the polyuria is due to other causes the decrease is seldom more than 30%.

**Frequent patient monitoring is essential because severe dehydration, possible neurologic complications, and even death could ensue.

THERAPEUTICS

- Patients should be hospitalized for the modified water deprivation test; the ADH trial is often performed as an outpatient procedure.

Activity

- Not restricted.

Diet

- Normal, with free access to water.

Client Education

- Review dosage of DDAVP and administration technique.
- Stress importance of having water available at all times.

Surgical Considerations

- Not available.

Drug(S) of Choice

CDI

- DDAVP (1–2 drops of the intranasal preparation in the conjunctival sac q. 12–24 h to control PU/PD); alternatively, the intranasal preparation may be given SC (2–5 µg q.12–24 h).
- An oral preparation of DDAVP is available in 0.1–0.2 mg tablets, with each 0.1 mg comparable to 1 large drop of the intranasal preparation.
- DDAVP is also available from compounding pharmacies as an oral 'chew' (0.1 and 0.2 mg), a 0.01% sterile and pH-adjusted ophthalmic solution, and a 0.01% sterile solution packaged in a vial designed for SC administration (1 µg equals 1 U on a 100 U insulin syringe).

NDI

- Hydrochlorothiazide (2–4 mg/kg PO q. 12 h).

Contraindications

- None

Precautions

- Overdose of DDAVP can cause water intoxication.

Alternative Drugs

- Chlorpropamide (Diabinese; 125–250 mg/day may reduce PU/PD in CDI).

Patient Monitoring

- Adjust treatment according to the patient's signs; the ideal dosage and frequency of DDAVP administration is based on water intake.
- Laboratory tests such as PCV, total solids, and serum sodium concentration to detect dehydration (inadequate DDAVP replacement) – usually not necessary.

Prevention/Avoidance

- Circumstances that might markedly increase water loss.

Possible Complications

- Anticipate complications of primary disease (pituitary tumor).

Expected Course and Prognosis

- The condition is usually permanent, except in rare patients in which the condition was trauma induced.
  - Prognosis is generally good, depending on the underlying disorder.
  - Without treatment, dehydration can lead to stupor, coma, and death.

Associated Conditions

- Not available.

Age-Related Factors

- Congenital CDI and NDI usually manifest before 6 months of age
- CDI related to pituitary tumors is usually seen in dogs >5 years old.

Zoonotic Potential

- Not available.

Pregnancy/Fertility/Breeding

- Not available.

Synonyms

- Central diabetes insipidus.
- Cranial diabetes insipidus.

- ADH-responsive diabetes insipidus.
- Nephrogenic diabetes insipidus.

See Also

- Hyposthenuria

Abbreviations

ADH   = Antidiuretic hormone
CDI   = Central diabetes insipidus
DDAVP = Brand name of desmopressin
DI   = Diabetes insipidus
MRI   = Magnetic resonance imaging
NDI   = Nephrogenic diabetes insipidus
PCV   = Packed cell volume
PU/PD = Polyuria/polydipsia

Suggested Reading

Feldman, E.C., Nelson, R.W. (2006) *Canine and Feline Endocrinology and Reproduction*, 3rd edition. Saunders, Philadelphia.

Mooney, C.T., Peterson, M.E. (2012) *BSAVA Manual of Canine and Feline Endocrinology*, 4th edition. British Small Animal Veterinary Association, Gloucester.

Author: Rhett Nichols DVM, ACVIM (Internal Medicine)

chapter 11

Canine Diabetes Mellitus

DEFINITION

- Diabetes mellitus is caused by absolute or relative insulin deficiency.
- Diagnosis: hyperglycemia and glucosuria.
- Diabetic dogs are dependent on exogenous insulin.

ETIOLOGY/PATHOPHYSIOLOGY

- In populations in which female dogs are routinely neutered, the majority of cases have type 1 diabetes mellitus caused by immune destruction of pancreatic β cells triggered and sustained by poorly understood genetic and environmental factors.
- Genetic predisposition has been determined in certain breeds of dogs including Samoyed, terriers (Australian, Tibetan), miniature schnauzers, and Labrador retrievers. The disease is associated with the DLA haplotype.
- Canine diabetes can also be due to extensive pancreatic damage from chronic pancreatitis. There is a high prevalence of concurrent diabetes and pancreatitis in dogs, and this increases the risk of complications such as diabetic ketoacidosis, insulin resistance, hypoglycemia, and exocrine pancreatic insufficiency (EPI). Glycemic control might be 'brittle' as a result of variation in the degree of pancreatic inflammation.
- In intact bitches, a form analogous to human gestational diabetes can occur during diestrus or pregnancy. If insulin therapy is initiated promptly, diabetic remission can sometimes be achieved following spay or whelping.
- Canine diabetes is also associated with other insulin-resistant states, including corticosteroid therapy, hyperadrenocorticism, or progesterone-induced acromegaly.
- Juvenile-onset diabetes is recognized rarely in dogs less than 12 months of age.
- Polyuria with compensatory polydipsia is the result of osmotic diuresis caused by persistent glucosuria.
- Weight loss, polyphagia, and lethargy occur because insulin deficiency results in decreased ability to metabolize nutrients.

Blackwell's Five-Minute Veterinary Consult Clinical Companion: Small Animal Endocrinology and Reproduction, First Edition. Edited by Deborah S. Greco and Autumn P. Davidson. © 2017 John Wiley & Sons, Inc. Published 2017 by John Wiley & Sons, Inc.
Companion Website: www.fiveminutevet.com/endocrinology

Systems Affected

- Endocrine/Metabolic – disorder of carbohydrate, protein, and fat metabolism.
- Pancreas/Hepatobiliary – β cell loss, endocrine hepatopathy.
- Ophthalmic – diabetic cataracts.
- Renal/Urologic – osmotic dieresis.

SIGNALMENT/HISTORY

- Onset typically occurs after 5 years of age with the highest prevalence between 8 and 12 years of age.
- Breed predisposition varies with geographic region. In the USA, breeds at increased risk include Miniature Schnauzer, Bichon Frise, Miniature Poodle, and Samoyed. In the UK, Samoyeds, Tibetan terriers, Cairn terriers, Miniature Schnauzers, Yorkshire terriers, Border terriers, and Labrador retrievers are over-represented. Breeds at reduced risk include Boxer, German Shepherd Dog, and Golden Retriever.

Risk Factors

- Intact females are at increased risk, especially if they are also overweight.
- The onset of diabetes can be associated with insulin resistance caused by drugs such as corticosteroids and progestins, or disease states such as hyperadrenocorticism.

Historic Findings

- The classic clinical signs of polydipsia, polyuria, polyphagia, lethargy, and weight loss typically have an insidious onset over weeks to months, and may initially be unnoticed or considered insignificant by the owner.

CLINICAL FEATURES

- Physical findings include hepatomegaly, poor hair coat, and reduced immunity.
- Approximately 30% will have diabetic cataracts at initial presentation. The majority of the remainder will develop cataracts within 5–6 months of diagnosis and, by 16 months, approximately 80% have significant cataract formation (Fig. 11.1).
- Any concurrent illness that causes inappetence or anorexia and vomiting is rapidly complicated by dehydration, depression, and ketosis. The majority of dogs that present with diabetic ketoacidosis have at least one concurrent disease, with acute pancreatitis the most common.

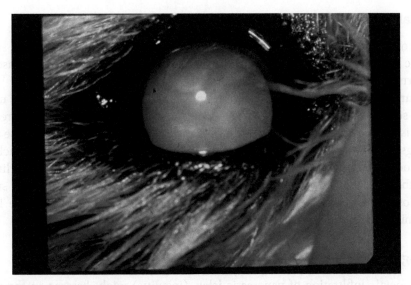

■ **Fig. 11.1.** Diabetic cataract in a dog.

 ## DIFFERENTIAL DIAGNOSIS

- Differential diagnoses for polydipsia and polyuria in dogs includes chronic renal failure, hypercalcemia, hyperadrenocorticism, and pyelonephritis. An important differential diagnosis in intact bitches is pyometron. Diabetes and hyperadrenocorticism share many clinical features and can occur concurrently.
- Glucosuria without hyperglycemia (blood glucose concentration <180 mg/dl; <10 mmol/l) occurs with renal glycosuria.

 ## DIAGNOSTICS

CBC/Biochemistry/Urinalysis

- Hyperglycemia (blood glucose concentration >200 mg/dl; >11 mmol/) and glucosuria.
- Increased serum liver enzyme activities and concentrations of cholesterol and triglycerides are common.
- Ketosis and ketonuria are also common.
- Acidosis and electrolyte abnormalities such as hypernatremia, hypokalemia, and hypophosphatemia indicate severe decompensation. Hypophosphatemia can cause hemolysis.
- Bacterial cystitis is common. Occult infections occur with no lower urinary tract signs and no inflammation evident on urine sediment examination.

Other Laboratory Tests/Imaging

- Diagnosis of concurrent pancreatitis can be difficult. Measurement of canine serum pancreatic lipase immunoreactivity (cPLI) is the most sensitive test whereas ultrasonography performed by a skilled operator is the most specific.
- Measurement of serum trypsin-like immunoreactivity (TLI) to diagnose EPI is most useful when severe insufficiency exists. The TLI concentration can be transiently increased when there is active pancreatic inflammation, in which case diagnosis of EPI may be missed.
- In dogs with poorly controlled diabetes, diagnosis of concurrent conditions such as hyperadrenocorticism or hypothyroidism can be challenging. Glycemia and the clinical signs of diabetes should be as well controlled as possible before performing tests such as the low-dose dexamethasone suppression test, the ACTH stimulation test, or free T4 assay to minimize false diagnoses of hyperadrenocorticism or hypothyroidism.

Pathological Findings

- Lymphocytic infiltration of pancreatic islets (insulitis) might be seen in the early stage of type 1 diabetes. The most prominent histologic finding in later stages is islet vacuolar degeneration.
- Chronic pancreatitis is characterized by fibrosis. In severe cases, there might be no detectable normal pancreatic tissue.

 # THERAPEUTICS

- The goals are to control the signs of diabetes (polydipsia/polyuria, weight loss, lethargy) and to avoid insulin-induced hypoglycemia.
- A consistent insulin dosing and feeding regimen is recommended. Insulin administration should be at strict 12-hour intervals, and it is generally safer to miss an occasional dose than to give injections less than 12 hours apart.

Drug(s) of Choice

- Exogenous insulin is the mainstay of treatment.
- Inappetent or anorexic diabetic dogs should be hospitalized and treated with short-acting insulin and intravenous fluids until recovered and eating well. Suitable preparations include regular insulin (e.g., Actrapid ®; Novo Nordisk) or lispro insulin (Humalog ®; Eli Lilly). Protocols involving either constant rate intravenous infusion (CRI) or intermittent intramuscular/subcutaneous injections are effective; however CRI protocols are simpler and less labor-intensive. The main constraint is that a separate fluid administration line and infusion pump is required in addition to those used for supportive fluid therapy.
- Diabetic dogs with a normal appetite may be managed as outpatients and treated with intermittent-acting insulin preparations administered at an initial dose rate of

0.25–0.5 U/kg SC q.12 h based on estimated ideal body weight. Suitable preparations include isophane/Neutral Protamine Hagedorn (NPH) insulin (e.g., Humulin N®; Eli Lilly and Protophane®; Novo Nordisk), pre-mixed combinations of 30% regular and 70% isophane/NPH insulin (e.g., Humulin 70/30®; Eli Lilly and Mixtard 30/70®; Novo Nordisk), and lente insulin (Vetsulin, when available in the USA) or elsewhere in the world Caninsulin®; MSD Animal Health).

- Although not typically recommended as first-choice therapy, longer-acting insulin preparations can be efficacious. Examples include protamine zinc insulin (PZI) (ProZinc®; Boehringer Ingelheim), glargine insulin (Lantus®; Sanofi Aventis), and detemir insulin (Levemir®; Novo Nordisk). Note that detemir insulin is much more potent and has a longer duration of action than the others, requiring a substantially lower initial dose rate (0.1–0.2 U/kg SC q.12 h) in dogs. Thus, its usefulness in small dogs is limited and daily blood glucose testing is recommended for all dogs managed with detemir insulin.
- Insulin dosing pens enable easier and less painful administration of insulin doses than syringes. They are also much more accurate and precise than syringes for small doses. Insulin syringes deliver on average a 10–20% greater volume than dosing pens at low doses. The potential clinical impact of the imprecision of using 0.3 ml or 0.5 ml insulin syringes is indicated by the range of doses delivered when intending to administer 1 U (0.65–2.80 U). Note that insulin dosing pens are designed for use with a specific insulin brand, and are not accurate with other insulin types.

Precautions/Interactions

- Insulin-induced hypoglycemia can cause neuroglycopenia. Signs range from mild behavioral changes and weakness to seizures, irreversible brain damage, or death.
- Insulin-induced hypoglycemia can also cause rebound hyperglycemia (Somogyi effect), which is usually characterized by a period of good diabetic control followed by worsening diabetic control despite increasing insulin doses. Hypoglycemia might be very brief, asymptomatic, and occur overnight when the dog is sleeping. The subsequent hyperglycemia can last for several days.
- Corticosteroids are the most common drugs that cause insulin resistance. Diabetic dogs usually require a higher insulin dose while receiving systemic or topical corticosteroids.
- Insulin resistance occurs during estrus and diestrus in intact bitches and resolves rapidly following spay.
- Insulin resistance also occurs with obesity and with most concurrent diseases.
- Diabetic dogs with hepatic insufficiency have increased risk of hypoglycemia.

Alternative Drugs

- Oral hypoglycemic drugs are not generally recommended for canine diabetes; however, starch blockers such as acarbose (Precose) may be used at a dosage of 1–2 mg/kg with meals to attenuate the post-prandial rise in blood glucose.

Appropriate Health Care

- The same health care recommendations apply for diabetic dogs as for non-diabetic dogs of the same life-stage. For example, many will benefit from regular dental health care.
- Urinary tract infections (UTIs) associated with clinical signs and/or pyuria require antibiotic treatment based on culture and susceptibility test results. Treatment of bacteriuria may not be necessary in diabetic dogs that have no clinical signs of UTI and no evidence of UTI on urine sediment examination.
- Assessment by an ophthalmologist is recommended for all diabetic dogs that develop cataracts. Prompt treatment of lens-induced uveitis is often required.

Nursing Care

- Intravenous fluid therapy is recommended for all sick diabetic dogs requiring hospitalization, and for those undergoing elective procedures under general anesthesia.
- Glucose monitoring is recommended for all hospitalized diabetic dogs. Venous or capillary blood testing using a veterinary glucose meter is appropriate. A real-time continuous glucose monitoring system (CGMS) will greatly simplify glucose monitoring of hospitalized patients.

Diet

- Insulin dosing needs to be matched to the feeding of consistent meals, with each meal containing the same quantity and type of ingredients. Meals should be timed so that maximal insulin activity occurs during the postprandial period. Thus, dogs should be fed within 1 hour of administration of lente or NPH insulin. A feasible compromise is to feed the dog just before or immediately following each insulin injection.
- Most diabetic dogs will readily consume meals twice-daily if the meals are highly palatable. Usually, the best approach is to feed standardized meals based on the dog's normal diet (see Table 11.1). In the majority of cases, the meal comprises a complete and balanced commercial dog food formulated for adult maintenance with <10% of the calories from treats or other foods. Consistency of amount and type of ingredients is crucial. The brand or flavor of the commercial food and treats should not be varied from day to day. Each meal should contain half the dog's daily caloric requirement.
- For finicky eaters, the meal should be fed at the time of insulin administration and remain available until the expected end of the period of maximal insulin activity (approximately 4 hours for lente and NPH insulin).
- If treats are fed, they should also be consumed during the expected period of maximal insulin activity. All treats containing high sugar or fat should be avoided.
- Clinical benefit for diabetic dogs of feeding a high-fiber diet compared with a typical adult maintenance diet has not been clearly demonstrated. Importantly, increased dietary fiber content in excess of that routinely recommended for healthy dogs might be associated with unwanted effects such as weight loss and inappetence.
- Dietary fat restriction should be considered for diabetic dogs with concurrent chronic pancreatitis or persistent hypertriglyceridemia.

TABLE 11.1. Macronutrient content of selected therapeutic dog foods suitable for treatment of diabetes mellitus.

Diet	Food form	Protein	Nutrient dry matter %			Metabolizable energy* %		
			CHO*	Fat	FIBER	Protein	CHO	Fat
Hill's Prescription Diet								
Canine	Canned	26	39	9	21	30	46	24
Canine	Dry	25	37	8	23	30	45	25
Canine	Canned	17	52	13	12	18	52	30
Canine	Dry	18	50	9	17	21	55	24
Purina Veterinary Diets								
DCO Canine Formula	Dry	26	48	12	8	24	46	29
OM Canine Formula	Canned	44	22	8	19	51	25	24
OM Canine Formula	Dry	31	44	7	10	34	48	18
Royal Canin								
Diabetic HF 18	Dry	22	55	8	15	23	51	25
Digestive Low Fat LF 20	Canned	36	50	7	7	25	60	15
Digestive Low Fat LF 20	Dry	22	68	4	5	32	53	15
Eukanuba								
Eukanuba Weight Loss	Dry	24	61	10	5	Not listed		

CHO, carbohydrate; *Nitrogen-free extract.

Activity

- Regular daily exercise, such as lead walking and visits to a dog park, is encouraged and appears to have minimal impact on diabetic control.
- Strenuous and sustained exercise can result in lowering of blood glucose concentration. Therefore a decreased insulin dose is recommended prior to such exercise and high-carbohydrate snacks may be fed before, during, and after exercise.

Surgical Considerations

- Half the usual dose of insulin should be administered in the morning when food is withheld prior to elective general anesthesia.
- Whenever possible, surgery for diabetic dogs should be scheduled early in the day, so if the procedure allows the patient can be recovered and discharged to the home environment before the next insulin injection and meal are due.
- CRI administration of insulin and glucose is recommended while the dog is hospitalized, with the goal of maintaining blood glucose concentration at 110–270 mg/dl (6–15 mmol/l).

COMMENTS

Client Education

- Success requires close rapport between the owner and the clinician with appropriate individualization of the dog's therapeutic and monitoring regimen. It is important to provide support and guidance while the owner becomes accustomed to and establishes a practical routine.

- Owners should keep detailed records of their dog's progress. Minimum home monitoring might include daily notes on demeanor and appetite, and weekly measurement of 24-hour water intake, body weight, and urine glucose and ketones. Note that if there is more than one pet drinking from the same water bowl, it is useful to measure the volume of water drunk by all the animals. The diabetic dog typically is the reason for most of the variation in water drunk in multi-pet households.

- If mild signs of hypoglycemia develop, the owner should feed a meal of the dog's usual food. If the dog is unwilling to eat, glucose syrup can be administered orally. When the dog recovers, a meal of the dog's usual food should be fed immediately. The owner should then contact their veterinarian before the next insulin injection is due, at which point dosage reduction is usually recommended.

Patient Monitoring

- The primary aim of therapy in diabetic dogs is to achieve resolution of clinical signs, so it is important to regularly monitor signs such as the volume of water drunk and body weight. If the dog drinks more than 60 ml/kg/day or is lethargic or losing weight, then an adjustment of the dog's insulin dose is probably required. If this occurs after a period of good control of clinical signs, hypoglycemia-induced hyperglycemia (Somogyi effect) should be suspected.

- Although assessment of clinical signs is valuable for identifying dogs with poor glycemic control, it is often not effective for detecting dogs at risk of hypoglycemia. Monitoring urine glucose at home can provide useful additional information as persistent negative glucosuria might indicate an increased risk of hypoglycemia. If urine glucose is consistently negative for 2 weeks, then it is often advisable to decrease the dog's insulin dose.

- Some owners are able to perform serial blood glucose concentration curves at home. Single, sporadic measurements provide little useful information for monitoring glycemic control, with the exception of measurements taken when there are signs suggesting hypoglycemia or vague clinical signs of unknown origin. Micromanagement with frequent adjustment of insulin dose should be avoided. Owners who choose home monitoring often need to be advised against over-zealous blood glucose measurement and interpreting the results themselves. As with blood glucose curves obtained in hospital, results must be related to the dog's clinical signs. A practical approach is to use knowledge of the dog's clinical signs to guide the timing of home-generated blood glucose curves. For example, if there is marked variability of 24-hour water intake, owners can be advised to perform a glucose curve during a period when the dog is not drinking much water and/or there is no glucosuria. This approach increases the chance of detecting hypoglycemia.

- CGMS can also be used in the home environment. Important advantages over intermittent blood glucose measurement are that they facilitate detection of brief periods of hypoglycemia and provide information overnight. One limitation is that the systems must be calibrated with blood glucose two to three times every 24 hours, so there is still a requirement for blood sampling during monitoring. Cost is another limitation, particularly the ongoing cost of the glucose sensors.
- Hospital-generated serial blood glucose curves are most useful in cases where the clinical history is inadequate and home glucose monitoring is not being performed. However, it is important to recognize that, if used alone, they can be an unreliable clinical tool for evaluation of insulin dose in individual diabetic dogs because of high day-to-day variability in results. Additional indicators of glycemic control, such as changes in water intake, appetite, body weight, and urine glucose concentrations, should always be considered when appraising insulin dose.
- Measurement of fructosamine is an additional method for assessing glycemic control. This is an approximate measure of average blood glucose concentration over the preceding 2–4 weeks. Measurement is most useful when there is little available information about recent clinical signs or when other glycemic results do not match the reported clinical signs. Monitoring the trends in serial measurements of fructosamine in an individual diabetic dog allows evaluation of response to management changes. A major limitation is that fructosamine represents average glycemia and gives no information about the degree of fluctuation around that average.

Prevention/Avoidance

- There is no information on the prevention of type 1 diabetes or chronic pancreatitis in dogs.
- Diestrus and gestational diabetes can be prevented by neutering of female dogs. For entire bitches, the risk of developing diabetes might be decreased by maintenance of lean body condition.

Possible Complications

- Cataract formation is the most common, and one of the most important, long-term complications associated with diabetes in dogs. They are irreversible and can progress quite rapidly. Mild or subclinical uveitis is present in most dogs with diabetic cataracts.
- Concurrent EPI is usually characterized by continued weight loss despite high calorie intake and good glycemic control. Affected dogs often will produce feces three or more times per day which may or may not be normal in appearance.

Expected Course and Prognosis

▪ Well-controlled diabetic dogs have a similar chance of survival to that of non-diabetic dogs of the same age, although death is more frequent during the first 6 months after diagnosis.
▪ The case-fatality rate of diabetic dogs seen at referral veterinary hospitals in North America is 5%.

Synonyms

▪ None.

Abbreviations

ACTH = Adrenocorticotropic hormone
CGMS = Continuous glucose monitoring system
CRI   = Constant rate infusion
cPLI = Canine pancreatic lipase immunoreactivity
EPI   = Exocrine pancreatic insufficiency
NPH = Neutral Protamine Hagedorn
T4   = Thyroxine
TLI   = Trypsin-like immunoreactivity
UTI   = Urinary tract infection

Suggested Reading

Cook, A.K. (2012) Monitoring methods for dogs and cats with diabetes mellitus. *J. Diabetes Sci. Technol.*, 6 (3), 491–495.
Fleeman, L.M., Rand, J.S. (2013) Canine Diabetes Mellitus, in *Clinical Endocrinology of Companion Animals* (eds J.S.Rand, E.J.Behrend, D.Gunn-Moore, M.L.Campbell-Ward), Wiley-Blackwell, pp.143–168.
Neissen, S.J., Powney, S, Guitian, J., *et al.* (2012) Evaluation of a quality-of-life tool for dogs with diabetes mellitus. *J. Vet. Intern. Med.*, 26 (4), 953–961.
Surman, S., Fleeman, L.M. (2013) Continuous glucose monitoring in small animals. *Vet. Clin. North Am. Small Anim. Pract.*, 43 (2), 381–406.
Watson, P. (2012) Chronic pancreatitis in dogs. *Top. Companion Anim. Med.*, 27 (3), 133–139.

Authors: Linda M. Fleeman BVSc, PhD, MANZCVS; Aline B. Vieira DVM, MSc, PhD

chapter 12

Feline Diabetes Mellitus

DEFINITION

- Relative or absolute insulin deficiency causes abnormalities in carbohydrate, fat, and protein metabolism leading to polyuria, polydipsia, polyphagia and weight loss.
- Commonly associated with obesity and other causes of insulin resistance that aggravates the relative insulin deficiency.

ETIOLOGY/PATHOPHYSIOLOGY

- The prevalence of diabetes mellitus (DM) in cats is about 1:80–100 (as of 2010).
- It is generally believed that the most common type of diabetes in cats is Type 2 diabetes, based on similarities to human Type 2 DM including the association with obesity, amyloid deposition in the islets of Langerhans, the typical middle age-older onset and some evidence of genetic predisposition.
- The exact pathogenesis of Type 2 DM is unknown in cats but it is characterized by decreased sensitivity of β cells to the stimulatory effect of glucose, leading to delayed and inadequate insulin secretion relative to the degree of hyperglycemia.
- A key feature of Type 2 DM is impaired β-cell function with residual but declining insulin secretion.
- Amylin is a hormone that is synthesized in β cells and is co-secreted with insulin. Secretion of amylin is regulated with the secretion of insulin, and both increase during insulin resistance.
- The incretin hormones GIP (glucose-dependent insulinotropic peptide) and GLP-1 (glucagon-like peptide-1) are secreted from the intestines in response to the presence of nutrients in the intestinal lumen. They increase the sensitivity of β cells to glucose so that in any given concentration of glucose more insulin will be secreted. The reduction in the incretin effect in DM and prediabetes is attributed to a decreased sensitivity of β cells to the effect of GIP or a decrease in GLP-1 secretion, or both.

- Incretin hormones also participate in the regulation of β cell differentiation, proliferation, and survival, overall contributing to increased β cell mass. Incretin hormones also affect glucagon secretion, slow the rate of gastric emptying, and increase satiety.
- Cats are obligate carnivores and are therefore adapted to ultra-low carbohydrate diets. Incretin secretion is not stimulated by glucose in cats, and their overall incretin effect in response to glucose is reduced. This means that a carbohydrate-rich meal will result in a relatively prolonged postprandial hyperglycemia.

Systems Affected

- Endocrine/Metabolic
  - Hyperglycemia.
  - Hyerlipidemia.
  - Metabolic acidosis.
  - Electrolyte depletion.
- Hemic/Lymphatic/Immune – Impaired immune system.
- Hepatobiliary – Hepatic lipidosis.
- Musculoskeletal – Muscle wasting and weakness.
- Nervous – Diabetic neuropathy.
- Renal/Urologic – Proteinuria, diabetic nephropathy, urinary tract infections.
- Skin/Exocrine – Dry, lusterless, unkempt haircoat.

 ## SIGNALMENT/HISTORY

- Age: 75% are 8–13 years old, 95% are over 5 years old, but DM can occur at any age.
- Predominant sex: Neutered males.

Risk Factors

- Obesity is a significant risk for developing DM in cats. Obese cats are 3.9-fold more likely to develop DM compared with normal cats.
- Other risk factors are increasing age, male sex, being neutered, physical inactivity, and glucocorticoid and progestin administration.

Historic Findings

- Polyuria – can be misinterpreted as pollakiuria.
- Weight loss.
- Lethargy.
- Decreased grooming behavior.
- Polydipsia and polyphagia are often overlooked by owners.
- Decreased ability to jump, hindlimb weakness and a plantigrade stance.

CLINICAL FEATURES

- Abnormalities on physical examination are often not present in the uncomplicated diabetic cat.
- Overweight (despite history of weight loss) but can present underweight.
- Dorsal muscle wasting.
- Dry, lusterless, unkempt hair coat.
- Hepatomegaly.
- Hind limb weakness and a plantigrade stance (with the hocks touching the ground) caused by diabetic neuropathy (Fig. 12.1).
- Sensitivity to touch (especially extremities) – in people, diabetic neuropathy is reported to cause numbness or tingling/burning feeling or sharp pain in the extremities, and it is possible that cats experience similar sensations.

 ## DIFFERENTIAL DIAGNOSIS

- Chronic kidney disease.
- Hyperthyroidism.
- Stress-related hyperglycemia.
- Hyperadrenocorticism.
- Acromegaly. Note: Hyperadrenocorticism and acromegaly should be considered as differential diagnoses for diabetic cats that are insulin-resistant and are difficult to regulate.

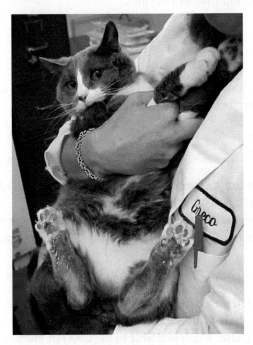

■ **Fig. 12.1.** Diabetic cat with signs of diabetic neuropathy. Note the hair worn off of the ventral aspect of the tarsus.

DIAGNOSTICS

- Persistent hyperglycemia: >150 mg/dl (8 mmol/l) on several occasions.
- Glycosuria: the absence of glycosuria cannot be used to rule out early diabetes mellitus because of the higher renal threshold (300 mg/dl) in cats.
- Increased serum fructosamine concentrations: >350 µmol/l.
- The magnitude of hyperglycemia is not useful, nor is the presence of glycosuria, for diagnosis of diabetes.
- Lack of clinical signs associated with diabetes should raise the suspicion of stress-related hyperglycemia. Glycosuria without hyperglycemia, if not stress-related, is more likely associated with renal tubular disorders.
- Serum fructosamine concentrations are useful for diagnosis of diabetes mellitus and ruling out stress-related hyperglycemia or glycosuria.
- Cats with recent onset of diabetes or with mild diabetes may have normal serum fructosamine concentrations.
- Female cats tend to have lower serum fructosamine concentrations compared to male cats. A high–normal fructosamine result might be consistent with recent-onset diabetes, especially in a female cat.
- Decreased serum total thyroxine (TT4) concentrations.
- Mild non-regenerative anemia.
- Stress leukogram.
- Mild-to-moderate elevation in liver enzymes.
- Hypercholesterolemia.
- Hypertriglyceridemia.
- Mild proteinuria.
- Azotemia.
- Bacteriuria is not uncommon in diabetics and should be followed up with a urine culture.
- Ketonuria can be present occasionally in stable diabetics.

 THERAPEUTICS

- The goals of treatment are to control the signs of diabetes (polydipsia/polyuria, weight loss, lethargy) and to avoid insulin-induced hypoglycemia.
- In newly diagnosed diabetic cats, remission of diabetes (no longer require insulin) should be a goal; however, remission may only occur in 50–70% of the cases.

Drug(s) of Choice

- Exogenous insulin: initial dose rate of 2 U per cat SC q. 12 h.
- Insulin preparations include (Table 12.1):
    - Lente insulin (Vetsulin; when available in the USA) or elsewhere in the world Caninsulin® (MSD Animal Health).

TABLE 12.1. Insulin types, frequency, and dose in cats.				
Lente	Caninsulin; Vetsulin	0.5 U/kg	BID	SQ
Protamine Zinc	PZI Vet	2 U per cat	BID	SQ
Glargine	Lantus	2 U per cat	BID	SQ

- Protamine zinc insulin (PZI) (ProZinc®; Boehringer Ingelheim).
- Glargine insulin (Lantus®; Sanofi Aventis).
- Insulin dosing pens enable easier and less painful administration of insulin doses than syringes. They are also much more accurate and precise than syringes for small doses. Insulin syringes deliver on average a 10–20% greater volume than dosing pens at low doses. The potential clinical impact of the imprecision of using 0.3 ml or 0.5 ml insulin syringes is indicated by the range of doses delivered when intending to administer 1 U (0.65 2.80 U). Note that insulin dosing pens are designed for use with a specific insulin brand and are not accurate with other insulin types.

Precautions/Interactions

- Insulin-induced hypoglycemia can cause neuroglycopenia. Signs range from mild behavioral changes and weakness to seizures, irreversible brain damage, or death.
- Corticosteroids are the most common drugs that cause insulin resistance. Diabetic dogs usually require a higher insulin dose while receiving systemic or topical corticosteroids.
- Insulin resistance also occurs with obesity and with most concurrent diseases.

Alternative Drugs

- Glipizide – 2.5 mg BID PO.
- Glimeperide – 1 mg q. 24 h PO.
- Acarbose – 12.5 mg BID with food.

Appropriate Health Care

- Urinary tract infections (UTIs) associated with clinical signs and/or pyuria require antibiotic treatment based on culture and susceptibility test results.
- Treatment of bacteriuria may not be necessary in diabetic cats that have no clinical signs of UTI and no evidence of UTI on urine sediment examination.

Nursing Care

- Intravenous fluid therapy is recommended for all sick diabetic cats requiring hospitalization, and for those undergoing elective procedures under general anesthesia.
- Glucose monitoring is recommended for all hospitalized diabetic cats. Venous or capillary blood testing using a veterinary glucose meter is appropriate. Real-time continuous glucose monitoring systems (CGMS) greatly simplify glucose monitoring of hospitalized patients.

TABLE 12.2. Nutrient (macro) composition (% dry matter) of feline prescription diets for diabetes mellitus.

Diet	Food form	Protein	CHO	Fat	Fiber
Hills m/d	Canned	52	15.7	19.4	6
Purina DM	Dry	51	15.1	21	6
	Canned	53	4.5	32.8	2.9
Royal Canin	Dry	47.8	30	12	6

Diet (see Table 12.2)

- Studies have shown that a low-carbohydrate, high-protein canned diet is associated with the highest remission rates.
- Canned food is preferred but the lowest carbohydrate content dry food is Purina DM.
- Addition of acarbose (12.5 mg BID) to dry food at mealtimes (meal feeding is mandatory) may decrease carbohydrate absorption.

Activity

- Regular daily exercise using cat play toys and perches is encouraged.

Surgical Considerations

- Half the usual dose of insulin should be administered in the morning when food is withheld prior to elective general anesthesia.
- Whenever possible, surgery for diabetics should be scheduled early in the day, so if the procedure allows the patient can be recovered and discharged to the home environment before the next insulin injection and meal are due.
- CRI administration of insulin and glucose is recommended while the cat is hospitalized, with the goal of maintaining blood glucose concentration at 110–270 mg/dl (6–15 mmol/l).

TABLE 12.3. Advantages and disadvantages of different monitoring parameters for diabetes mellitus.

Monitoring parameter	Advantages	Disadvantages
Urine glucose	Can be done at home	Insensitive to small changes
Blood glucose curves	Can be done at home	Not reproducible
Serum fructosamine	Average of blood glucose over several weeks	Cannot be used for day to day regulation

COMMENTS

Client Education

- Thorough client education includes complete explanation of:
  - Diet – low-carbohydrate diets have been shown to be more effective.
  - Insulin administration – clients should be instructed to inject insulin behind the last rib, below the costochondral junction, and to rotate the site of injection.
  - Consistent exercise.
  - Clinical signs of hypoglycemia.
  - Urine glucose and/or blood glucose monitoring.

Patient Monitoring

Urinary glucose

- Urinary glucose monitoring may be performed at home by owners, is not affected by stress, and may indicate insulin-induced hyperglycemia (Somogyi effect).
- Urine glucose is a measure of trends in blood glucose and should not be used alone to adjust insulin dosages. However, urine glucose should decrease to trace or 1+ with appropriate therapy. Consistently high urine glucose indicates the need for blood glucose evaluation.
- It is vitally important that the client monitor the urine sugar to determine *if and when* the cat is ready to go off insulin.
- The following schedule may be used to taper the insulin dose using urine glucose measurements:
  - Start monitoring urine glucose daily with urine glucose strips (e.g., Bayer).
  - Starting insulin dose: 2 U per cat.
  - When urine glucose becomes negative for 2 days in a row, reduce insulin dose to 1 U BID.
  - The next time urine glucose becomes negative for 2 days in a row, reduce the insulin dose to 1 U once daily.
  - The next time urine glucose becomes negative, stop insulin injections and bring cat in for veterinary evaluation (fructosamine, blood glucose, etc.).

Blood glucose curves

- Glucose monitors designed for home monitoring in people are inexpensive, accurate, rapid, and require only a drop of blood. Although reasonably accurate in the blood glucose range of 60–120 mg/dl (4–12.5 mmol/l), these monitors are designed to read lower than the actual value as glucose approaches the hypoglycemic range.
- Altitude, oxygen therapy, patient hematocrit, shock, dehydration, severe infection, and out-of-date or improperly stored test strips, can all affect the monitors' accuracy.
- A veterinary glucose monitor marketed as the Abbott AlphaTRAK has the highest correlation to clinical laboratory sample glucose analysis.
- It is very rare to obtain a perfect glucose curve in a single patient. In fact, blood glucose curves are good for identifying trends in blood glucose during the day.

- The glucose nadir is the lowest concentration of blood glucose on the curve, and should occur approximately halfway through the dosing interval.
- The time of the glucose nadir indicates the time of peak insulin action, and the ideal blood glucose curve should have a nadir of 100–150 mg/dl (5–8 mmol/l).
- The duration of insulin action is related to both the time of the glucose nadir and the absolute concentration of the glucose nadir, in that you cannot determine insulin duration until achieving the target glucose nadir concentration of 80–120 mg/dl (4–7 mmol/l).
- The glucose differential is the difference between the absolute concentration of glucose at the nadir and the absolute concentration of glucose before the next insulin dose. The glucose differential should be less than 150–200 mg/dl (8–11 mmol/l) in cats.
- Generally, *atypical* blood glucose curves can be differentiated by the curve's characteristics and the insulin dosage (per dosing interval). If the patient is receiving >2.2 U/kg of insulin per dose, insulin resistance should be investigated. Causes of insulin resistance in cats can include high-carbohydrate diets, incorrect insulin administration (injecting in scruff of neck), hyperthyroidism, hyperadrenocorticism, acromegaly, drug therapy, and infections. If concurrent disease is ruled out, corrective actions include increasing the insulin dose and/or changing to longer-acting insulin.
- If the patient is receiving <2.2 U/kg per dose, the blood glucose curve usually is indicative of one of the following: insufficient dosage of insulin; short duration of action of insulin; or insulin overlap seen with prolonged insulin action. Corrective actions include reduction of the insulin dose by 25%, or changing to a shorter-duration insulin or a mixture of insulin types.

Continuous glucose monitors

- Recently, continuous glucose monitors have been developed by Abbott and other companies for remote interstitial glucose monitoring at home or in the veterinary hospital. These small devices are inserted between the shoulder blades and contain a glucose sensor combined with a transmitter device. The receiver and monitor obtain messages from the sensor and display continuous glucose concentrations throughout the day. The monitor may be attached to the animal's collar or to a cage.

Fructosamine

- Fructosamine is the product of a non-enzymatic and irreversible reaction between glucose and plasma proteins. Serum fructosamine concentrations typically reflect glycemic control over the course of 2–3 weeks, although massive changes in blood glucose concentrations can increase serum fructosamine concentrations within a few days. Serum fructosamine concentrations are also indicated for routine monitoring of the treated diabetic.
- Small changes in glycemic control might not be apparent clinically but could still be reflected by changes in serum fructosamine concentrations. Thus, it is recommended to obtain serum fructosamine concentrations on diagnosis and every time a change is made in therapy: before (for baseline) and 3 weeks after making the change. Serum fructosamine concentrations are affected by the half-life of serum proteins. Thus, when protein turnover is increased (e.g., hyperthyroidism, protein-losing enteropathy), serum fructosamine

Algorithm: Monitoring with serum fructosamine

Measure blood glucose (BG) and serum fructosamine (FR)

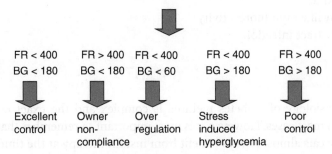

FR < 400	FR > 400	FR < 400	FR < 400	FR > 400
BG < 180	BG < 180	BG < 60	BG > 180	BG > 180
Excellent control	Owner non-compliance	Over regulation	Stress induced hyperglycemia	Poor control

concentrations can be falsely decreased. Hemolysis (either *in vivo* or *in vitro*) affects the laboratory's ability to analyze fructosamine concentrations and should be avoided.

■ Glycosylated blood proteins are indicative of mean glucose concentrations in serum over an extended period of time, and may be used to monitor long-term insulin therapy. These proteins are particularly useful in monitoring diabetic cats that may be stressed by hospitalization and serial blood glucose curves.

■ Fructosamine concentrations less than 400–450 µmol/l are associated with good to excellent glycemic control; concentrations of 450–550 µmol/l indicate fair to good control; and serum fructosamine >550 µmol/l indicates poor glycemic control. Relative changes in serum fructosamine may be more helpful than absolute values in some cases. An algorithm for monitoring diabetes mellitus in cats with serum blood glucose and fructosamine is shown in Fig. 12.2.

Prevention/Avoidance

■ Obesity is a precursor to diabetes in cats; therefore, avoidance of obesity in middle-aged cats is advised.

Possible Complications

■ Diabetic neuropathy.
■ Diabetic nephropathy.

Expected Course and Prognosis

■ Between 50% and 70% of newly diagnosed cats may go into remission with a correct diet and insulin/oral hypoglycemic therapy; however, the remission may not be lifelong.

Synonyms

■ None.

Abbreviations

ACTH = Adrenocorticotropic hormone
CGMS = Continuous glucose monitoring system

CRI   = Constant rate infusion
cPLI   = Canine pancreatic lipase immunoreactivity
EPI   = Exocrine pancreatic insufficiency
T4   = Thyroxine
TLI   = Trypsin-like immunoreactivity
UTI   = Urinary tract infection

 COMMENTS

- The pathophysiology of diabetes mellitus is complex and the exact etiology cannot be determined in most cases. However, it is most important to remember that regardless of the exact etiology cats almost always benefit from insulin therapy at the time of diagnosis and that with appropriate diet and insulin therapy many of them become insulin-dependent.

See Also

Hypersomatotropism or Acromegaly – Cats
Diabetic Hepatopathy
Glucosuria
Hyperadrenocorticism (Cushing's Syndrome) – Cats
Hyperglycemia
Hyperlipidemia
Hyperosmolarity
Polydipsia/polyuria
Diabetes Feline Dietary therapy
Insulin Therapy
Oral hypoglycemics
Expanded Monitoring: Diabetes Feline and Canine

Suggested Reading

Kahn, S.E., Prote, D. (2003) The Pathophysiology and Genetics of Type 2 Diabetes Mellitus, in *Ellenberg and Rifkin's Diabetes Mellitus*, 6th edition (eds D.Porte, R.S.Sherwin, A.Baron), The McGraw-Hill Companies Inc., pp. 331–366.

Gilor, C., Graves, T.K., Gilor, S., *et al.* (2011) The incretin effect in cats: comparison between oral glucose, lipids, and amino acids. *Domest. Anim. Endocrinol.*, **40** (4), 205–212.

Reusch, C.E. (2010) Feline Diabetes Mellitus, in *Textbook of Veterinary Internal Medicine*, 7th edition. Elsevier, St Louis pp. 1796–1816.

Mazzaferro, E., Greco, D.S., Turner, A.S., Fettman, M.J. (2003) Treatment of feline diabetes mellitus using an alpha-glucosidase inhibitor (acarbose) and a high protein, low carbohydrate diet. *J. Fel. Med. Surg.*, **5** (3), 183–190.

Bennett, N., Greco, D.S., Peterson, M.E., Kirk, C.E., Mathes, M., Fettman, M.E. (2006) Comparison of a low carbohydrate vs high fiber canned diet for the treatment of diabetes mellitus in cats. *J. Fel. Med. Surg.*, **8** (2), 73–84.

Suliman, A.G., Langston, C., Greco, D.S., *et al.* (2011) Microalbuminuria in diabetic cats. *Top. Companion Anim. Med.*, **26**, 154-157.

Author: Chen Gilor DVM, PhD, DACVIM

chapter 13

Diabetes Mellitus with Ketoacidosis

DEFINITION

- A true medical emergency secondary to absolute or relative insulin deficiency, characterized by hyperglycemia, ketonemia, metabolic acidosis, dehydration, and electrolyte depletion.

ETIOLOGY/PATHOPHYSIOLOGY

- Insulin deficiency causes an increase in lipolysis, which results in excessive ketone body production and acidosis; an inability to maintain fluid and electrolyte homeostasis causes dehydration, prerenal azotemia, electrolyte disorders, obtundation, and death.
- Many diabetic ketoacidosis patients have underlying conditions such as infection, inflammation, or heart disease that cause stress hormone (e.g., glucagon, cortisol, growth hormone, and epinephrine) secretion; this probably contributes to the development of insulin resistance and diabetic ketoacidosis by promoting lipolysis, ketogenesis, gluconeogenesis, and glycogenolysis.
- Dehydration and electrolyte abnormalities result from osmotic diuresis promoting the loss of total body water and electrolytes.

Systems Affected

- Endocrine/metabolic.
- Gastrointestinal.
- Hematologic (cats).

Genetics

- None

Incidence/Prevalence

- Unknown

Blackwell's Five-Minute Veterinary Consult Clinical Companion: Small Animal Endocrinology and Reproduction, First Edition. Edited by Deborah S. Greco and Autumn P. Davidson. © 2017 John Wiley & Sons, Inc. Published 2017 by John Wiley & Sons, Inc.
Companion Website: www.fiveminutevet.com/endocrinology

SIGNALMENT/HISTORY

Species

- Dogs and cats

Breed Predilections

- Dogs – miniature poodle and dachshund.
- Cats – none.

Mean Age and Range

- Dogs – mean age 8.4 years.
- Cats – median age 11 years (range: 1–19 years).

Predominant Sex

- Dogs – females 1.5 times males.
- Cats – males 2 times females.

CLINICAL FEATURES

- Polyuria.
- Polydipsia or adipsia.
- Diminished activity.
- Anorexia.
- Weakness.
- Vomiting.
- Lethargy and depression.
- Muscle wasting and weight loss.
- Unkempt haircoat.
- Tachypnea.
- Dehydration.
- Thin body condition.
- Hypothermia.
- Dandruff.
- Thickened bowel loops.
- Hepatomegaly.
- Ketone odor on breath.
- Icterus.

Causes

- Insulin-dependent diabetes mellitus.
- Infection (e.g., skin, respiratory, urinary tract, prostate gland, pyelonephritis, pyometra, and pneumonia).
- Concurrent disease (e.g., heart failure, pancreatitis, renal insufficiency or failure, asthma, neoplasia, acromegaly, and estrus).
- Idiopathic.
- Medication non-compliance.
- Stress.
- Surgery.

Risk Factors

- Any condition that leads to an absolute or relative insulin deficiency.
- History of corticosteroid or β-blocker administration.

DIFFERENTIAL DIAGNOSIS

- Hyperosmolar non-ketotic coma.
- Acute hypoglycemic coma.
- Uremia.
- Lactic acidosis.

DIAGNOSTICS

CBC/Biochemistry/Urinalysis

- Leukocytosis with mature neutrophilia.
- Hyperglycemia – blood glucose usually >250 mg/dl.
- High liver enzyme activity.
- Hypercholesterolemia and lipemia.
- Azotemia.
- Hypochloremia.
- Hypokalemia.
- Hyponatremia.
- Hypophosphatemia.
- High anion gap – anion gap = (sodium + potassium) – (chloride + bicarbonate); normal is 16 ± 4.
- Glucosuria and ketonuria.
- Variable urinary specific gravity with active or inactive sediment.

- Hyperproteinemia.
- Heinz body anemia (cats).

Other Laboratory Tests

- Metabolic acidosis – venous TCO_2 <15 mEq/l caused by ketosis.
- Hyperosmolarity (>330 mOsm/kg).
- Bacterial culture of urine and blood.

Diagnostic Procedures

- ECG may help evaluate potassium status; prolonged Q-T interval in some patients with hypokalemia; tall, tented T waves in some patients with hyperkalemia.

Pathologic Findings

- Pancreatic islet cell atrophy.

 # THERAPEUTICS

Appropriate Health Care

- If the animal is bright, alert, and well-hydrated, intensive care and intravenous fluid administration are not required; start subcutaneous administration of insulin (short- or intermediate-acting insulin), offer food, and supply constant access to water; monitor closely for signs of illness (e.g., anorexia, lethargy, vomiting).
- Treatment of 'sick' diabetic ketoacidotic dog or cat requires inpatient intensive care; this is a life-threatening emergency; goals are to correct the depletion of water and electrolytes, reverse ketonemia and acidosis, and increase the rate of glucose use by insulin-dependent tissues.

Nursing Care

- Fluids – necessary to ensure adequate cardiac output and tissue perfusion and to maintain vascular volume; also reduce blood glucose concentration.
- IV administration of 0.9% saline supplemented with potassium is the initial fluid of choice.
- Volume determined by dehydration deficit plus maintenance requirements; replace over 24–48 hours.

Activity

- Not available.

Diet

▪ A low-fat, high-fiber, high-complex-carbohydrate diet is recommended once the patient is stabilized.

Client Education

▪ Serious medical condition requiring lifelong insulin administration in most patients

Surgical Considerations

▪ Not available.

MEDICATIONS

Drug(s) of Choice

Insulin

▪ Necessary to inhibit lipolysis, inhibit hepatic gluconeogenesis, and promote peripheral glucose uptake.
▪ Regular insulin is the insulin of choice.
▪ Initial dosage – 0.2 U/kg IM (or SC if hydration is normal).
▪ Subsequent dosage 0.1–0.2 U/kg given 3–6 hours later – may be given hourly if patient is closely monitored; response to previous insulin dosage should be considered when calculating subsequent dosages. Ideally, glucose concentration should drop to 50–100 mg/dl/hour.
▪ Regular insulin can also be administered as a continuous-rate infusion via a designated catheter. For dogs, place 2.2 U/kg into 250 ml of 0.9% NaCl fluid. For cats, place 1.1 Units/kg into 250 ml 0.9% NaCl fluid. Then, allow 50 ml of the dilute insulin to flow through the IV tubing and discard. If blood glucose is >250 mg/dl, administer at 10 ml/hour. If blood glucose is between 200 and 250 mg/dl, administer at 7 ml/hour. If blood glucose is between 150 and 200 mg/dl, administer at 5 ml/hour. If blood glucose is between 100 and 150 mg/dl, administer at 5 ml/hour and add 2.5% dextrose to the IV crystalloid fluids. If blood glucose is <100 mg/dl, discontinue IV insulin infusion and continue 2.5–5% dextrose in IV crystalloid infusion.
▪ Check blood glucose every 1–3 hours with Chemstrip BG reagent strips and an automated test strip analyzer (Accu-Chek III, Boehringer Mannheim; Alpha Trak glucometer, Abbott Laboratories).
▪ Monitor urine glucose and ketones daily.
▪ Start administering longer-acting insulin when the patient is eating, drinking, and no longer receiving IV fluids and ketosis is resolved or greatly diminished; the dosage is based on that of short-acting insulin given in hospital.

Potassium Supplementation

▪ Total body potassium is depleted and treatment (e.g., fluids and insulin) will further lower serum potassium; potassium supplementation is always necessary.

- If possible, check potassium concentration before initiating insulin therapy to guide supplementation dosage; if it is extremely low, insulin therapy may need to be delayed (hours) until serum potassium concentration increases.
- Refractory hypokalemia may indicate magnesium depletion, requiring magnesium replacement at 0.75–1 mEq/kg/day as magnesium chloride or magnesium sulfate as a continuous-rate infusion.
- If potassium concentration is unknown, add potassium (40 mEq/l) to the IV fluids, obtain results of pretreatment biochemical analysis ASAP, and draw blood for follow-up biochemical analysis 24 hours after treatment is initiated.

Dextrose Supplementation
- Must give insulin, regardless of the blood glucose concentration, to correct the ketoacidotic state.
- Whenever blood glucose is <200–250 mg/dl, 50% dextrose should be added to the fluids to produce a 2.5% dextrose solution (increase to 5% dextrose if needed). Discontinue dextrose once glucose is maintained above 250 mg/dl.
- Do not stop insulin therapy.

Bicarbonate Supplementation
- Controversial; to be considered if the patient's venous blood pH is <7.0 or total CO_2 is <11 mEq/l; bicarbonate is of no benefit if the pH is >7.0.
- Dosage – body weight (kg) × 0.3 × base deficit (base deficit = normal serum bicarbonate – patient's serum bicarbonate); *slowly* administer one-quarter to one-half of the dose IV and give the remainder in fluids over 3–6 hours.
- Re-check blood gas or serum TCO_2 before further supplementation.

Phosphorus Supplementation
- Pretreatment serum phosphorus usually is normal; however, treatment of ketoacidosis reduces phosphorus, and serum concentrations should be checked every 12–24 hours once supplementation is initiated.
- Dosage – 0.01–0.03 mmol/kg/h for 6–12 hours in IV fluids (may need to increase dose to 0.03–0.06 mmol/kg/h).

Contraindications

- If the patient is anuric or oliguric or if potassium is >5 mEq/l, do not supplement potassium until urine flow is established or potassium concentration decreases.

Precautions

- Use bicarbonate with caution in patients without normal ventilation because of their inability to excrete carbon dioxide created during treatment.

Possible Interactions

- None

Alternative Drug(s)

- None

Patient Monitoring

- Attitude, hydration, cardiopulmonary status, urine output, and body weight.
- Blood sugar q.1–3 h initially; q.6 h once stable.
- Electrolytes q.4–8 h initially; q.24 h once stable.
- Acid–base status q. 8–12 h initially; q.24 h once stable.

Prevention/Avoidance

- Appropriate insulin administration

Possible Complications

- Hypokalemia.
- Hypoglycemia.
- Hypophosphatemia.
- Cerebral edema.
- Pulmonary edema.
- Renal failure.
- Heart failure.

Expected Course and Prognosis

- Guarded

Miscellaneous/Associated Conditions

- Pancreatitis.
- Hyperadrenocorticism.
- Diestrus.
- Bacterial infection.
- Electrolyte depletion.

Age-Related Factors

- Not available.

Zoonotic Potential

- Not available.

Pregnancy/Fertility/Breeding

- Risk of fetal death may be relatively high.
- Glucose regulation is often difficult.

Synonyms

- Not available.

See Also

- Diabetes Mellitus without Complication – Cats
- Diabetes Mellitus without Complication – Dogs

Abbreviations

TCO_2 = total carbon dioxide.

Suggested Reading

Brady, M.A., Dennis, J.S., Wagner-Mann, C. (2003) Evaluating the use of plasma hematocrit samples to detect ketones utilizing urine dipstick colorimetric methodology in diabetic cats and dogs. *J. Vet. Emerg. Crit. Care*, **13** (1), 1–6.

Connally, H.E. (2002) Critical care monitoring considerations for the diabetic patient. *Clin. Tech. Small Anim. Pract.*, **17**, 73–78.

Duarte, R., Simoes, D.M.N., Franchini, M.L., Marquezi, M.L., Ikesaki, J.H., Kogika, M.M., Alves, F.O. (2002) Serum beta-hydroxybutyrate concentrations in the diagnosis of diabetic ketoacidosis in 116 dogs. *J. Vet. Intern. Med.*, **16**, 411–417.

Durocher, L.L., Hinchcliff, K.W., DiBartola, S.P., Johnson, S.E. (2008) Acid base and hormonal abnormalities in dogs with naturally occurring diabetes mellitus. *J. Am. Vet. Med. Assoc.*, **232** (9), 1310–1320.

Feldman, E.C., Nelson, R.W. (1996) Diabetic ketoacidosis, in *Canine and Feline Endocrinology and Reproduction*, 2nd edition. Saunders, Philadelphia, pp. 392–421.

Fincham, S.C., Drobatz, K.J., Gillespie, T.N., Hess, R.S. (2004) Evaluation of plasma ionized-magnesium concentration in 122 dogs with diabetes mellitus: a retrospective study. *J. Vet. Intern. Med.*, **18**, 612–617.

Hume, D.Z., Drobatz, K.J., Hess, R.S.(2006) Outcome of dogs with diabetic ketoacidosis: 127 dogs (1993–2003). *J. Vet. Intern. Med.*, **20** (3), 547–555.

Kerl, M.E. (2001) Diabetic ketoacidosis: treatment recommendations. *Comp. Cont. Educ. Pract. Vet.*, **23**, 330–339.

Kerl, M.E. (2001) Diabetic ketoacidosis: pathophysiology and clinical and laboratory presentation. *Comp. Cont. Educ. Pract. Vet.*, **23**, 220–228.

Koenig A., Drobatz K.J., Beale A.B., King L.G. (2004) Hyperglycemic, hyperosmolar syndrome in feline diabetics: 17 cases (1995–2001). *J. Vet. Emerg. Crit. Care*, **14** (1), 30–40.

Nichols, R., Crenshaw, K.L. (1995) Complications and concurrent disease associated with diabetic ketoacidosis and other severe forms of diabetes mellitus, in *Small Animal Practice Current Veterinary Therapy XII* (ed. J.B.Bonagura). Saunders, Philadelphia, pp. 384–386.

Parsons, S.E., Drobatz, K.J., Lamb, S.V., Ward, C.R., Hess, R.K. (2002) Endogenous serum insulin concentrations in dogs with diabetic ketoacidosis. *J. Vet. Emerg. Crit. Care*, **12**, 147–152.

Sieber-Ruckstuhl, N.S., Klev, S., Tschuor, F., Zini E., Ohlerth S., Boretti F.S., Reusch C.E. (2008) Remission of diabetes mellitus in cats with diabetic ketoacidosis. *J. Vet. Intern. Med.*, **22** (6), 1326–1332.

Zeugswetter, E., Paqitz, M. (2009) Ketone measurements using dipstick methodology in cats with diabetes mellitus. *J. Small Anim. Pract.*, **50** (1), 4–8.

Author: Elisa M. Mazzaferro MS, DVM, PhD, DACVECC

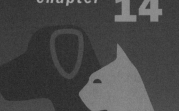

chapter 14

Disorders of Sexual Differentiation (DSD)

DEFINITION

- Errors in the establishment of chromosomal, gonadal, or phenotypic/genitalia sex cause abnormal sexual differentiation.
- Variety of patterns from ambiguous genitalia to apparently normal genitalia with sterility.

ETIOLOGY/PATHOPHYSIOLOGY

- Sexual differentiation is a sequential process – chromosomal sex established at fertilization (dog: 78,XX or 78,XY; cat: 38,XX or 38,XY), development of gonadal sex, and finally development of phenotypic/genitalia sex.
- Testis differentiation normally determined by sex chromosome constitution; *SRY* (on the Y chromosome) and *SOX9* (autosomal gene), expressed by Sertoli cells, are critical for testis differentiation.
- Ovarian differentiation – once considered a passive process; now recognized as an active process involving *WNT4/RSPO1* and β-catenin.
- Phenotypic sex differentiation (tubular reproductive tract and external genitalia) depends on gonadal sex – basic embryonic plan is female; male phenotype results if testes are capable of secreting anti-Müllerian hormone (AMH) and testosterone at the correct time during embryogenesis, and functional androgen receptors (X-linked gene) are present on genital tissues.
- Consensus terminology for categorizing Disorders of Sexual Development recently revised. Previous nomenclature also noted.

Sex Chromosome DSD

- Defects in number or structure of sex chromosomes – chromosomal non-disjunction during meiosis causes trisomy, monosomy; mitotic non-disjunction of a single zygote causes mosaicism; fusion of zygotes leads to chimerism.
- XXY (Klinefelter) syndrome – 79,XXY (dog); 39,XXY (cat); hypoplastic testes; phenotypic male (normal to hypoplastic genitalia); sterile; some tortoiseshell male cats.

Blackwell's Five-Minute Veterinary Consult Clinical Companion: Small Animal Endocrinology and Reproduction, First Edition. Edited by Deborah S. Greco and Autumn P. Davidson. © 2017 John Wiley & Sons, Inc. Published 2017 by John Wiley & Sons, Inc.
Companion Website: www.fiveminutevet.com/endocrinology

- XO (Turner) syndrome – 77,XO (dog); 37,XO (cat); dysgenetic ovaries; phenotypic female; infantile genitalia; sterile.
- XXX syndrome – 79,XXX (dog); hypoplastic ovaries, usually without follicles or corpora lutea; anestrus to irregular estrous cycles; female phenotype; high FSH and LH; somatic abnormalities common in XXX women.
- True hermaphrodite chimera – XX/XY or XX/XXY; ovarian and testicular tissue; phenotypic sex depends on amount of testicular tissue; dogs and cats.
- XX/XY chimera with testes and XY/XY chimera with testes – vary from phenotypic female with abnormal genitalia to male with possible fertility; dogs and cats (some tortoiseshell males).

XY DSD

Disorders of Testicular Development
- Complete or Partial Testicular Dysgenesis – SRY-positive 78,XY dog; genitalia incompletely masculinized: (enlarged clitoris); testes undescended or perivulvar; Müllerian and Wolffian duct derivatives variably present.
- Ovotesticular DSD – (XY sex reversal, true hermaphrodite).
  - SRY-positive 38,XY true hermaphrodite cat (one report); ovotestes in ovarian position; Müllerian and Wolffian duct derivatives present; penis.
  - 78,XY (SRY status unknown) dog; ambiguous female genitalia (enlarged clitoris, os clitoris); abdominal ovary (hypoplastic) and testis (Sertoli cell tumor, no spermatogenesis).

Disorders in Androgen Synthesis or Action
- Complete Androgen Insensitivity Syndrome – 38,XY cat; testes at caudal pole of kidneys; no Wolffian or Müllerian duct derivatives; blind-ended vagina; vulva.
- Partial Androgen Insensitivity Syndrome – 78,XY dog; vulva; perivulvar scrotal-like swellings at 6 months of age; blind vaginal pouch; hypoplastic testes; epididymides, partially developed vasa deferentia; vulvar fibroblasts unable to bind dihydrotestosterone.
- Persistent Müllerian duct syndrome (Male Pseudohermaphrodite) – XY; testes (50% are unilateral or bilateral cryptorchid); epididymides, vasa deferentia, prostate, oviducts, uterus, cervix, cranial vagina; penis, prepuce, and scrotum usually normal; dogs and cats.
- Isolated Hypospadias – incomplete masculinization of urogenital sinus during urethral development causing abnormal location of urinary orifice from glans penis (mild) to perineum (severe); external genitalia unambiguous; testes (cryptorchid or scrotal) or bifid scrotum (cats) with spermatogenesis.

XX DSD

Ovotesticular DSD and Testicular DSD
- Canine XX DSD (Sex Reversal) – SRY-negative 78,XX reported in 28 dog breeds, not in cats; the autosomal gene causing testis induction presently unknown; not due to mutation of genes involved with sex reversal in polled goats and humans; two phenotypes:
  - Ovotesticular DSD, XX true hermaphrodite (90% of cases) – ovotestis (at least one); masculinized female phenotype; varies from normal to abnormal vulva, normal or

enlarged clitoris (os clitoris possible), uterus, oviducts, epididymides, and vasa deferentia; rarely fertile.
- Testicular DSD, XX males (10% of cases) – testes (usually cryptorchid); epididymides, vasa deferentia, prostate; bicornuate uterus, no oviducts; hypoplastic penis and prepuce; hypospadias common.

Androgen Excess

- Fetal origin – single report of congenital adrenal hyperplasia in a phenotypic male cat (38,XX, ovaries, oviducts, epididymides, vasa deferentia, bicornuate uterus); due to 11 β-hydroxylase deficiency; ACTH, testosterone, progesterone, 17-OH-progesterone, androstenedione, deoxycorticosterone, 11-dexoycorticosterone elevated.
- Maternal origin (Female Pseudohermaphrodite) – XX; ovaries; masculinized genitalia (mild clitoral enlargement to nearly normal male genitalia); oviducts, uterus, cranial vagina; prostate variable; caused by sex steroid administration during pregnancy; rare in dogs and cats.

Systems Affected

- Reproductive – anomalies of the gonads, tubular tract, and external genitalia.
- Renal/Urologic – occasionally affected (e.g., agenesis, incontinence, hematuria, cystitis).
- Skin/Exocrine – perivulvar dermatitis (hypoplastic vulva); perineal or peri-preputial dermatitis (hypospadias); hyperpigmentation (Sertoli cell tumor).

Genetics

- Chromosomal sex abnormalities – usually caused by random events during gamete formation or early embryonic development.
- XX DSD – autosomal recessive trait in American cocker spaniels and likely in Beagles, German shorthaired pointers; familial in English cocker spaniels, Chinese pugs, Kerry blue terriers, Norwegian elkhounds, Weimaraners; other reported breeds include soft-coated Wheaten terriers, Vizslas, Walker hounds, Doberman pinschers, Basset hounds, American pit bull terriers, Border collies, Afghan hounds.
- PMDS – autosomal recessive trait in miniature schnauzers in the US, Basset hounds in the Netherlands, and possibly Persian cats; expression limited to XY individuals.
- Hypospadias familial in Boston terriers.
- Failure of androgen-dependent masculinization (predominantly cats) probably X-linked.

Incidence/Prevalence

- Generally rare.
- In affected breeds – may be common within families or within the breed as a whole.

SIGNALMENT/HISTORY

Species

- Dogs and cats.

Breed Predilections

- Dogs (see Suggested Reading).

Mean Age and Range

- All are congenital disorders, but individuals with normal external genitalia may not be identified until breeding age or a routine gonadectomy.

Predominant Sex

- Phenotypic females and males.

CLINICAL HISTORY

- Depends on type of disorder.
- Listed are possible findings for any of the conditions; not all occur with each specific disorder.

Historic Findings

- Failure to cycle.
- Infertility and sterility.
- Vulva, clitoris, prepuce, or penis – abnormal size, shape, or location.
- Urine stream – abnormal location.
- Affected phenotypic males attractive to other males.
- Urinary incontinence.
- Vulvar discharge.
- PU/PD or polakiuria.

Physical Examination Findings

- Vulva normal or hypoplastic; sometimes preputial in appearance.
- Clitoris normal or enlarged; os clitoris.
- Perivulvar dermatitis and vulvar discharge.
- Testes scrotal, unilateral or bilateral cryptorchid; bifid scrotum.
- Penis and prepuce normal or hypoplastic.

- Urethral meatus normal or abnormal location.
- Dermatologic signs of hyperestrogenism in males.
- Abdominal mass.

Causes

- Congenital – heritable or non-heritable.
- Exogenous steroid hormone administration during gestation.

Risk Factors

- Androgen or progestagen administration during pregnancy (Female Pseudohermaphrodite).

 ## DIFFERENTIAL DIAGNOSIS

Individuals with Unambiguous Genitalia

- Female infertility–male infertility; mistimed breeding; subclinical cystic endometrial hyperplasia/endometritis; hypothyroidism.
- Failure to cycle (female) – silent heat; hypothyroidism; hyperadrenocorticism; previous gonadectomy.
- Male infertility–female infertility; mistimed breeding; exogenous drug use affecting fertility; orchitis or epididymitis; testicular degeneration or hypoplasia; prostatitis.

 ## DIAGNOSTICS

CBC/Biochemistry/Urinalysis

- Usually normal.
- Neutrophilia; normochromic, normocytic anemia; hyperglobulinemia, hyperproteinemia; azotemia; high ALT, ALP with pyometra (PMDS).
- Urinalysis – may reveal evidence of cystitis with anatomic abnormalities that affect the location of the urethral meatus.

Other Laboratory Tests

- Sex steroid hormones (progesterone, testosterone, and estradiol) – generally below the normal range; may be normal if disorder mild and patient not sterile.
- Detect testicular tissue – GnRH or hCG simulation test; resting serum AMH (see Cryptorchidism, Ovarian remnant syndrome, Hyperestrogenism).
- Karyotyping – required to define chromosomal sex (Molecular Cytogenetics Laboratory, Texas A&M University, 979-458-0520; call first).
- Polymerase chain reaction test for *SRY* – not commercially available.
- Androgen-binding studies on genital fibroblasts – testicular feminization-not commercially available.

Imaging

- Routine radiography and ultrasonography – may be of diagnostic value for suspected abdominal mass (e.g., testicular neoplasia with PMDS, testicular feminization, or XX DSD); males with signs referable to pyometra (Female Pseudohermaphrodite or PMDS).
- Contrast studies of the lower urogenital tract – may be useful in diagnosing Female Pseudohermaphrodites.

Pathologic Findings

Gross

- Precisely describe the genitalia: size and location of the vulva or prepuce; presence and appearance of the clitoris, penis, scrotum, prostate, caudal vagina, or os clitoris; position of the urinary orifice (identifies the phallic structure as penis or clitoris).
- Most patients with no identified chromosomal abnormalities – exploratory laparotomy to determine the location and morphology of the gonads and internal genitalia.

Histopathologic

- Examination of all tissues removed – necessary to define the type of disorder.
- Gonads – vary from nearly normal architecture to dysgenetic or a combination of ovary and testis (ovotestis).
- Essential to describe the components of the Müllerian and/or Wolffian duct system, if found.

 THERAPEUTICS

Appropriate Health Care

- Usually outpatient.
- Inpatient – exploratory laparotomy.

Nursing Care

- Phenotypic females with a hypoplastic vulva and perivulvar dermatitis and males with hypospadias – local therapy to improve dermatologic sequelae (see Episioplasty).

 COMMENTS

Client education

- Advise client to sterilize affected individuals.
- Advise client to remove carriers of known or suspected heritable disorders from the breeding program.

Surgical Considerations

- Gonadectomy and hysterectomy (if a uterus is found) – recommended.
- Amputation of an enlarged clitoris – recommended if the mucosal surface is repeatedly traumatized.
- Reconstructive surgery of the prepuce and malformed penis – dogs; may be necessary with testicular DSD, XX males, or hypospadias.

Medications

- Not available.

Contraindications

- Avoid androgen or progestagen use during pregnancy.

Patient Monitoring

Prevention/Avoidance
- Sterilize individuals with heritable disorders.
- Remove carriers of heritable disorders from the breeding program.

Possible Complications

- Infertility.
- Sterility.
- Urinary tract problems – incontinence; cystitis.
- Testicular neoplasia.
- Pyometra.

Miscellaneous

Age-Related Factors
- Patients not diagnosed at an early age – pyometra (e.g., PMDS; female pseudohermaphrodite); testicular neoplasia (e.g., PMDS; any DSD with cryptorchidism).

Synonyms

- Hermaphrodites.
- Intersexes.
- Klinefelter syndrome.
- Pseudohermaphrodites.
- Sex reversal.
- Turner syndrome.

See Also

Breeding, Timing
Cryptorchidism
Infertility, Female – Dogs
Infertility, Male – Dogs
Episioplasty

Abbreviations

ALP   = Alkaline phosphatase
ALT   = Alanine aminotransferase
AMH   = Anti-Müllerian hormone
DSD   = Disorders of Sexual Development
FSH   = follicle-stimulating hormone
GnRH = gonadotropin-releasing hormone
hCG   = human chorionic gonadotropin
LH   = luteinizing hormone
PMDS = persistent Müllerian duct syndrome
PU/PD = polyuria/polydipsia

Internet Resources

Meyers-Wallen, V.N. (2001) Inherited abnormalities of sexual development in dogs and cats, in *Recent Advances in Small Animal Reproduction* (eds P.W. Concannon, G. England, J. Verstegen, III, C. Linde-Forsberg). International Veterinary Information Service, Ithaca NY. Available at: www.ivis.org, 2001; A1217.0901.

Suggested Reading

Meyers-Wallen, V.N. (2012) Gonadal and sex differentiation abnormalities of dogs and cats. *Sex. Dev.*, 6, 46–60.
Christensen, B.W. (2012) Disorders of sexual development in dogs and cats. *Vet. Clin. Small Anim.*, 42, 515–526.

Acknowledgment: The author and editors acknowledge the previous contribution of Vicki N. Meyers Wallen to *Blackwell's Five-Minute Veterinary Consult: Canine and Feline*, on which this topic is based.

Author: Sarah K. Lyle DVM, PhD, DACT

chapter 15

Dystocia

DEFINITION

- Although many bitches and queens deliver in the home or kennel/cattery setting without difficulty, requests for veterinary obstetrical assistance are becoming more common. The increased financial and emotional value of stud dogs, brood bitches, toms, queens and their offspring to the pet fancier makes the preventable loss of even one neonate undesirable. Breeding colonies in academic, scientific and industrial facilities need to maximize neonatal survival for financial and ethical reasons. Veterinary involvement in canine and feline obstetrics has several goals: to increase live births (minimizing stillbirths resulting from the difficulties in the birth process); to minimize morbidity and mortality in the dam; and to promote increased survival of neonates during the first week of life. Neonatal survival is directly related to the quality of labor. Optimal management of whelping/queening requires an understanding of normal labor and delivery in the bitch and queen, as well as the clinical ability to detect abnormalities in the birthing process.

- Dystocia is defined as difficulty in the normal vaginal delivery of a neonate from the uterus. Dystocia must be diagnosed in a timely fashion for medical or surgical intervention to improve outcome. Additionally, the etiology of dystocia must be identified for the best therapeutic decisions to be made.

Normal Parturition

Gestation

- Clinicians are commonly asked to ascertain if a bitch or queen is at term pregnancy, ready chronologically to deliver a litter, and then to intervene if labor has not begun. An accurate determination of gestational length can be difficult, especially if numerous copulations occurred and no ovulation timing was performed. Prolonged gestation is a form of dystocia. Gestation in the bitch is more challenging to calculate than in the cat, because bitches are spontaneous ovulators. Normal gestation in the bitch is 56–58 days from the first day of diestrus (detected by serial vaginal cytologies, defined as the first day that cytology returns to ≤50% cornified/superficial cells), 64–66 days from the initial rise in progesterone from baseline (generally >2 ng/ml), or 58–72 days from the first instance

Blackwell's Five-Minute Veterinary Consult Clinical Companion: Small Animal Endocrinology and Reproduction, First Edition. Edited by Deborah S. Greco and Autumn P. Davidson. © 2017 John Wiley & Sons, Inc. Published 2017 by John Wiley & Sons, Inc. Companion Website: www.fiveminutevet.com/endocrinology

that the bitch permitted breeding. Predicting gestational length without prior ovulation timing is difficult because of the disparity between estrual behavior and the actual time of conception in the bitch, and the length of time semen can remain viable in the bitch reproductive tract (often up to >7 days). Breeding dates and conception dates do not correlate closely enough to permit very accurate prediction of whelping dates.

- Additionally, clinical signs of term pregnancy are not specific: radiographic appearance of fetal skeletal mineralization varies at term, fetal size varies with breed and litter size, and the characteristic drop in body temperature (typically less than 99 °F) may not be detected in all bitches, and varies in many. Breed, parity and litter size can also influence gestational length.

- Because the queen is an induced ovulator (ovulation follows coitus by 24–36 hours), gestational length can be predicted more accurately from breeding dates, assuming that copulation provided adequate coital stimulation for the LH surge and subsequent ovulation, and a limited number of copulations were permitted. The gestational length of queens ranges from 52 to 74 days from the first to last breeding. The mean gestational length is 65–66 days. Because of the poor outcome with the delivery of premature puppies and kittens, elective intervention is best delayed until stage I labor has begun, or prolonged gestation confirmed.

Labor and Delivery

- Bitches typically enter stage I labor within 24 hours of a decline in serum progesterone to below 2–5 ng/ml, which occurs in conjunction with elevated circulating prostaglandins and is commonly associated with a transient drop in body temperature, usually to <100 °F (33.7 °C). Queens typically enter stage I labor 24 hours after serum progesterone levels fall to less than 2 ng/ml.

- Monitoring serial progesterone levels for impending labor is problematic due to the fact that in-house canine kits enabling rapid results are inherently less accurate between 2–5 ng/ml, and a rapid decline in progesterone levels can occur over a period of a few hours. Commercial laboratories offering quantitative progesterone by chemiluminescence typically have a 12- to 24-hour turnaround time, which is not rapid enough to enable decisions about an immediate indication for obstetrical intervention.

- Stage I labor in the bitch normally lasts from 12 to 24 hours, during which time the uterus has myometrial contractions of increasing frequency and strength, associated with cervical dilation. No abdominal effort (visible external contractions) is evident during stage I labor. Bitches may exhibit changes in disposition and behavior during stage I labor, becoming reclusive, restless, and nesting intermittently, often refusing to eat and sometimes vomiting. Panting and trembling may occur. Vaginal discharge is clear and watery.

- Normal stage II labor in the bitch is defined to begin when external abdominal efforts can be seen, accompanying myometrial contractions to culminate in the delivery of a neonate. Presentation of the fetus at the cervix triggers the Ferguson reflex, promoting the release of endogenous oxytocin from the hypothalamus. Typically, these efforts should not last longer than 1–2 hours between puppies, although great variation exists. The entire delivery

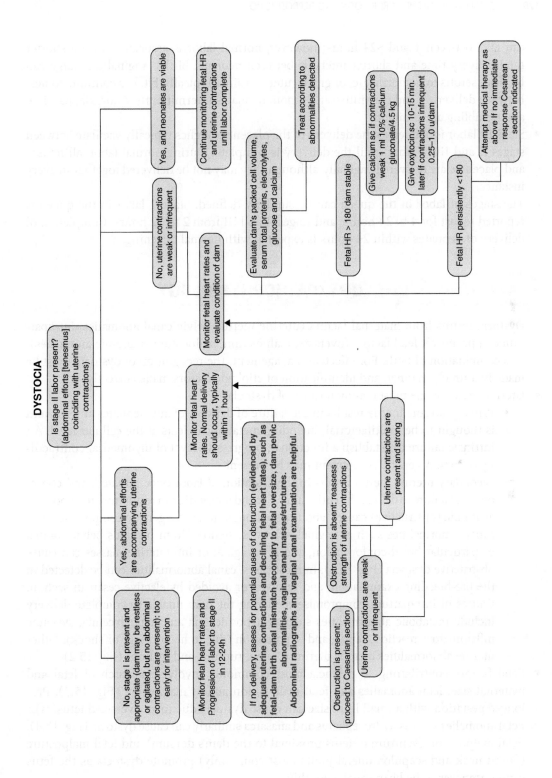

DYSTOCIA

Is stage II labor present? (abdominal efforts [tenesmus] coinciding with uterine contractions)

No, stage I is present and appropriate (dam may be restless or agitated, but no abdominal contractions are present): too early for intervention

Monitor fetal heart rates and Progression of labor to stage II in 12-24h

Yes, abdominal efforts are accompanying uterine contractions

Monitor fetal heart rates. Normal delivery should occur, typically within 1 hour

If no delivery, assess for potential causes of obstruction (evidenced by adequate uterine contractions and declining fetal heart rates), such as fetal-dam birth canal mismatch secondary to fetal oversize, dam pelvic abnormalities, vaginal canal masses/strictures. Abdominal radiographs and vaginal canal examination are helpful.

Obstruction is present: proceed to Caesarian section

Obstruction is absent: reassess strength of uterine contractions

Uterine contractions are weak or infrequent

Uterine contractions are present and strong

No, uterine contractions are weak or infrequent

Monitor fetal heart rates and evaluate condition of dam

Yes, and neonates are viable

Continue monitoring fetal HR and uterine contractions until labor complete

Evaluate dam's packed cell volume, serum total proteins, electrolytes, glucose and calcium

Treat according to abnormalities detected

Fetal HR > 180 dam stable

Give calcium sc if contractions weak 1 ml 10% calcium gluconate/4.5 kg

Give oxytocin sc 10-15 min. later If contractions infrequent 0.25–1.0 u/dam

Fetal HR persistently <180

Attempt medical therapy as above If no immediate response Cesarean section indicated

119

can take between 1 and >24 hours; however, normal labor is associated with a shorter total delivery time and shorter intervals between neonatal births. Vaginal discharge can be clear, serous to hemorrhagic, or green (uteroverdin). Typically, bitches continue to nest between deliveries, and may nurse and groom neonates intermittently. Anorexia, panting, and trembling are common.

- Stage III labor is defined as the delivery of the placenta. Bitches typically vacillate between stages II and III of labor until the delivery is complete. During normal labor, all fetuses and placentae are delivered vaginally, although they may not be delivered together in every instance.

- The stages of labor in the queen can be similarly defined. Stage 1 labor in the queen is reported to last for 4 to 24 hours, and stages II and III from 2 to 72 hours. Completion of delivery of neonates within 24 hours is expected with normal queening.

ETIOLOGY/PATHOPHYSIOLOGY

- Dystocia results from maternal factors (uterine inertia, pelvic canal anomalies, intrapartum compromise), fetal factors (oversize, malposition, malposture, anatomic anomalies), or a combination of both. For effective management, the recognition of dystocia must be made in a timely manner, and identification of etiologic factors made correctly.
- Uterine inertia is the most common cause of dystocia.
  - Primary uterine inertia results in the failure of delivery of any neonates at term, and is thought to be multifactorial, including metabolic defects at the cellular level. An intrinsic failure to establish a functional, progressive level of myometrial contractility occurs. A genetic component may be present.
  - Secondary uterine inertia results in the cessation of labor once initiated, and consequential failure to deliver the entire litter. Secondary inertia can result from metabolic or anatomic (obstructive) causes, and is also thought to have a genetic component. Birth canal abnormalities such as vaginal strictures, stenosis from previous pelvic trauma or particular breed conformation, and intravaginal or intrauterine masses can cause obstructive dystocia (Fig. 15.1). In most cases, canal abnormalities can be detected in the pre-breeding examination, and resolved or avoided by elective cesarean section. Causes of intrapartum compromise rendering the dam unable to complete delivery include metabolic abnormalities such as hypocalcemia and hypoglycemia, systemic inflammatory reaction, sepsis, and hypotension (due to hemorrhage or shock). Other uterine abnormalities include uterine torsion, rupture, and hydrops (Fig. 15.2).
- Fetal factors contributing to dystocia most commonly involve mismatch of fetal and maternal size, fetal anomalies and fetal malposition and/or malposture (Fig. 15.3). Prolonged gestation with a small litter size can cause dystocia due to an oversized fetus(es).
- Fetal anomalies such as hydrocephalus and anasarca similarly can cause dystocia (Fig. 15.4).
- Fetal malposition (ventrum of fetus proximal to the dam's dorsum) and fetal malposture (flexed neck and scapulohumeral joints most commonly) promote dystocia as the fetus cannot transverse the birth canal smoothly.

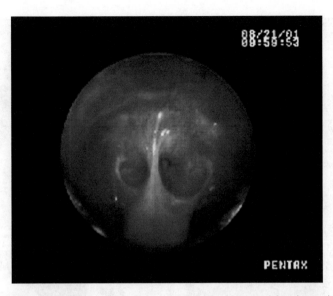

■ **Fig. 15.1.** Septate vaginal stricture seen with vaginoscopy, positioned just cranial to the urethral papilla.

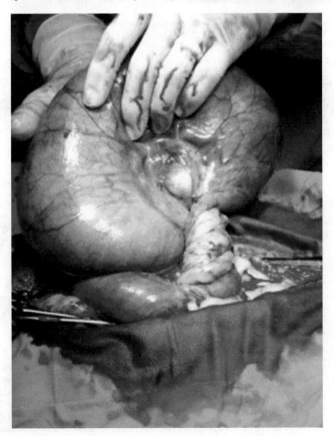

■ **Fig. 15.2.** Uterine torsion.

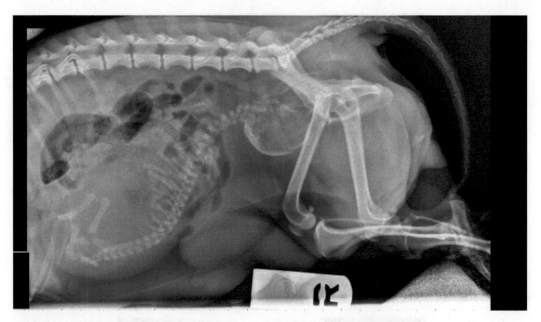

■ **Fig. 15.3.** Fetal maternal mismatch; singleton fetus the size of which has caused a dystocia.

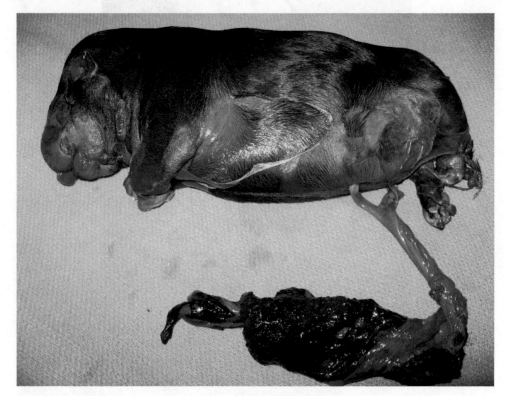

■ **Fig. 15.4.** Anasarca often results in fetal maternal mismatch and dystocia.

DIAGNOSTICS

- An efficient diagnosis of dystocia is dependent upon taking an accurate history and performing a thorough physical examination in a timely manner. The clinician must quickly obtain a careful reproductive history detailing breeding dates, any ovulation timing performed, historical and recent labor, as well as a general medical history.
- The physical examination should address the general status of the patient, as well as include a digital and/or vaginoscopic pelvic examination for patency of the birth canal, evaluation of litter and fetal size (radiography most useful), assessment of fetal viability (Doppler or real-time ultrasound ideally), and uterine activity (tocodynamometry most useful).
- A novel approach to veterinary obstetrical monitoring in use in the United States involves the use of external monitoring devices using tocodynamometry (Healthdyne Inc., Marietta, GA, USA) and a hand-held Doppler (Sonicaid, Oxford Instruments, England) to detect and record uterine activity and fetal heart rates. These devices can be used either in the home setting or at the veterinary clinic. Their use requires that the hair coat be lightly clipped caudal to the ribcage, over the gravid area of the lateral flanks, to allow good contact of the uterine sensor and fetal Doppler (Fig. 15.5).
  - The uterine sensor detects changes in intrauterine and intra-amniotic pressures. The sensor is strapped over the lightly clipped area of the bitch's/queen's caudolateral abdomen using an elasticized strap. The sensor's recorder is worn in a small backpack placed over the caudal shoulder area. Bitches/queens are at rest in the whelping/ queening box or in a crate or cage during the monitoring sessions. The monitoring equipment is well tolerated (Fig. 15.5). Subsequent to each recording session, data is transferred from the recorder via a modem using standard telephones.

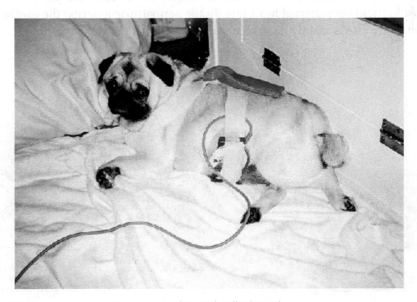

■ **Fig. 15.5.** Tocodynamometry; uterine sensor in place and well tolerated.

- Fetal Doppler monitoring is performed bilaterally with a hand-held unit with the bitch/queen in lateral recumbency, using acoustic coupling gel. Directing the Doppler perpendicularly over a fetus results in a characteristic amplification of the fetal heart sounds, distinct from maternal arterial or cardiac sounds, which enables determination of fetal heart rates (Fig. 15.6).
- Interpretation of the contractile pattern in strips produced by the uterine monitor requires training and experience. Data is transferred by modem to obstetrical personnel capable of interpretation, who subsequently consult with the attending veterinary clinician and client. Recordings are made on a twice-daily, hour-long basis when home monitoring is performed, then intermittently on bitches or queens at home as indicated during active labor, or on site in the veterinary clinic for shorter periods of time (minimally 20 minutes) when patients are being evaluated for suspected dystocia.
- The canine and feline uterus each have characteristic patterns of contractility, varying in frequency and strength before and during different the stages of labor.
- Serial tocodynamometry in the bitch and queen permits evaluation of the progression of labor. During late term, the uterus may contract once or twice an hour before actual stage I labor is initiated. During stage I and II labor, uterine contractions vary in frequency from 0 to 12 per hour, and in strength from 15 to 40 mmHg, with spikes up to 60 mmHg. Contractions during active labor can last 2–5 minutes in duration. Recognizable patterns exist during pre-labor and active (stages 1–3) labor. Aberrations is uterine contractility can be detected during monitoring. Abnormal, dysfunctional labor patterns can be weak or prolonged, and often are associated with fetal distress. Additionally, the completion of labor (or lack thereof) can be evaluated via tocodynamometry.
- The presence of fetal distress is reflected by sustained deceleration of the heart rates. Normal canine and feline fetal heart rates at term are from 170 to 230 beats per minute (bpm), or at least fourfold the maternal heart rate. In the periparturient period the cardiac output of the fetus/neonate is mainly dependent on heart rate, as the right ventricle is relatively

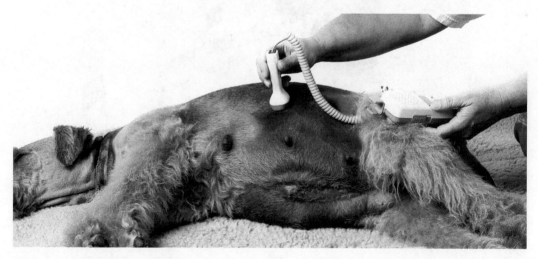

■ Fig. 15.6. Doppler monitoring of fetal heart rates.

stiff (low compliance) and the autonomic nervous system is immature (minimal inotropic response to catecholamines). Decelerations associated with uterine contractions suggest mismatch in size between the fetus and dam, or fetal malposition or malposture. Transient accelerations occur with normal fetal movement. Fetal heart rates of ≤150–160 bpm indicate stress. Fetuses with heart rates ≤130 bpm have poor survival if not delivered within 2–3 hours, and fetuses with heart rates ≤100 bpm are an indication for immediate intervention to hasten delivery (medical or surgical) before their demise.

 THERAPEUTICS

- The use of uterine and fetal monitors allows the veterinary clinician to detect and monitor labor, as well as manage labor medically or surgically with insight instead of guesswork.
  - Medical therapy for dystocia, based on the administration of oxytocin and calcium gluconate, can be directed and tailored based on the results of monitoring. Generally, the administration of oxytocin increases the frequency of uterine contractions, while the administration of calcium increases their strength.
  - Oxytocin, 10 USP u/ml (American Pharmaceutical Partners Inc., Los Angeles, California, USA) is effective at mini doses, starting with 0.25 units SC or IM to a maximum dose of 4 units per bitch or queen. Higher doses of oxytocin or intravenous boluses can cause tetanic, ineffective uterine contractions that can further compromise fetal oxygen supply by placental compression. The frequency of oxytocin administration is dictated by the labor pattern, and it is generally not given more frequently than hourly.
  - Calcium gluconate 10% solution with 0.465 mEq Ca^{2+}/ml (Fujisawa Inc., USA) is given SC at 1 ml/5.5 kg body weight as indicated by the strength of uterine contractions, generally no more frequently than every 4–6 hours. Calcium is given before oxytocin in most cases, improving contraction strength before increasing frequency. Additionally, the action of oxytocin appears to be improved when given 15 minutes subsequent to calcium. Most bitches/queens are eucalcemic, suggesting that the benefit of calcium administration is at a cellular or subcellular level.
- Surgical intervention (cesarean section) is indicated if a bitch or queen fails to respond to medical management, or if fetal distress is evidenced despite adequate to increased uterine contractility (suggesting mismatch of maternal birth canal to fetal size, or fetal malposition or malposture incompatible with vaginal delivery), or if aberrant contractile patterns are noted by uterine monitoring. Well-orchestrated cesarean sections result when anesthetic and neonatal resuscitative protocols are established and coordinated, and the preoperative preparation of the dam optimized.

See Also

Cesarean Section Elective and Emergency.
Uterine Inertia/Uterine Irritability.

Neonatal Resuscitation and Postpartum Neonatology.
Canine Breeding Management.
Feline Prebreeding Examination and Breeding Husbandry.
Pregnancy Diabetes.
Pregnancy Ketosis.

Suggested Reading

Davidson, A.P. (2003) Obstetrical monitoring in dogs. *Vet. Med.*, 6, 508.

Davidson, A.P. (2016) Dystocia management, in *Kirk's Veterinary Therapy, XIV* (ed. J.D.Bonagura), W.B. Saunders Co., Philadelphia, PA, pp. 992–998.

Davidson, A.P. (2001) Uterine and fetal monitoring in the bitch, in (ed. A.P. Davidson), Vet Clin N Am. 31 (2), W.B. Saunders Co., Philadelphia, PA.

Davidson, A.P. (2014) Clinical Conditions of the Bitch and Queen, in *Small Animal Internal Medicine*, 5th edition (eds R.W.Nelson, C.G.Couto), Elsevier, St Louis, MO, pp. 915–944.

Author: Autumn P. Davidson DVM, MS, DACVIM (Internal Medicine)

Chapter 16

Eclampsia

DEFINITION

- Eclampsia (also called puerperal tetany or postparturient hypocalcemia) is associated with ionized calcium depletion in the extracellular compartment of the body. It appears mainly during the first month of lactation, but can occur at any time of lactation or even during late gestation. Signs include restlessness, muscle tremors, panting, dilated pupils, and hyperthermia. Treatment consists of balancing body calcemia. If untreated during the first hours of clinical signs, eclampsia can progress to tetany and death.

ETIOLOGY/PATHOPHYSIOLOGY

- Eclampsia is a consequence of hypocalcemia and depletion of membrane-bound calcium, increasing membrane permeability and resulting in spontaneous muscle depolarization.
- Hypocalcemia is a common metabolic disorder during the first month of lactation (milk production is at its peak).

Systems Affected

- Cardiovascular.
- Musculoskeletal.
- Nervous.
- Neuromuscular.
- Ophthalmic.
- Skin.
- Respiratory.

SIGNALMENT/HISTORY

- Hypocalcemia occurs more commonly in toy breeds, older bitches (aged >7 years) and malnourished females. It is very uncommon in queens and in large-breed dogs.

Blackwell's Five-Minute Veterinary Consult Clinical Companion: Small Animal Endocrinology and Reproduction, First Edition. Edited by Deborah S. Greco and Autumn P. Davidson. © 2017 John Wiley & Sons, Inc. Published 2017 by John Wiley & Sons, Inc.
Companion Website: www.fiveminutevet.com/endocrinology

- Clinical signs include agitation, nervousness, dysorexia, panting, moaning, trembling, staggering, stiffness, fever, dry mucous membranes, changes in heart rate (tachycardia and bradycardia), tachypnea, facial pruritus and mydriasis with delayed response to light.
- If hypocalcemia is left untreated, within hours the above signs can progress to recumbency, hypersalivation, dyspnea, extensor rigidity, tetany resulting from cerebral edema, and death.

Risk Factors

- Nutrition seems to have a role in the onset of eclampsia, but other unknown factors appear to be involved.
- Excess calcium intake during pregnancy may induce eclampsia secondary to an iatrogenic atrophy of the parathyroid glands; under the demands of lactation hypocalcemia results; inadequate mobilization of skeletal calcium and regulation of renal loss occurs.
- Home-made diets rich in phytates (rice, corn, soybean) limit the intestinal absorption of calcium and can promote hypocalcemia.

Historic Findings

- Decreased appetite and apathy are often the first signs described by attentive (alert) owners, followed by agitation, nervousness, panting, moaning and trembling.
- Frenetic face rubbing is sometimes reported by owners, but is rarely the reason for consultation, unless the client has been educated to watch for this sign.

 CLINICAL FEATURES

- Hyperthermia.
- Dry mucous membranes.
- Tachycardia or bradycardia.
- Tachypnea.
- Mydriasis and/or delayed response to light stimulation.
- Muscle rigidity.
- Tetany.

 DIFFERENTIAL DIAGNOSIS

- Hypoglycemia (does not cause muscle rigidity and hyperthermia).
- Seizure activity: toxicosis, epilepsy, and other neurologic disorders. The history of recent parturition aids in the diagnosis of eclampsia.

 DIAGNOSTICS

- Ionized calcium ≤80 mg/dl.
- Corrected total serum calcium <7 mg/100 ml (less reliable). Early in the course of the disease (dysorexia, agitation), females may have a normal *total* calcium concentration.

Pathological Findings

- None

THERAPEUTICS

- Immediate calcemia restoration.
- Reduce calcium loss.
  Optimize calcium intestinal absorption.
- Restore glycemia, hypoglycemia is commonly concurrent.
- Reduce hyperthermia.
- Treat tetany and prevent cerebral edema and associated complications.

Drug(s)

- 10% calcium chloride solution or 10% calcium gluconate solution.
- Vitamin D.
- Oral calcium carbonate tablets.

Procedures

- Acute eclampsia with tetany
  - Slow intravenous calcium injection
  - Concurrent cardiac (ECG, stethoscope) and frequent ionized calcium monitoring.
  - 10% calcium gluconate solution: 0.2–0.5 ml/kg in 5–10 minutes.

or

- CRI calcium solution: 2/3 5% dextrose + 1/3 NaCl 0.9%, 20 mEq/l K^+, 40 mEq/l Ca^{2+}. 10 ml/kg/h.
- Eclampsia (without tetany)
  - SC/IM injections.
  - Calcium gluconate solution 10%/NaCl 0.9% solution, 50/50) : rapidly effective, prolonged duration of action (8 hours).
- Discrete hypocalcemia/Prevention (at the time of discharge)
  - Oral supplementation
    - 50–100 mg/kg/day calcium tablets (carbonate or gluconate).
    - 500 mg of calcium carbonate balance 200 mg of calcium.
  - ± Vitamin D: 1000–2500 IU/day.
- Complementary treatments :
  - Reduce/stop milk production by limiting neonates suckling. Consider antiprolactin therapy if neonates are weaned: Cabergoline 5 µg/kg/day PO.
  - Balance glycemia.
  - Control hyperthermia: cool perfusion, cool shower, alcohol soaks (footpads).

- Prevent/control cerebral edema: mannitol perfusions, intravenous glucocorticoids (but promote calciuria), diazepam administration IV.
- Correct dietary imbalance. The calcium/phosphorus ratio in the prenatal and post-natal diet should be 1:1–1.2:1.

 ## COMMENTS

- Commercial calcium solutions vary widely in their concentrations of elemental calcium.
- For example, 10% calcium gluconate solution contains 9.3 mg/ml of calcium, and 10% calcium chloride solution contains 27.2 mg/ml of calcium (i.e., threefold more).

Expected Course and Prognosis

- Untreated hypocalcemia leads rapidly to death (in a few hours).
- Hypocalcemia may recur in the current lactation period, and again in future pregnancies. Re-checking serum ionized calcium levels and close owner monitoring for clinical signs is important if puppies continue to nurse.
- The owner needs to understand that excessive calcium intake during pregnancy does not prevent eclampsia but, on the contrary, increases its risk.

See Also

Dystocia.
Hypercalcemia.
Hypocalcemia.
Hypoglycemia.
Nutrition in Pregnancy and Lactation Bitch Queen.
Uterine Inertia/Uterine Irritability.
Parturition.

Suggested Reading

Davidson, A. (2010) Clinical approach to abnormal pregnancy, in *BSAVA Manual of Canine and Feline Reproduction and Neonatalogy*, 2nd edition (eds G.England, A. VonHeimendahl). BSAVA, Gloucester, pp. 116–117.
Drobatz, K.J., Casey, K.K. (2000) Eclampsia in dogs: 31 cases (1995–1998). *J. Am. Vet. Med. Assoc.*, **217** (2), 216–219.
Johnston, S.D., Kustritz, M.V.R., Olson, P.N.S. (2001) Periparturient disorders in the bitch, in *Canine and Feline Theriogenology*. WB Saunders, Philadelphia, pp. 141–143.
Levy, X. (2012) Quel est votre diagnostic ? *PratiqueVet*, **47**, 12–14.

Author: Xavier Lévy DVM, DECAR

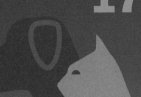

chapter 17

Episioplasty/Vulvoplasty in the Bitch and Queen

DEFINITION

- Episioplasty is a surgical procedure used to eliminate redundant perivulvar skin folds and vulvar recession that produce perivulvar dermatitis and urine pooling, and also predispose to urinary tract infections (Fig. 17.1).

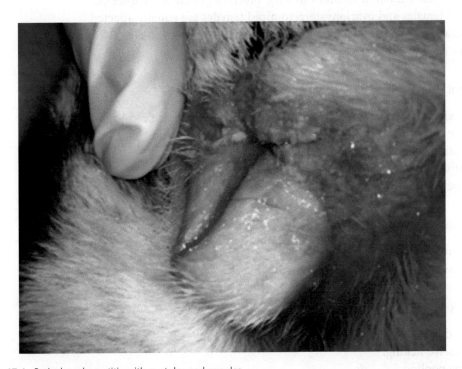

■ **Fig. 17.1.** Perivulvar dermatitis with pustules and papules.

Blackwell's Five-Minute Veterinary Consult Clinical Companion: Small Animal Endocrinology and Reproduction, First Edition. Edited by Deborah S. Greco and Autumn P. Davidson. © 2017 John Wiley & Sons, Inc. Published 2017 by John Wiley & Sons, Inc.
Companion Website: www.fiveminutevet.com/endocrinology

ETIOLOGY/PATHOPHYSIOLOGY

- Perivulvar folds are prone to accumulate vaginal secretions and urine, which create a stimulus for ulceration and bacterial growth.
- Bacterial overgrowth produces perivulvar dermatitis and can produce an ascending urinary tract infection.
- A redundant dorsal vulvar fold can cause urine pooling and signs of incontinence.

SIGNALMENT/HISTORY

- Multiple breeds of dogs, mixed-breed dogs and cats are affected.
- Occurs more often in medium to large-breed dogs and obese queens.
- Intact females and ovariohysterectomized females are equally affected.
- Median age of presentation is approximately 4–4.5 years of age.
- Dogs aged less than 1 year can be affected.

Clinical Signs

- Malodorous vulvo-vaginal area due to dermatitis and vestibulo-vaginitis.
- Urine and salivary staining of the perivulvar area/pelvic limbs.
- Scooting, excoriation of the perineal area.
- Painful perineal area.
- Urine pooling.

Risk Factors

- Obesity.
- Juvenile vulva with cranial placement (Fig. 17.2).

Historic Findings

- Malodor.
- Excessive licking.
- Urine pooling.
- Repeated urinary tract infections.

CLINICAL FEATURES

- Recessed vulva/redundant perivulvar folds with perivulvar dermatitis.
- May observe vaginal discharge.
- Vaginal area often painful upon palpation.
- Urine and saliva stains in the perineal area and on the pelvic limbs.

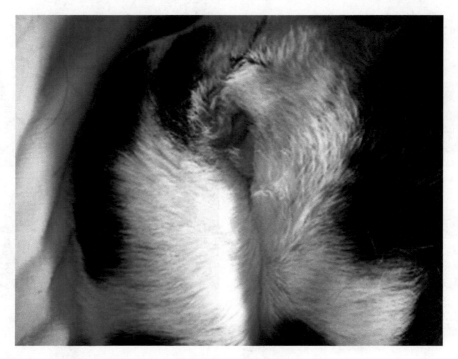

■ **Fig. 17.2.** Juvenile canine vulva with cranial asymmetric placement.

DIFFERENTIAL DIAGNOSIS

- Extension of generalized pyoderma.
- Incontinence/urine pooling can be produced by urethral sphincter incompetence, a pelvic bladder, ectopic ureters, or urethral and vestibular diverticula.
- Cystitis and urethritis can cause incontinence.

DIAGNOSTICS

- Physical examination of perineal area can require sedation. Manual reduction of the skin fold is necessary to evaluate the area (Fig. 17.3a–f).
- Complete blood count to determine the severity of infection.
- Serum chemistry panel to determine renal function, evidence of pyelonephritis, or other metabolic disease predisposing to urinary tract infection.
- Urinalysis/culture and sensitivities to check for urinary tract infection and organisms present.
- Abdominal ultrasound, contrast radiography, uroendoscopy, CT and MRI can be employed to rule out other causes of urinary tract infection and incontinence.
    - Incontinence produced by a recessed or hooded vulva is episodic, not continuous.

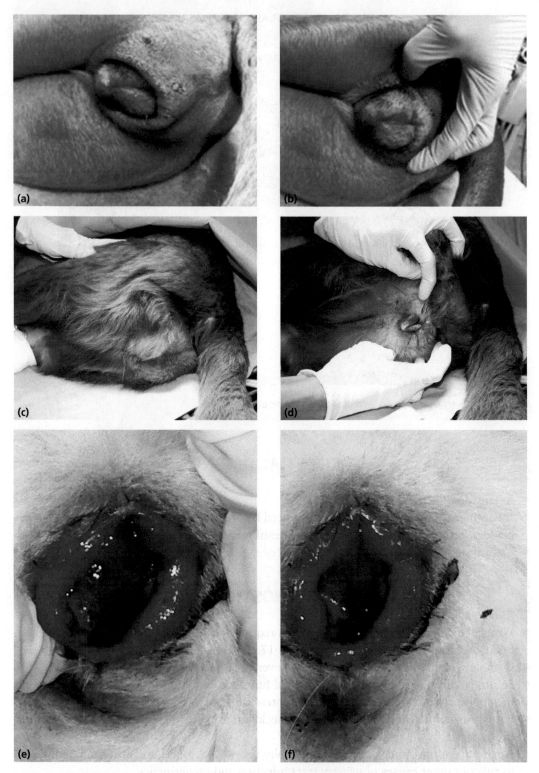

■ **Fig. 17.3.** (a,c) Recessed or hooded vulva in bitches with perivulvar dermatitis, becoming visible with retraction of the skin fold (b,d). (e,f) Obese queen with recessed vulva and perivulvar dermatitis.

THERAPEUTICS

- The goal of therapy is to excise the redundant perivulvar skin folds and elevate the recessed vulva to produce a free urine stream that avoids contact with the skin.
- Medical management of perivulvar dermatitis with the administration of antibiotics or topical treatments such as antibiotic ointments or drying agents only produces temporary and brief relief of signs.
- Episioplasty:
  - A horse-shoe or crescent-shaped section of skin is removed from the dorsal and lateral aspects of the vulva (Figs. 17.4 and 17.5).
  - The area of the skin removed is thicker dorsally and tapers laterally.
  - Absorbable suture material in a simple interrupted pattern is used to appose the subcutaneous and subcuticular layers.
  - The skin is closed with suture material or staples (Fig. 17.6).
  - Surgical morbidity and complications are very low. Scooting and self-excoriation must be prevented during healing for optimal results (Fig. 17.7a,b)

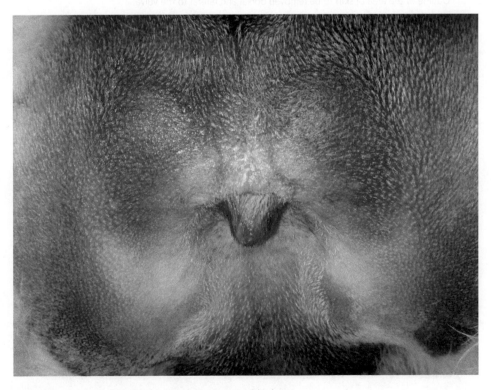

■ **Fig. 17.4.** Recessed or hooded vulva in a dog prior to episioplasty.

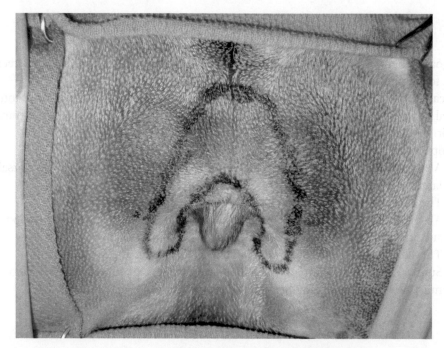

■ **Fig. 17.5.** Outline of the area of skin to be removed dorsal and lateral to the vulva.

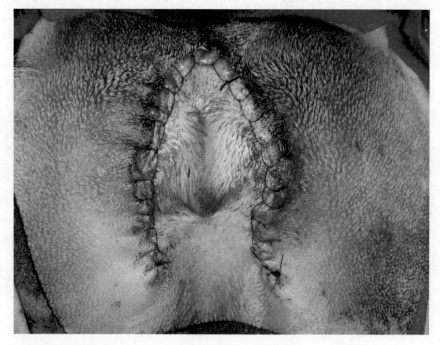

■ **Fig. 17.6.** Completed episioplasty.

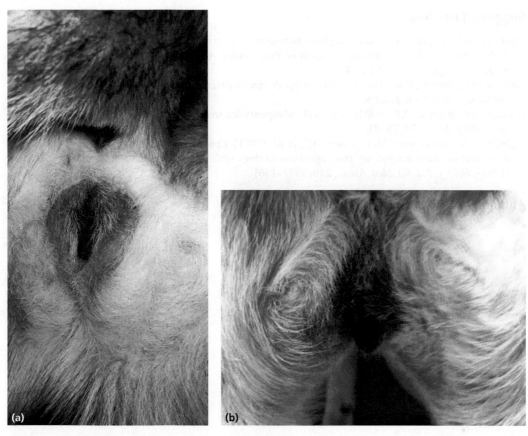

■ **Fig. 17.7.** Bitch at (a) 4 and (b) 12 weeks post episioplasty.

 # COMMENTS

- Episioplasty is often performed in combination with the application of a hydraulic urethral occluder for the control of sphincter incontinence.
- Expected course and progress:
- Episioplasty has been reported to control perivulvar dermatitis in up to 93% of bitches.
- Episioplasty has been reported to control urinary tract infections in 50–100% of bitches.

See Also

Vulvovaginal malformations.

Suggested Reading

Chon, E., Mehl, M., et al. (2006) Episioplasty as treatment for recurrent urinary tract infections in bitches with excessive perivulvar skin folds. Scientific Presentation Abstracts. American College of Veterinary Surgeons Symposium. *Vet. Surg.*, **35**, E4.

Gourley, I.M., Gregory, C.R. (1992) Perivulvar pyoderma, in *Atlas of Small Animal Surgery*. Gower Medical Publishing, New York, p. **22**.5.

Hammel, S.P., Bjorling, D.E. (2002) Results of vulvoplasty for treatment of recessed vulvas in dogs. *J. Am. Anim. Hosp. Assoc.*, **38**, 79–83.

Lightner, B.A., McLoughin, M.A., Chew, D.J., *et al.* (2001) Episioplasty for the treatment of perivulvar dermatitis for recurrent urinary tract infections in dogs with excessive perivulvar skin folds: 31 cases (1983–2000). *J. Am. Vet. Med. Assoc.*, **219**, 1577–1581.

Author: Clare Gregory DVM, DACVS

chapter 18

Estrous Cycle Abnormalities

(Prolonged Proestrus/Estrus, Prolonged Anestrus, Short Interestrous Interval)

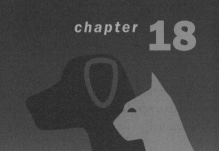

 ## DEFINITION/OVERVIEW

Prolonged Proestrus/Estrus

- Either or both stages of the cycle last longer than 30 days.
- Associated with split heat cycles where the bitch fails to ovulate during the first proestrus and then a short time later (days to weeks) begins the cycle again, with the second estrus culminating in normal ovulation and fertility.
- Alternatively can be associated with follicular ovarian cysts or functional ovarian tumors elaborating estrogen (see Ovarian remnant syndrome/Hyperestrogenism).
- Rule out exogenous estrogen exposure.

Prolonged Anestrus

- An extended period of time between the end of diestrus and the onset of the next proestrus.
  - Normal anestrus period is 4 months.
  - Considered prolonged when it lasts more than 10–18 months from the previous cycle.
- Delayed puberty is a prolongation from the normal expected range for onset of puberty for a particular breed.
  - The larger the breed, the later in life puberty is expected to start. Toy, small and medium breeds: 6–8 months of age; large and giant breeds: 6–16 months of age.

Silent Heat

- Few to no outward signs of proestrus or estrus.
- There is minimal to no bloody vulvar discharge or vulvar edema.
- Often no receptive behavior from the bitch and reduced interest from males.

Shortened Interestrous Interval (IEI)

- The time period between two ovulations is less than normal for the particular breed.
- Most breeds have a normal IEI of 5–6 months.

Blackwell's Five-Minute Veterinary Consult Clinical Companion: Small Animal Endocrinology and Reproduction,
First Edition. Edited by Deborah S. Greco and Autumn P. Davidson. © 2017 John Wiley & Sons, Inc.
Published 2017 by John Wiley & Sons, Inc.
Companion Website: www.fiveminutevet.com/endocrinology

- Certain breeds may have a normal IEI of 4 months (German Shepherd, Akitas, Labrador Retriever, Rottweiler, Cocker Spaniel, Basset Hound), while other breeds cycle only once annually (Basenji, Tibetan Mastiff).

 ## ETIOLOGY/PATHOPHYSIOLOGY

Prolonged Proestrus/Estrus

- May be variations of normal cyclicity.
- Failure to ovulate as a result of abnormal follicular development, abnormal LH receptors, inadequate or complete lack of LH release.
- Follicular cysts, ovarian neoplasia.
- Confused with vaginitis, cystitis or vaginal foreign bodies if there is prolonged vulvar discharge or male interest.
- Confused with split heat if the interval between cycles is short.

Prolonged Anestrus

- This may be normal variation of length of IEI.
- Rule out prolonged luteal phase due to luteal cysts or progesterone-secreting neoplasia.
- Following a pregnancy by delaying onset of the next cycle by 2–3 or more months as a means to allow the bitch's body to recover from the physiologic stress of pregnancy and lactation.
- Poor body condition or systemic disease.
- Hypothyroidism.
- Premature ovarian failure.
- Silent heat may be confused with prolonged anestrus, but it is not a true prolonged anestrus.
  - Failure of the observation by the owner.
  - Pooling of blood in the cranial vagina.
  - Fastidious cleaning.

Delayed Puberty

- Normal variation amongst breeds.
- Poor nutrition, parasitism, systemic disease.
- Exogenous hormone administration (purposeful or inadvertent).
- Hyperadrenocorticism, stress.
- Hypothyroidism.
- Luteal cysts.
- Silent heat.
- Abnormal sexual differentiation, ovarian agenesis/aplasia/hypoplasia.
- Immune-mediated oophoritis.
- Prior ovariectomy.

Prolonged Diestrus

- Clinically appear not to cycle.
- Differentiated from prolonged anestrus by documenting elevated progesterone (>1 ng/ml) for longer than 70 days.
- Often accompanied by cystic endometrial hyperplasia/pyometra.
- Luteal ovarian cysts.
- Progesterone-secreting ovarian neoplasia.

Shortened IEI

- Ovulation failure.
- Short luteal period (non-pregnant cycle or hypoluteoidism).
- Short anestrus.
- Uterine pathology may result in early release of PGF2α and a shortened diestrus.

SYSTEMS AFFECTED

- Reproductive – abnormal estrus cycles may result in subfertility, infertility, conception failure, small litter size, CEH.
- Skin/Exocrine – conditions of prolonged estrogen secretion may result in bilateral symmetrical non-pruritic alopecia, hyperpigmentation, lichenification, hyperkeratosis.
- Hemic/Lymphatic/Immune – conditions of prolonged estrogen secretion may result in bone marrow suppression with anemia, leukopenia and thrombocytopenia.

SIGNALMENT/HISTORY

- Anovulatory cycles – more common in older bitches, but can occur at any age. Occurs in 1.2% of bitches presenting for ovulation timing.
- Follicular cysts are more common in nulliparous bitches.
- Split or silent heats – most common on the pubertal estrus.
- Silent heat, prolonged anestrus – cycle irregularity occurs more commonly in aged bitches.
- Silent heat is more common when there is no intact male in the kennel, but can occur even when bitches are housed directly with males.
- Shortened IEI – may have a history of resorption, abortion or conception failure.

CLINICAL FEATURES

- Prolonged proestrus/estrus – vulvar edema and bloody vulvar discharge, ± signs of estrogen toxicity, prolonged male interest and receptivity.
  - Anovulatory cycles – failure of progesterone to exceed 10 ng/ml (often in the range of 3–6 ng/ml).

- Prolonged diestrus – appear not to cycle.
- Prolonged anestrus, delayed puberty – may have infantile or ambiguous genitalia, small stature, thin body condition.
- Shortened IEI – may be associated with inflammatory vulvar discharge indicative of uterine pathology.

DIAGNOSTICS

Prolonged Proestrus/Estrus, Silent Heat, Split Heat

- Vaginal cytology, speculum examination and progesterone measurement.
- Ultrasound may be used to assess follicle size and determine when ovulation occurs (color-flow Doppler helpful) or may be attempted to be induced; also to evaluate for presence of ovarian pathology (Fig. 18.1).

Prolonged Diestrus

- Progesterone measurement.
- Abdominal ultrasound (Fig. 18.1).

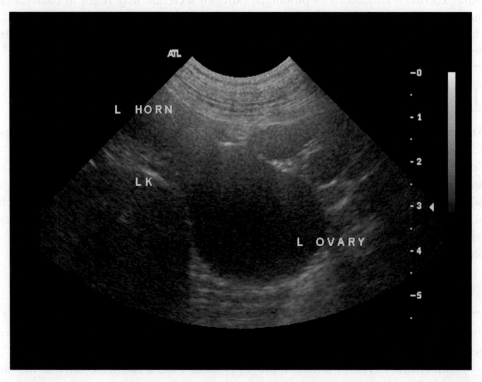

■ **Fig. 18.1.** Hypoechoic follicular ovarian cyst (L) at the cranial pole of the left ovary. Image courtesy of T.W. Baker.

Prolonged Anestrus

- Karyotype.
- Serum chemistry and adrenal challenge testing.
- Progesterone measurement to differentiate from prolonged diestrus.
- Thyroid evaluation.
- Ultrasound.

Shortened IEI

- Progesterone level during luteal phase.
- Ultrasound uterus to look for CEH or endometritis.
- Uterine biopsy.

PATHOLOGICAL FINDINGS

Prolonged Proestrus/Estrus

- Large, singular or multiple follicular cysts may be found.
  - Structures >0.8 cm in toy, small or medium breed bitches, or >1.0 cm in large or giant breed bitches are considered pathologic.
- Ovarian neoplasia – granulosa cell tumors tend to be multiloculated but can be cystic or solid; cystadenoma tend to be more solid, luteomas often cystic (Figs 18.2 and 18.3).

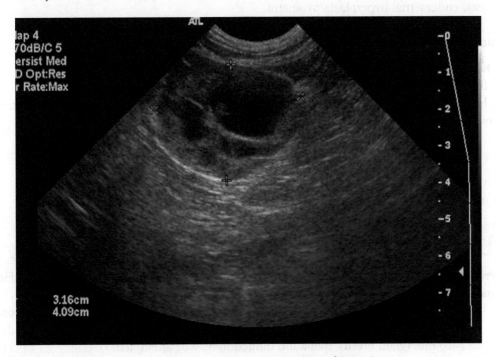

■ Fig. 18.2. Luteoma (cursors) causing prolonged diestrus. Image courtesy of T.W. Baker.

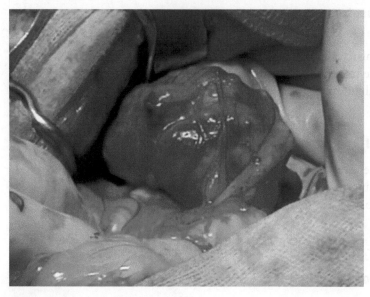

■ **Fig. 18.3.** Intraoperative image of luteoma.

Prolonged Diestrus

■ Ovarian luteal cyst or progesterone-producing neoplasia.
■ Cystic endometrial hyperplasia/pyometra.

Prolonged Anestrus

■ Ovarian senescence.
■ Clinical signs of systemic disease.
■ Chromosomal abnormalities may present with abnormal external genitalia and reproductive tract abnormalities of hypoplasia or aplasia, ovotestes, or gonadal dysgenesis.

Shortened IEI

■ Cystic endometrial hyperplasia.
■ Endometritis.

 THERAPEUTICS

■ Prolonged proestrus/estrus – can attempt to medically induce ovulation as described for anovulatory cycles, if signs of maximum estrogen production are present.
  • Anovulatory cycles – once cytology reaches >70% anucleated squames and majority of follicles are >4–5 mm (toy and small breed); 5–7 mm (medium–large breed); 7–10 mm (giant breed), ovulation induction may be attempted.
    □ GnRH – 1.1–2.2 µg/kg IM or IV repeated for 1–3 days.
    □ hCG 500–1000 IU/bitch IM; may repeat in 2–3 days if ovulation does not occur.

- ☐ GnRH and hCG concurrently (same doses as above).
  - ☐ Ovuplant (deslorelin acetate) – place implant in vulvar mucosa following lidocaine block; remove implant once ovulation documented.
  - Split heats – breed on second heat.
- Prolonged diestrus – can attempt luteolysis with prostaglandins, but most luteal cysts are not responsive; ovariectomy can be performed with histopathology.
- Prolonged anestrus – once silent heat is refuted and ensure an appropriate IEI, can try to induce estrus, if karyotype normal.
  - Cabergoline 5 µg/kg PO QD until proestrus begins (average 10–14 days).
  - Bromocriptine 50–100 µg/kg PO BID until proestrus begins (average 10–14 days). May cause nausea, vomiting, diarrhea.
  - Ovuplant – estrus within 2–7 days, ovulation within 7–10 days. Higher incidence of anovulation and hypoluteoidism.
  - Silent heat – breed once ovulation is documented.
  - Delayed puberty – improve nutrition, deworm, treat systemic disease appropriately, discontinue exogenous hormones, PGF2α for luteal cysts. No treatment for chromosomal abnormalities, ovarian dysgenesis, immune-mediated oophoritis.
- Shortened IEI – suppress estrus with mibolerone or deslorelin acetate (Suprelorin® 4.7 or 9.4 mg implants, 6 or 12 months suppression, respectively).
  - Mibolerone – 0.5–12 kg, 30 µg/day; 12–23 kg, 60 µg/day; 23–45 kg, 120 µg/day; >45 kg or any German Shepherd-type breed, 180 µg/day.
  - Documented hypoluteoidism during pregnancy may be treated with Regumate® 0.088 mg/kg PO QD; progesterone in oil 2 mg/kg IM q. 48–72 hours; or Prometrium® 10 mg/kg PO divided BID. If using progesterone in oil or Prometrium®, the dose should be tailored based on serum progesterone testing to produce a normal progesterone profile in late pregnancy. All progesterone supplementation should be discontinued at least 2–3 days prior to the expected due date to allow for free whelping. May have decreased mammary development and poor mothering behaviors in bitches treated with progestogens during pregnancy. Do not initiate therapy before day 35 of pregnancy to avoid masculinization of female fetuses (see Disorders of Sexual Differentiation/Premature Labor). Consider tocolytic therapy as an alternative to progestogens.

 ## COMMENTS

Expected Course and Prognosis

- Prolonged proestrus/estrus – breeding once ovulation occurs is associated with normal fertility, fertility should be normal if follicular cysts can be treated or neoplastic ovary is removed.
  - Anovulatory cycles – approximately 50% of bitches with anovulatory follicles can be induced to ovulate; 40–50% will recur on a subsequent cycle.
  - Split heats – normal fertile second heat.
  - Silent heat – normal fertility if cycle documented and bred during fertile period.
- Prolonged diestrus – guarded prognosis for fertility due to endometrial changes secondary to prolonged progesterone exposure.

- Prolonged anestrus – if due to neoplasia or luteal cyst prognosis is good once removed/treated. Fertility is normal for silent heat if documented and bred post-ovulation. No treatment for premature ovarian failure.
  - Delayed puberty – if poor body condition, nutrition, parasitism, fertility should be normal once normal condition is established. No successful treatment for chromosomal abnormalities, ovarian dysgenesis, immune-mediated oophoritis. Bitches with adrenal disease should not be bred due to potential complications during pregnancy. Fertility following treatment for luteal cysts should be normal.
- Shortened IEI – if the IEI can be prolonged and the primary cause treated; fertility may be acceptable.

Abbreviations

IEI   = Interestrous interval
GnRH = Gonadotropin-releasing hormone
hCG   = Human chorionic gonadotropin
PGF2α = Prostaglandin F2α
CEH   = Cystic endometrial hyperplasia

See Also

Canine Breeding Management
Medical Manipulation of the Estrous Cycle

Suggested Reading

Johnston, S.D., Root Kustritz, M.V., Olsen, P.N.S. (2001) *Canine and Feline Theriogenology*. WB Saunders, Philadelphia, pp. 16–32; 193–242; 257–273.
England, G.C.W. (2010) Clinical Approach to Infertility in the Bitch, in *BSAVA Manual of Canine and Feline Reproduction and Neonatology*. BSAVA, Waterwells, pp. 51–69.

Author: Cheryl Lopate MS, DVM, DACT

Genetic Disease Counseling in the Pre-Breeding Examination

chapter 19

DEFINITION

- Genetic counseling is used to assist breeders with a breeding plan: whether to breed an individual animal and who to breed that animal to. When discussing genetic counseling, there are several terms that are commonly used:
  - Allele – an alternate form of the same region in the DNA. For example, a single base change in the DNA can cause up to four different alleles for that region (one for each nucleotide: A, C, G, or T). Two alleles form a genotype.
  - Congenital disorder – a disease or disorder that is present at birth, whether hereditary or not. Example: umbilical hernia is a congenital defect, although it is yet unclear whether it is hereditary.
  - DNA (genotypic) test – a test that identifies the genotype for a specific trait.
    - Marker test – a test that uses a genetic marker that is associated with a trait in order to predict the genotype. This test is usually performed when the specific causative alleles have yet to be identified. There is a possibility for false results (both negative and positive) with this test due to recombination events.
    - Mutation test – a test that directly tests for the presence of alleles for a desired trait and therefore identifies the genotype.
  - Genotype – The genetic make-up leading to a certain phenotype, for a specific trait. A genotype in dogs and cats is composed of two copies of the same region of DNA (unless dealing with a sex-linked trait). Each copy is termed an allele.
  - Heterozygous – A genotype that is composed of two different alleles. Heterozygous individuals may be referred to as 'carriers' when referring to a recessive trait.
  - Hereditary disorder – a disease or disorder that can be passed from parent to offspring, whether or not it is present at time of birth. Example: Generalized progressive retinal atrophy which is not detected at birth but is hereditary.
  - Homozygous – A genotype that is composed of two identical alleles.
  - Mode of inheritance – The pattern in which a trait or disease is inherited.
    - Autosomal – The pattern of inheritance is independent of the sex of the individual. Example: Progressive retinal atrophy in Cornish Rex cats.

Blackwell's Five-Minute Veterinary Consult Clinical Companion: Small Animal Endocrinology and Reproduction, First Edition. Edited by Deborah S. Greco and Autumn P. Davidson. © 2017 John Wiley & Sons, Inc. Published 2017 by John Wiley & Sons, Inc. Companion Website: www.fiveminutevet.com/endocrinology

- □ Sex-linked – The inheritance pattern is dependent on the sex of the individual carrying the trait. Example: Hemophilia A in dogs.
- □ Recessive – Two alleles that cause the trait have to be present for the trait (phenotype) to be evident. Example: Hyperuricosuria in English Bulldogs.
- □ Dominant – Only one of the causative alleles has to be present for the trait (phenotype) to be evident. Example: Polycystic kidney disease in Persian cats.
- □ Co-Dominant (incomplete dominance) – the phenotype of the heterozygous state has an intermediate phenotype, differing from the phenotype of either homozygous type. Example: The Siamese and Burmese cat point coat color.
- □ Monogenic – a trait that is caused by a change in a single gene. Example: Spinal Muscular atrophy in Maine Coon cats.
- □ Polygenic – a trait that is caused by a change in two or more genes. Example: coat color of Labrador Retriever dogs.
- □ Multi-factorial – a trait that is controlled by genetic and environmental factors. Example: Hip dysplasia in dogs.
- □ Epistasis – a genotype of a certain gene masks the genotype and the phenotypic effect of another gene. An example is the yellow coat color of Labrador retrievers that is controlled by a different gene than that of the black or chocolate color. When the dog is homozygous recessive for the yellow gene, the dog will be yellow, no matter what the genotype is at the black/brown gene. If the dog is heterozygous or homozygous for the dominant allele at the yellow gene, the dog will show the coat color, as determined by the black/brown gene.
- Phenotype – An observable characteristic or trait. Example: hip dysplasia (observed on radiographs) or coat color.
- Phenotypic test – A test that identifies the presence of a trait based on the presence of a phenotype. Example: PennHIP and CERF examinations.
- Recombination – The process of rearrangement of genetic material. This process can occur naturally and may lead to false association between a genetic marker and a mutation causing a trait.

INDICATIONS

- Although genetic diseases can occur in all dogs and cats, whether purebred or mixed breed, genetic testing is commonly performed in purebred animals. There are two reasons to genetically test an animal:
  - In preparation for planned breeding – with the main goal to avoid a breeding that will produce individuals affected with diseases common in the breed. Ideally, genetic counseling would also reduce the production of animals that carry undesirable alleles.
  - To determine if an individual has a genetic disease that its breed is predisposed to – identifying such an individual will allow the owner to take appropriate precautions and management measures. Examples of such cases include testing herding dogs

to identify Ivermectin sensitivity, finding out if a Maine Coon or a Ragdoll cat is genetically predisposed to hypertrophic cardiomyopathy, and identifying a Doberman Pincher that has von Willebrand's disease.

EQUIPMENT

- Cytology buccal swab.
- EDTA blood collection tube, refrigerated until sent and mailed overnight to testing facility.

PROCEDURE

- Determine common heritable or genetic diseases in the breed by searching the following websites:
    - The breed's national website
    - Canine Health Information Center (CHIC) – http://www.caninehealthinfo.org
    - Feline Advisory Bureau (FAB-UK) – http://www.fabcats.org/breeders/inherited_disorders/index.php
- For each disease:
    - Determine mode of inheritance.
    - Determine the ramifications of producing an affected animal.
- Treatability of the disease.
- Expense of treatment.
- Quality of life of affected animal.
- Age of onset – specifically whether the disease can be identified before breeding age.
    - Determine how prevalent the disease is in the breed
- If common (mutation frequency ≥0.09% affected in breed) – may be necessary to breed carrier and/or affected animals to prevent a significant decrease in genetic diversity.
- If uncommon – may not need to test both sire and dam or may be able to only breed 'clear' animals (animals that do not have even a single copy of the mutation) and still preserve good genetic diversity.
- If a genetic test for a disorder is available for the breed:
    - Type of test – mutation versus marker test.
    - Whether the test is published/peer reviewed – tested in the breed and a correlation has been established between the test and disease.
    - Test the animal that is being examined and offer to test the animal it is being bred to.
    - Results will help predict the percentage of offspring, if any, that will be affected (based on mode of inheritance).
- If a genetic test is not available for a disorder:
    - Determine if the animal has a history of the disease in their pedigree.
    - If a phenotypic test is available, recommend testing the phenotype with the understanding that a normal phenotypic test will not guarantee normal progeny.

- Recommend breeding to a dog or cat from a distant line and that does not have this disease in the pedigree.
- Mars Veterinary offers the Optimal Selection™ Genetic Breeding Analysis test which may assist dog breeders in identifying the overall genetic similarity of breeding animals.
- Breeding Scenarios and General Recommendations for traits with a simple Mendelian inheritance – these recommendations should be amended based on the considerations listed above.
- Autosomal Recessive Disorders – the undesirable allele is recessive. An affected individual has to be homozygous recessive.
- Ideal breeding:
  - Two 'normal' (homozygous dominant) individuals bred to each other – all offspring will be normal and no carriers (heterozygotes) will be produced.
- Acceptable breeding:
  - A 'normal' to a carrier breeding – all offspring will be unaffected, but ~50% will carry the recessive allele (undesirable).
- If possible, steer clear of the following:
  - An affected (homozygous recessive) to a 'normal' breeding – all progeny will be unaffected but all of them will carry the recessive allele.
  - Two 'carriers' bred to each other – ~75% of the offspring will be unaffected, however two-thirds of them (50% of the total) will carry the trait. ~25% of the progeny will be affected.
- Avoid the following:
  - Two affected individuals bred to each other – 100% of the progeny will be affected.
  - Affected to carrier breeding – 50% of the progeny will be affected and 50% will be unaffected but will carry the undesirable allele.
  - Autosomal Dominant Disorders – the undesirable trait is dominant. An affected individual can be heterozygous or homozygous dominant.
- Ideal breeding:
  - Two unaffected (homozygous recessive) individuals bred to each other – 100% of the progeny will be unaffected.
- Acceptable breeding:
  - An unaffected individual to a heterozygous individual breeding – ~50% of the progeny will be unaffected and 50% will be affected but will only have a single undesirable allele (will be heterozygous).
- Avoid the following:
  - Two homozygous dominant individuals bred to each other – 100% of the progeny will be affected and will only have the undesirable allele.
  - A homozygous dominant individual to a heterozygote – 100% of the progeny will be affected, but ~50% of them will carry the desirable allele.
  - Sex-Linked Disorders – the mutation is on the X-chromosome, and most commonly recessive. Therefore, the disorder is more common in males than females. Affected females have to be homozygous recessive and males have only a single allele.

- Ideal breeding:
  - Unaffected male to homozygous dominant female – 100% of progeny will be unaffected, 100% of females will be homozygous dominant.
- Acceptable breeding:
  - Affected male to homozygous dominant female – 100% of the progeny will be unaffected, with ~50% of the females being heterozygous.
- If possible, steer clear of the following:
  - Unaffected male to heterozygous female – ~50% of males will be affected; 100% of females will be unaffected, with ~50% of the females being heterozygous.
- Avoid the following:
  - Affected male to affected (homozygous recessive) female – 100% of progeny will be affected, females will be homozygous recessive.
  - Affected male to heterozygous female – ~50% of the males will be affected. ~50% of the females will be affected (homozygous recessive) and 50% will be heterozygous unaffected.
  - Unaffected male to homozygous recessive female – 100% of males will be affected, 100% of females will be unaffected heterozygotes.

 ## COMMENTS

- A list of available genetic tests and testing labs is compiled and updated by:
  - World Small Animal Veterinary Association: http://research.vet.upenn.edu/DNAGeneticsTestingLaboratorySearch/tabid/7620/Default.aspx
- To date, in the United States, genetic test results are confidential and are not reported to any entity other than the person that paid to run the test and, in some cases, their veterinarian. However, in an effort to reduce the occurrence of genetic disease, owners and breeders are encouraged to share test results.
- Genetic registries have been established in order to advance genetic disease control. All registries have the limitation of being voluntary and that in cases in which the animal has an easily observable defect, it is unlikely that the owners will elect to officially test or register the animal. As of yet, there is no American cat registry. The following are the main American dog registries:
  - Canine Eye Registry Foundation (CERF) – currently is a closed database that will show only normal eye exam results. In the near future, the database will include information on dogs that did not pass the exam, if their owners request the test results to show.
- http://web.vmdb.org/home/CERF.aspx
  - Orthopedic Foundation for Animals (OFA) – a semi-open domain (only normal results are automatically made public) but owners have the option of making it an open domain, allowing normal and abnormal results to be publically available. As of September, 2012, the OFA now includes an eye certification registry in addition to its orthopedic, thyroid, cardiac disease and genetic testing registries.

- http://offa.org/
  - Canine Health Information Network (CHIC) – an open registry for purebred dogs. Owners can apply for a CHIC number for their dog if the dog fulfills the phenotypic and genotypic testing requirement, as set by the national breed club. A CHIC number is issued to all dogs that have been tested, whether the results were normal or abnormal and the results will be made public. The premise for the CHIC database is health awareness, not health perfection because as the number of available tests increases, it becomes less likely for any animal to test normal for all of the tests.
- http://www.caninehealthinfo.org/
- To date, there are no health requirements for breeding animals. The burden is an ethical one and the breeder is the one that has to elect to test their cat or dog and to share the information. Breeders can elect to breed an affected animal and the only obligation of the veterinarian is to make them aware of the potential problems that may arise from such a breeding.
- Some states have a 'lemon law': a law meant to protect owners in the face of purchasing a dog or cat that is sick, in some cases with a genetic disease and others with infectious disease. Each state has different criteria pertaining to the length of time after the purchase that the buyer has to identify the illness, what testing is required in order to verify the dog or cat is sick, as well as to what the compensation would be in the case that they are sick. In most states, the lemon law targets commercial establishments or 'puppy-mills' but not hobby breeders. Please refer to the law in the state from which the puppy was purchased.

See Also

Feline Pre-Breeding Examination and Breeding Husbandry
Canine Breeding Management

Suggested Reading

Bell, J.S. (2012) *Veterinary Medical Guide to Dog and Cat Breeds*. Teton NewMedia, Jackson, WY.
Metallinos, D.L. (2001) Canine molecular genetic testing. *Vet. Clin. North Am. Small Anim. Pract.*, **31**, 421–431

Author: Nili Karmi PhD, DVM

chapter 20

Glucagonoma

 ## DEFINITION

- Glucagonoma is a rare tumor arising from alpha cells in the pancreatic islets. Alpha cells secrete glucagon which is responsible for the catabolism of amino acids to glucose.
- Glucagonoma may be considered a subtype of tumor in the larger classification of APU-Doma. APUDomas arise from cells responsible for amine precursor uptake and decarboxylation. Most of the cells possessing these characteristics arise in the gut, CNS, thyroid and parathyroid. APUDomas are named for the endocrine product they secrete (i.e., glucagonomas secrete glucagon).
- Excess circulating glucagon results in increased protein/amino acid catabolism, lipolysis, gluconeogenesis, and glycogenolysis. The culmination of these biochemical changes results in hyperglycemia, hypoaminoacidemia, anemia, diarrhea and weight loss.
- Patients with glucagonomas frequently exhibit a characteristic dermatopathy, most frequently referred to as Necrolytic Migratory Erythema (NME) or Superficial Necrolytic Dermatopathy (SND). This syndrome is not pathognomonic for glucagonoma, however, and can occur more frequently with advanced liver disease (hepatocutaneous syndrome).
- Surgery, if possible, is the treatment of choice for patients with glucagonoma.

 ## ETIOLOGY/PATHOPHYSIOLOGY

- The etiology of glucagonoma has not been elucidated. Glucagonomas can be a part of multiple endocrine neoplasia syndrome.
- Glucagonoma is typically first recognized by the presence of dermatologic changes, consistent with SND/NME.
- SND/NME is characterized by erosive to ulcerative, erythematous, hyperkeratotic lesions at the footpads, mucocutaneous junctions or pressure points.
- The pathogenesis of the skin lesions associated with NME is thought to be related to a direct or indirect role of hyperglucagonemia, as well as disturbances in amino acids, but is not fully understood.
- Patients with glucagonoma may exhibit diabetes mellitus due to the excess production of glucose in the face of normal insulin production.

Blackwell's Five-Minute Veterinary Consult Clinical Companion: Small Animal Endocrinology and Reproduction, First Edition. Edited by Deborah S. Greco and Autumn P. Davidson. © 2017 John Wiley & Sons, Inc. Published 2017 by John Wiley & Sons, Inc.
Companion Website: www.fiveminutevet.com/endocrinology

Systems Affected

- Endocrine/metabolic – diabetes mellitus, polyuria/polydipsia.
- Skin/exocrine – dermatitis.
- Gastrointestinal – diarrhea, weight loss.

 # SIGNALMENT/HISTORY

- Dogs – rare; middle-aged to older animals.
- Cats – no reports to date.

Risk Factors

- No known risk factors.

Historic Findings

- Dermatitis, primarily involving foot pads, mucocutaneous junctions or pressure points.
- Weight loss.
- Diarrhea.
- Polyuria/polydipsia.

 # CLINICAL FEATURES

- The hallmark sign of glucagonomas reported in dogs is a characteristic dermatopathy most commonly called NME or Necrolytic Migratory Erythema. This has also been reported in the veterinary literature as metabolic epidermal necrosis, superficial necrolytic dermatitis (SND), hepatocutaneous syndrome and diabetic dermatopathy.
- Skin lesions include erythema, erosions and crusting generally located around mucocutaneous junctions (perineum, face and genitalia), distal extremities and footpads. Lesions are frequently hyperkeratotic and can be associated with painful, fissured footpads. In many cases, footpads are the only affected area.
- Other systemic signs may include lethargy, polyuria/polydipsia, diarrhea, secondary bacterial and/or yeast skin infections and weight loss.

 # DIFFERENTIAL DIAGNOSIS

- Glucagonoma should always be added to the differential list when the presence of skin lesions consistent with NME are found. More common differentials associated with NME should include non-specific, often advanced, liver disease.
- NME has been associated with diabetes, pancreatic tumors in cats, and hepatic disease. Other dermatologic differentials include pemphigus foliaceus, systemic lupus erythematosus, vasculitis, vitamin A responsive dermatosis, and zinc-responsive dermatosis.

- Mild-moderate hyperglucagonemia can be seen secondary to non-glucagonoma diseases such as liver disease, pancreatic disease, chronic renal failure, starvation, bacteremia, diabetic ketoacidosis and hyperadrenocorticism.

DIAGNOSTICS

CBC/Biochemistry/Urinalysis

- CBC – may be normal or mild non-regenerative, normocytic, normochormic anemia.
- Chemistry – liver enzyme elevations, persistent hyperglycemia and/or hypoalbuminemia may be noted.
- Bile acid and liver function tests are generally within normal limits.
- Urinalysis – decreased urine specific gravity is possible. If secondary diabetes mellitus is present, glucosuria may be present.

Other Laboratory Tests

- Plasma glucagon levels are generally extremely elevated (i.e., >1000 pg/ml); however, normal to mildly elevated glucagon levels do not rule out glucagonoma.
- Plasma amino acid levels are generally reduced and are thought to be pathophysiologically associated with the development of NME.
- Sensitivity and specificity of plasma glucagon and plasma amino acids is unknown in dogs.
- Fructosamine may be elevated in patients with secondary diabetes mellitus.

Imaging

- Similar to insulinoma, it can be difficult to identify the primary mass with abdominal ultrasound. Ultrasound is useful to screen for changes within the liver and pancreas, however. The 'honey-comb' pattern identified in the liver of patients with hepatocutaneous syndrome has not been documented in a canine patient with glucagonoma. Computed tomography may have utility in identifying small masses. Radiolabeled octreotide scintigraphy and endoscopic ultrasound are used to facilitate diagnosis in humans. Radiolabeled octreotide scintigraphy has been demonstrated in canine patients with insulinoma; it has not been reported in a canine patient with glucagonoma. Three-view thoracic radiographs should be performed for preoperative staging.

Pathologic Finding

- Histopathologically, skin biopsies taken from affected glucagon-associated NME lesions typically exhibit severe superficial to mid-epidermal edema, diffuse parakeratotic hyperkeratosis, and irregular epidermal hyperplasia. This triad of histopathologic findings is commonly referred to as a 'red, white and blue' pattern.
- Histopathology of the primary mass (or metastases) is necessary to confirm glucagonoma. Histopathologically, these samples exhibit pleomorphic islet cells with fine cytoplasmic

granules. Immunohistochemical glucagon expression (and often other secretory hormones) can help confirm glucagonoma.

 # THERAPEUTICS

- Surgical excision of non-metastatic primary pancreatic glucagonoma represents the best chance for cure. Unfortunately, there is a high rate of postoperative morbidity and mortality reported in dogs, as well as a high rate of metastasis at the time of diagnosis.
- Surgery may be helpful in palliating patients with metastatic disease (i.e., decreasing intensity of skin lesions).
- Hepatic arterial chemoembolization has been reported in human patients with hepatic metastasis.

Drugs

- In patients with unresectable and/or metastatic glucagonoma, the use of octreotide may be beneficial. Octreotide is a somatostatin analog that inhibits the conversion of preproglucagon to glucagon. Numerous side effects have been reported with human use of octreotide, including injection-site pain, vomiting, diarrhea, and cholestasis. The effective dosage of octreotide (or long-acting lanreotide) is uncertain in dogs; however, 10–20 µg/dog SC q.8–12 h has been reported, as well as a one-time safe dose of 50 µg/dog SC reported in healthy dogs. Octreotide is often cost-prohibitive in canine patients.
- Various chemotherapeutics have also been utilized in human glucagonoma patients, including dacarbazine, streptozotocin and 5-fluorouracil. The use of streptozotocin as an islet-cell lytic agent has been reported previously in a small number of dogs with insulinoma, but has not been reported to date in dogs with glucagonoma.
- Intravenous amino acids (500 ml of 10% amino acid solution (Aminosyn®, Abbott) given over 8–12 hours in a large central vein (due to potential for phlebitis) has shown variable improvement in skin lesions in dogs. Treatments may be repeated every 1–2 weeks if effective until clinical signs abate or resolve.
- Secondary skin infections should be treated appropriately.

Diet/Alternative Treatments

- Oral protein/amino acid supplementation (egg yolks have been suggested as a source of high-quality protein), zinc supplementation and fatty acid supplements may be beneficial.

 # COMMENTS

Patient Monitoring

- Serial blood work should be performed postoperatively to ensure the prior hyperglucagonemia (and any other abnormalities) is resolving and continues to be within normal limits.

- Serial ultrasounds and three-view thoracic radiographs to monitor for metastasis should be considered postoperatively.

Contraindications/Patient Monitoring

- Glucocorticoids may be beneficial for skin lesions, but they exacerbate hyperglycemia if secondary diabetes mellitus is present. Pancreatitis and thromboembolic disease are possible surgical complications.

Expected Course and Prognosis

- Prognosis is generally poor due to advanced disease often being present at time of diagnosis and degree of postoperative complications. Only a small number of cases have been reported in veterinary medicine, however.

Abbreviations

CT   = computed tomography
NME = necrolytic migratory erythema
SC   = subcutaneous
SND = superficial necrolytic dermatopathy

See Also

APUDoma
Diabetic Hepatopathy

Suggested Reading

Allenspach, K., Arnold P., Glaus T., Hauser B., *et al.* (2000) Glucagon-producing neuroendocrine tumour associated with hypoaminoacidemia and skin lesions. *J. Small Anim. Pract.*, **41**, 402–406.

Feldman, E.C., Nelson, R.W. (2004) Gastrinoma, Glucagonoma and Other APUDomas, in *Canine and Feline Endocrinology and Reproduction*, 3rd edition (eds E.D. Feldman, R.W. Nelson), Saunders, St Louis, pp. 654–655.

Kasper, C.S., McMurry, K. (1991) Necrolytic migratory erythema without glucagonoma versus canine superficial necrolytic dermatitis: Is hepatic impairment a clue to pathogenesis. *J. Am. Acad. Dermatol.*, **25** (3), 534–541.

Langer, N.B., Jergens, A.E., Miles, K.G. (2003) Canine glucagonoma. *Compendium*, **25** (1), 56–63.

Lunn, K., Page, R. (2013) Tumors of the Endocrine System, in *Small Animal Clinical Oncology*, 5th edition (eds S.J. Withrow, D.M. Vail, R.L. Page), Elsevier, St Louis, p. 521.

Mizuno, T., Hiraoka, H., Yoshioka, C., *et al.* (2009) Superficial necrolytic dermatitis associated with extrapancreatic glucagonoma in a dog. *Vet. Dermatol.*, **20** (1), 72–79.

Author: Virginia Gill DVM, DACVIM (Oncology)

chapter 21

Canine Hyperadrenocorticism (Cushing's syndrome)

DEFINITION

- Spontaneous hyperadrenocorticism (HAC) is a disorder caused by excessive production of cortisol by the adrenal cortex.
- Iatrogenic HAC results from excessive exogenous administration of glucocorticoids of any form or by any route.
- In either instance, clinical signs are due to deleterious effects of elevated circulating glucocorticoid concentrations on multiple organ systems.

ETIOLOGY/PATHOPHYSIOLOGY

- Approximately 80–85% of cases of naturally occurring HAC are due to bilateral adrenocortical hyperplasia resulting from pituitary corticotroph tumors or hyperplasia with oversecretion of ACTH.
- In the remaining 15–20% of cases, cortisol-secreting adrenocortical neoplasia is present; approximately one-half of these are malignant.
- Rarely caused by ectopic ACTH secretion from a non-pituitary tumor.
- Iatrogenic HAC results from excessive administration of exogenous glucocorticoids.

Systems Affected

- The degree to which each system is involved varies considerably; signs referable to one system may predominate or several systems may be involved to a comparable degree.
- Signs referable to the urinary tract or skin often predominate.
- Endocrine/Metabolic – hyperglycemia; diabetes mellitus occurs in 10%.
- Cardiovascular – hypertension (usually mild).
- Gastrointestinal – polyphagia.
- Hemic/Lymphatic/Immune – stress leukogram; immunosuppression; mild erythrocytosis and thrombocytosis.

Blackwell's Five-Minute Veterinary Consult Clinical Companion: Small Animal Endocrinology and Reproduction, First Edition. Edited by Deborah S. Greco and Autumn P. Davidson. © 2017 John Wiley & Sons, Inc. Published 2017 by John Wiley & Sons, Inc.
Companion Website: www.fiveminutevet.com/endocrinology

- Hepatobiliary – hepatopathy due to glycogen deposition; increased serum ALP activity due to production of corticosteroid-induced isoenzyme.
- Neuromuscular – muscle weakness; CNS signs including anorexia, ataxia, disorientation and, uncommonly, seizures if pituitary macroadenoma present.
- Renal/Urologic – polyuria/polydipsia in 90% of cases; proteinuria; UTI common.
- Reproductive – testicular atrophy and anestrus.
- Respiratory – panting; pulmonary thromboembolism possible due to a hypercoaguable state.
- Skin – bilaterally symmetric alopecia common; comedones; hyperpigmentation; recurrent pyoderma.

Genetics

- No genetic basis known.

Incidence/Prevalence

- No exact figures available.
- Considered one of most common endocrine disorders in dogs.

 SIGNALMENT/HISTORY

Species

- Dogs.

Breed Predilections

- Poodles, dachshunds, Boston terriers, German Shepherd dogs, and beagles.

Mean Age and Range

- Generally a disorder of middle-aged to old animals; pituitary-dependent HAC (PDH) can very rarely be seen in dogs as young as 1 year.

Predominant Sex

- No predilection for PDH in dogs; possible predilection for female dogs to have an adrenal tumor.

CLINICAL FEATURES

General Comments

- Severity varies greatly, depending on duration and severity of cortisol excess.
- In some cases, the physical presence of the neoplastic process (pituitary or adrenal) contributes.

Historical and Physical Examination Findings

- Polyuria and polydipsia.
- Polyphagia.
- Pendulous abdomen.
- Increased panting.
- Hepatomegaly.
- Hair loss (Fig. 21.1).
- Cutaneous hyperpigmentation (Fig. 21.2).
- Thin skin. (Fig. 21.3).
- Muscle weakness.
- Obesity.
- Lethargy.
- Muscle atrophy.

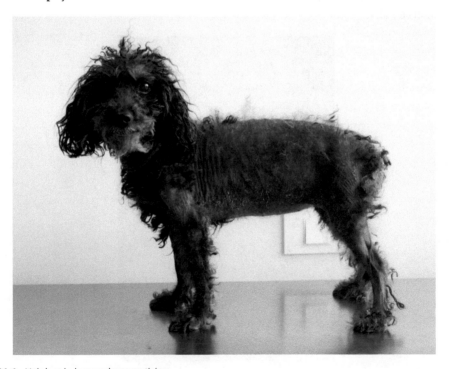

■ **Fig. 21.1.** Hair loss in hyperadrenocorticism.

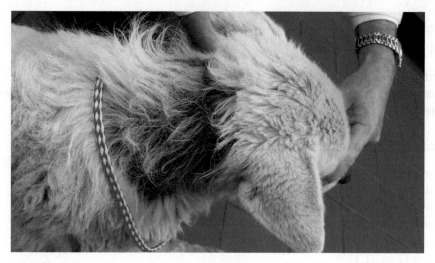

■ **Fig. 21.2.** Cutaneous hyperpigmentation in hyperadrenocorticism.

- Comedones.
- Bruising.
- Testicular atrophy
- Anestrus.
- Calcinosis cutis (Fig. 21.4).
- Facial nerve palsy.

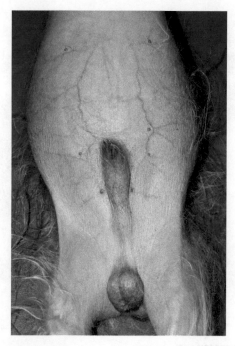

■ **Fig. 21.3.** Thin skin in hyperadrenocorticism.

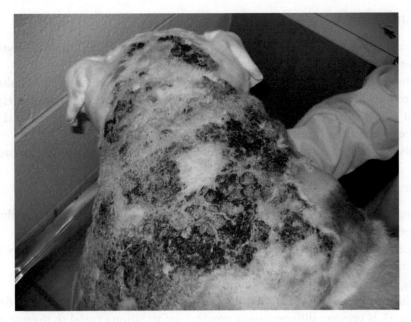

■ **Fig. 21.4.** Calcinosis cutis in hyperadrenocorticism.

Causes

- Pituitary-dependent – adenoma most common; adenocarcinomas rare; anterior pituitary involved in approximately 80% of cases, intermediate lobe in remaining cases; exact incidence of pituitary macroadenomas (i.e., >1 cm diameter) unknown, may be 10–25%.
- Adrenal tumor – adenoma or carcinoma (50/50).
- Ectopic ACTH secretion – rare.
- Iatrogenic – due to glucocorticoid administration.

Risk Factors

- None known for spontaneous disease.
- Presence any condition that leads to exogenous glucocorticoid administration is a risk factor for iatrogenic HAC.

 DIAGNOSIS/DIFFERENTIAL DIAGNOSIS

- Depends on clinical and laboratory abnormalities displayed.
- Includes hypothyroidism, sex hormone dermatoses, Alopecia X, sex hormone-secreting tumors, acromegaly, diabetes mellitus, hepatopathies, renal disease, and other causes of polyuria/polydipsia.

CBC/Biochemistry/Urinalysis

- Hemogram may show eosinopenia, lymphopenia, leukocytosis, neutrophilia, erythrocytosis and/or thrombocytosis.
- Serum chemistry may show high liver enzymes, cholesterol, and total CO_2; alkaline phosphatase activity high in approximately 90% and ALP elevations are proportionately greater than that for ALT; hyperglycemia common but only about 10% of dogs with HAC have concurrent diabetes mellitus.
- Urinalysis may reveal low specific gravity, proteinuria, hematuria, pyuria and/or bacteriuria.

Other Laboratory Tests

- Endocrine testing required in dogs with history, clinical signs, and laboratory abnormalities suggestive of HAC.
- Do not perform testing for HAC in sick dogs unless clinical signs consistent with HAC are present.
- Screening tests are designed to determine if HAC is present or not.
- Once a diagnosis of HAC is made, a differentiation test should be performed to determine if PDH or AT is present; differentiation provides information crucial to therapeutic decisions and an accurate prognosis.
- Differentiation tests should never be performed before a diagnosis of HAC is made via screening tests.
- See the end of the chapter for endocrine test protocols.
- To convert cortisol concentration in nmol/l to μg/dl, divide by 27.6.
- All cortisol concentrations below used for illustration purposes; check with your own laboratory for its normal ranges and cut-off values.

Screening Tests

Urine Cortisol:Creatinine Ratio (UC:Cr)
- Urine cortisol excretion increases as a reflection of augmented adrenal secretion of the hormone, whether PDH or AT is present.
- An elevated UC:Cr is a sensitive marker of HAC, present in 90–100% of affected dogs.
- Should be measured in a sample collected at home when the pet not stressed.
- False-positive results common; only about 20% of dogs with an elevated UC:Cr have HAC.
- A normal ratio makes the diagnosis of HAC very unlikely (≤10% chance).
- Elevated ratio consistent with a diagnosis of HAC, but since the chance of a false-positive result is great, an ACTH stimulation test or low-dose dexamethasone suppression test must always be done to confirm the presence of HAC.

Low-Dose Dexamethasone Suppression Test (LDDST) (Fig. 21.5a)
- Lack of suppression 8 hours after an injection of a low dose of dexamethasone consistent with a diagnosis of HAC.
- Sensitivity approximately 95% in dogs.

- In dogs, there is a relatively high chance of a false-positive result, up to 50%, if non-adrenal illness is present.
- Lack of suppression at 4 hours but with full suppression at 8 hours is technically not consistent with HAC but is suspicious for its presence; further testing warranted.

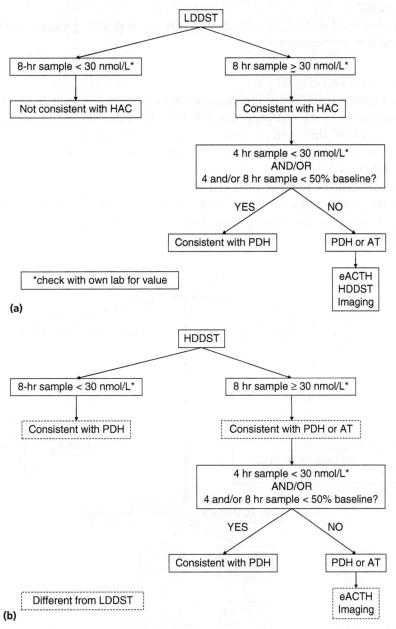

■ **Fig. 21.5.** (a) Low-dose dexamethasone suppression test (LDDST). (b) High-dose dexamethasone suppression test (HDDST).

- With certain results, the LDDST may also serve as a differentiation test; if the 8-hour sample is >30 nmol/l, the result is consistent with HAC; if, in addition, there is suppression to <30 nmol/l at 4 hours post-dexamethasone (i.e., an 'escape' at 8 hours post-dexamethasone) or the 4- and/or 8-hour post-dexamethasone samples are <50% of baseline, the results are consistent with PDH; if criteria for PDH not met, chances are still approximately 50/50 for PDH versus AT.
- If baseline values close to 30 nmol/l or suppression just at 50%, presence of PDH should be confirmed by other means.

ACTH Stimulation Test (Fig. 21.6)

- A response greater than normal is consistent with a diagnosis of spontaneous HAC.
- Overall sensitivity of the test approximately 80%; for PDH, sensitivity is approximately 87%, while for HAC due to an AT, sensitivity is approximately 61%.
- More specific in dogs than the LDDST (only 15% chance of a false-positive result with non-adrenal illness).
- Can never differentiate between PDH and AT.
- Only test that can diagnose iatrogenic HAC; a diagnosis is made with a history of glucocorticoid exposure by any route, presence of consistent clinical signs and a post-ACTH cortisol concentration below the reference range.

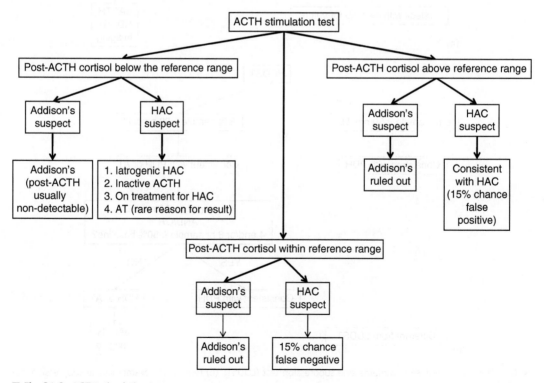

■ **Fig. 21.6.** ACTH stimulation test.

■ Cortrosyn is the recommended form of ACTH to use; if using compounded ACTH, collect samples before and at 1 and 2 hours post-ACTH administration so peak response not missed.

Differentiating Tests

High-Dose Dexamethasone Suppression Test (HDSST) (Fig. 21.5b)

■ Two responses consistent with PDH; if there is suppression to <30 nmol/l at 4 and/or 8 hours post-dexamethasone, or the 4- and/or 8-hour post-dexamethasone samples are <50% of baseline, PDH is present.

■ If baseline values close to 30 nmol/l or suppression just at 50%, presence of PDH should be confirmed by other means.

■ Can *never* confirm presence of an AT; if criteria for diagnosis of PDH not met, there is a 50/50 chance the patient has PDH or an AT.

Endogenous ACTH Concentration

■ Requires only a single blood sample, but special handling needed.

■ In patients with PDH, endogenous ACTH (eACTH) concentration is normal to increased; with AT, eACTH concentration is below normal.

■ Can be used to confirm the presence of an AT.

■ A gray zone exists in the results; if the patient's eACTH concentration falls into this zone, results not diagnostic.

■ With repeat testing when the original concentration measured is in the gray zone (about 15% chance), approximately 96% have definitive differentiation.

■ There is no way to predict when eACTH concentration will be in the gray zone.

Imaging

■ Abdominal radiographs may differentiate PDH from AT; approximately 40–50% of canine ATs are visualized; adrenal mineralization is highly suspicious for the presence of an AT.

■ Chest radiographs indicated in patients with an AT to check for metastases.

■ Ultrasonography, CT, and MR – useful for differentiating PDH from AT and for staging AT; abdominal ultrasonography can never be used as a screening test as bilateral adrenal enlargement may be seen due to chronic non-adrenal illness; AT can be small and may be difficult to see with ultrasonography; vena caval, hepatic or renal invasion is an indicator of malignancy; adrenal atrophy can be difficult to determine with ultrasonography.

■ CT and MRI – often useful for demonstrating pituitary macroadenomas.

■ Since radiation therapy, a treatment modality required for a pituitary macroadenoma, is more effective for smaller tumors, some authors advocate routine pituitary imaging in all dogs when PDH diagnosed; follow-up and treatment recommendations vary depending on tumor size.

DIAGNOSTICS

- Adrenal biopsy (usually performed on AT obtained via adrenalectomy) often needed to differentiate benign versus malignant tumor.

Pathologic Findings

- PDH – gross examination reveals normal-to-enlarged pituitary and bilateral adrenocortical enlargement.
- Microscopically, pituitary adenoma, adenocarcinoma, or corticotroph hyperplasia of pars distalis or pars intermedia and adrenocortical hyperplasia.
- AT – gross examination reveals variable-sized adrenal mass, atrophy of contralateral gland (rarely bilateral tumors), and metastasis in some patients with adrenal carcinoma; invasion into vena cava or vena caval thrombosis may be seen with malignant tumors.
- Microscopically, see adrenocortical adenoma or carcinoma.
- With any form HAC, general changes of cortisol excess may be seen such as cutaneous atrophy and glomerulopathy.

Treatment/Appropriate Health Care

- Dictated by severity of clinical signs, patient's overall condition, and any complicating factors (e.g., diabetes mellitus, pulmonary thromboembolism).

Nursing Care

- Variable as above.

Activity

- No alteration of activity necessary.

Diet

- Usually no need to alter; use appropriate diet if diabetes mellitus concurrent.

COMMENTS

Client Education

- If using medical therapy, lifelong therapy required.
- If adverse reaction to mitotane or trilostane occurs – discontinue drug, give prednisone, and have veterinarian re-evaluate next day; if no response to prednisone noted in a few hours, veterinarian should evaluate immediately.

Surgical Considerations

- Hypophysectomy – described, but generally not available in the United States.
- Bilateral adrenalectomy not used for treatment of PDH in dogs.
- Surgery treatment of choice in dogs with adrenocortical adenomas and small carcinomas unless the patient is a poor surgical risk; appropriate personnel and facilities required as this is a technically demanding surgery and intensive postoperative management is required.
- Depending on patient status, medical control of HAC may be desirable prior to surgery, if possible.

 THERAPEUTICS

Drug(s) Of Choice

Mitotane

- Mitotane (o,p′-DDD; Lysodren®) is one of two main drugs used for medical management of PDH in dogs; it selectively destroys glucocorticoid-secreting cells of the adrenal cortex; it may be a drug of choice for medical management of AT as it may destroy tumor cells as well as block control cortisol secretion (Figs 21.7).

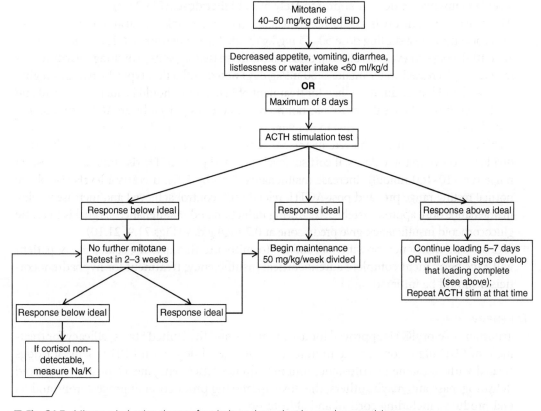

■ **Fig. 21.7.** Mitotane induction therapy for pituitary-dependent hyperadrenocorticism.

- PDH – give an initial loading dose of 40–50 mg/kg divided twice daily; evaluate efficacy with ACTH stimulation test after 8 days or sooner if decreased appetite, vomiting, diarrhea, listlessness or decreased water intake (<60 ml/kg/day) noted; goal is for both basal and post-ACTH cortisol concentration to be in ideal range of 30–150 nmol/l; continue induction with repeat testing as necessary until adequate response seen, then initiate maintenance therapy at 50 mg/kg/week divided into two to three doses; dosage adjustments based on ACTH stimulation testing (maintain basal and post-ACTH cortisol levels within ideal range); if serum cortisol concentration pre- or post-ACTH <30 nmol/l, stop administering mitotane and administer physiological doses of prednisone (0.1 mg/kg, q.12 h); cannot administer prednisone within 12 hours before ACTH stimulation test; perform ACTH stimulation tests every 7–14 days initially; cortisol secretion usually recovers in weeks to a couple months but can take longer; once cortisol concentration is in ideal range, discontinue prednisone and begin maintenance therapy; if had been on maintenance therapy when became cortisol deficient, restart maintenance at 25% lower dose; if relapse occurs at any time while on maintenance therapy, as indicated by cortisol levels above ideal range, dose adjustment required; if post-ACTH serum cortisol concentration 150–300 nmol/l, increase maintenance dose 25% and re-evaluate in 4 weeks; if post-ACTH serum cortisol concentration >300 nmol/l, reload for 5–7 days and do an ACTH stimulation test; continue loading until cortisol concentration is in ideal range, then re-initiate weekly maintenance dose at approximately 50% higher dose. (Fig 21.8)
- AT – goal of mitotane use is low-to-non-detectable (i.e., <30 nmol/l) basal and post-ACTH cortisol concentrations; starting dose 50–75 mg/kg divided daily; perform ACTH stimulation test after 10–14 days to evaluate efficacy, or sooner if decreased appetite, vomiting, diarrhea, listlessness or decreased water intake (<60 ml/kg/day) noted; induction typically requires higher doses and is of longer duration than for treatment of PDH; dose should be increased by 50 mg/kg/day every 10–14 days if control has not been achieved, as judged by an ACTH stimulation test; if adverse effects develop due to mitotane, administration should continue at highest tolerable dose; once control achieved, maintenance therapy should begin at 75–100 mg/kg/week divided into two to three doses; if cortisol levels pre- and post-ACTH rise into normal resting range (i.e., 10–160 nmol/l), increase maintenance dose by 50%; if cortisol levels rise above normal resting range pre- and post-ACTH, reload until control achieved and increase weekly maintenance dose approximately 50%; during induction and maintenance, as goal is to create glucocorticoid insufficiency, give prednisone at 0.2 mg/kg/day (Figs 21.9, 21.10)
- Aldosterone deficiency possible secondary to mitotane therapy; if occurs, likely patient will have permanent complete adrenocortical insufficiency; treatment for hypoadrenocorticism should be initiated.

Trilostane

- Trilostane (Vetoryl®) is approved for use in Europe and the United States; efficacy for treatment of PDH high, comparable to mitotane; survival of dogs with PDH is same for dogs treated with mitotane or trilostane; inhibits adrenocortical enzyme 11-β-hydroxysteroid dehydrogenase and maybe others, thereby suppressing production of progesterone and its end-products, including cortisol and aldosterone.

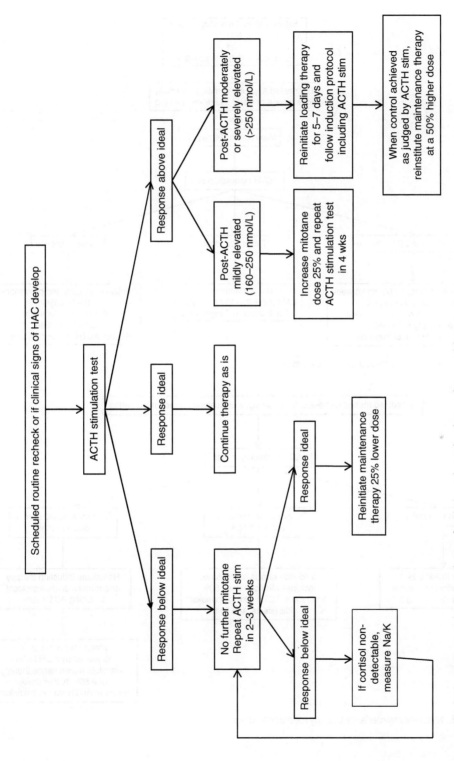

Scheduled routine recheck or if clinical signs of HAC develop

ACTH stimulation test

Response below ideal

No further mitotane
Repeat ACTH stim
in 2–3 weeks

Response ideal

Reinitiate maintenance
therapy 25% lower dose

Response below ideal

If cortisol non-
detectable, measure Na/K

Response ideal

Continue therapy as is

Response above ideal

Post-ACTH
mildly elevated
(160–250 nmol/L)

Increase mitotane
dose 25% and repeat
ACTH stimulation test
in 4 wks

Post-ACTH moderately
or severely elevated
(>250 nmol/L)

Reinitiate loading therapy
for 5–7 days and
follow induction protocol
including ACTH stim

When control achieved
as judged by ACTH stim,
reinstitute maintenance therapy
at a 50% higher dose

■ Fig. 21.8. Mitotane maintenance therapy for pituitary-dependent hyperadrenocorticism.

171

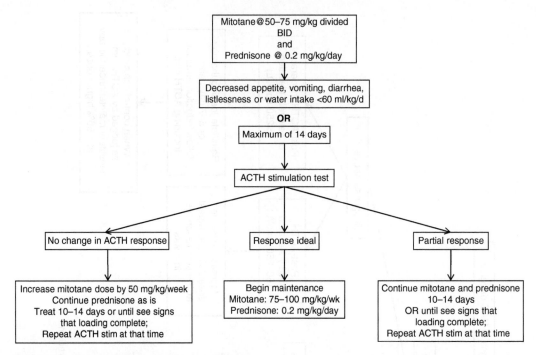

■ **Fig. 21.9.** Mitotane induction therapy for adrenal tumor.

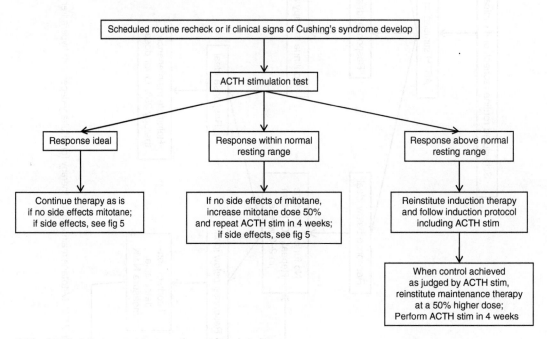

■ **Fig. 21.10.** Mitotane maintenance therapy for adrenal tumor.

- Initial dose is 2.2–6.7 mg/kg PO q.24 h or divided q.12 h; if minor side effects are seen (i.e., anorexia, vomiting, diarrhea), stop the drug for 3–5 days and then restart q.48 h for one week before continuing with initial dosing scheme; an ACTH stimulation test should be performed beginning 4–6 hours post-pill at 10–14 days, 30 days, and 90 days after being on a full dose; if at the 10–14-day re-check any improvement is seen, do not increase the dose even if cortisol concentrations above ideal, but wait until the 30-day re-check and change the dose then if needed. If post-ACTH cortisol concentration is <40 nmol/l and the patient feels well, stop the trilostane for 48–72 hours and then either restart at a lower dose, or, ideally, an ACTH stimulation test should be performed and trilostane not re-instituted until cortisol secretion has recovered; if the post-ACTH cortisol concentration is 40–150 nmol/l and clinical signs have resolved, the dose should continue as is; if the post-ACTH cortisol concentration is 150–250 nmol/l, increase the trilostane dose if clinical signs are present or, if the clinical signs have resolved, leave as is but monitor carefully for signs of recurrence; if the post-ACTH serum cortisol concentration is >250 nmol/l, increase once-daily dose or twice-daily therapy should be used; the same dose given once-daily should be divided and given twice (e.g., if giving 60 mg once-daily then give 30 mg q.12 h); if post-ACTH serum cortisol concentration is 40–150 nmol/l but clinical signs are continuing, use twice-daily therapy; once the dog's clinical condition and dose have stabilized, an ACTH stimulation test should be performed every 3–6 months and serum potassium concentration measured to check for hyperkalemia (Fig. 21.11).
- Since trilostane can suppress aldosterone secretion, an Addisonian crisis can occur; adrenocortical necrosis secondary to trilostane administration may be more common than previously believed; hypocortisolemia secondary to trilostane administration usually resolves within 48–72 hours of discontinuing drug administration, but temporary suppression of weeks to months and even permanent suppression can occur.
- Can be used to treat AT and will control clinical signs, at least transiently, but not the drug of choice; for AT, mitotane is the drug of choice as it is truly chemotherapeutic and may kill tumor cells.

L-Deprenyl

- L-Deprenyl (selegiline hydrochloride; Anipryl®) is FDA-approved for treatment of PDH; decreases pituitary ACTH secretion by increasing dopaminergic tone in the hypothalamic–pituitary axis, thus decreasing serum cortisol concentrations; indicated only for treating uncomplicated PDH; not recommended for dogs with concurrent illnesses such as diabetes mellitus; cannot be used to treat AT; initiate therapy with 1 mg/kg daily and increase to 2 mg/kg/day after 2 months if response inadequate; if higher dose also ineffective, give alternative therapy; no objective monitoring; assessment of efficacy based on subjective evaluation of remission of clinical signs.
- Efficacy questionable; one study found 20% efficacy and another judged L-deprenyl ineffective.
- Adverse effects such as anorexia, lethargy, vomiting, and diarrhea uncommon (<5% of dogs) and usually mild; disadvantages include need for lifelong daily administration and medication expense.

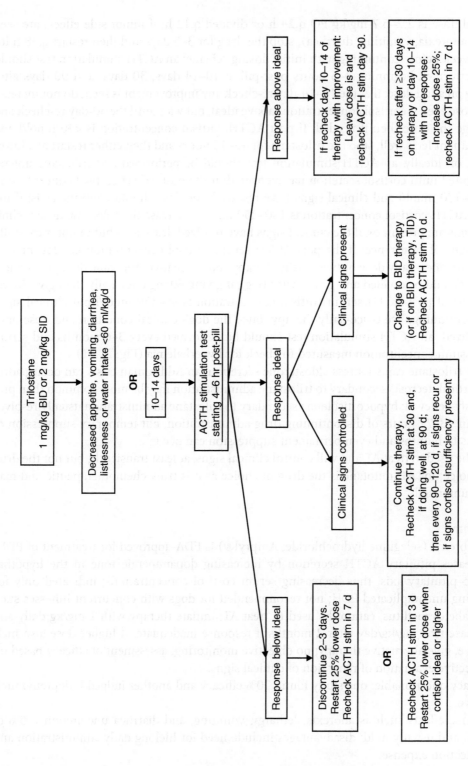

■ **Fig. 21.11.** Trilostane therapy for hyperadrenocorticism.

Ketoconazole

- Ketoconazole (10 mg/kg PO q.12 h initially; up to 20 mg/kg PO q.12 h in some dogs) inhibits enzymes responsible for cortisol synthesis; indicated for dogs unable to tolerate mitotane at doses necessary to control HAC; may be useful for palliation of clinical signs of HAC in dogs with AT; monitoring done by performance of ACTH stimulation tests with same goals as for mitotane; efficacy approximately 50% or less; adverse effects include anorexia, vomiting, diarrhea, lethargy, thrombocytopenia and idiosyncratic hepatopathy.

Contraindications

- Do not use non-steroidal anti-inflammatory agents in dogs with uncontrolled HAC.
- Drugs that increase blood pressure or coagulation should be used with caution.

Precautions

- Side effects of mitotane not uncommon; mild in most dogs; include lethargy, weakness, anorexia, vomiting, diarrhea, ataxia, and iatrogenic hypoadrenocorticism.
- Side effects more common in dogs with AT given high doses of mitotane.
- For mitotane, use with caution in patients with renal insufficiency and primary hepatic disease.
- Side effects of ketoconazole seem to be less common; include anorexia, vomiting, diarrhea, thrombocytopenia, and hepatopathy.
- For ketoconazole, use with caution in patients with primary hepatic disease or thrombocytopenia; effect on breeding ability unknown.
- Side effects of L-deprenyl uncommon.
- Side effects of trilostane include anorexia, lethargy, vomiting and diarrhea; may occur in approximately 60% of patients; Addisonian crisis and adrenocortical necrosis have been reported.
- For trilostane, use with caution in patients with renal insufficiency and primary hepatic disease; contraindicated in pregnancy.
- For all drugs, if using on a diabetic patient, careful monitoring needed; insulin needs can decrease rapidly with control of HAC.

Alternative Drug(s)

- Radiation therapy required for animals with pituitary macroadenomas; ACTH levels may take several months to decrease; control HAC with above drugs in the interim.

 ## COMMENTS

Patient Monitoring

- Response to therapy – use periodic ACTH stimulation testing to assess mitotane, ketoconazole, or trilostane efficacy (see above for details); once on maintenance mitotane therapy, test at 1, 3, and 6 months and every 3–6 months thereafter, or if clinical signs of HAC recur; adequacy of any necessary mitotane reloading period is checked with an ACTH stimulation test before higher maintenance mitotane dose initiated; adequacy of ketoconazole or trilostane dose checked with an ACTH stimulation test after any dose alteration; with trilostane, ACTH stimulation test should be performed starting 4–6 hours post-pill, while with mitotane and ketoconazole, post-pill timing does not matter; clinical signs of HAC resolve several days to months after control achieved; evaluate efficacy of L-deprenyl therapy solely on the basis of resolution of clinical signs of HAC.

Prevention/Avoidance

- For prevention of recurrence, regular administration of medications with appropriate follow-up required.

Possible Complications

- Hypertension.
- Proteinuria.
- Recurrent infection.
- Urinary calculi (calcium oxalate).
- Diabetes mellitus.
- Pulmonary thromboembolism.
- Neurological signs secondary to a pituitary macroadenoma.

Expected Course and Prognosis

- Untreated HAC – generally a progressive disorder with a poor prognosis.
- Treated PDH – usually a good prognosis; median survival time with mitotane or trilostane treatment approximately 2 years; at least 10% survive 4 years; dogs living longer than 6 months tend to die of causes unrelated to HAC.
- Macroadenomas and neurologic signs – poor-to-grave prognosis; macroadenomas with no or mild neurologic signs – fair-to-good prognosis with radiation and medical therapy.
- Adrenal adenomas – usually good-to-excellent prognosis; small carcinomas (not metastasized) fair-to-good prognosis overall, good-to-excellent with surgical resection.
- Large carcinomas and AT with widespread metastasis – generally poor-to-fair prognosis, but impressive responses to high doses of mitotane occasionally seen.

Associated Conditions

- Neurologic signs in dogs with large pituitary tumors; glucose intolerance or concurrent diabetes mellitus; pulmonary thromboembolism; increased incidence of infections, especially urinary tract and skin; hypertension; proteinuria/glomerulopathy.

Age-Related Factors

▪ Not available.

Zoonotic Potential

▪ Not available.

Pregnancy/Fertility/Breeding

▪ Not available.

Synonyms

▪ Cushing's disease; Cushing's syndrome

See Also

Hyperadrenocorticism (Cushing's syndrome) – Cats

Abbreviations

AT   = adrenal tumor
ACTH   = adrenocorticotropic hormone
ALP   = alkaline phosphatase
ALT   = alanine aminotransferase
CNS   = central nervous system
CT   = computed tomography
eACTH = endogenous ACTH
HAC   = hyperadrenocorticism
HDDST = high-dose dexamethasone-suppression test
LDDST = low-dose dexamethasone-suppression test
MRI   = magnetic resonance imaging
PDH   = pituitary-dependent hyperadrenocorticism
UC:Cr = urine cortisol:creatinine ratio
UTI   = urinary tract infection

Internet Resources

www.dechra.com: good information on use of trilostane.

Suggested Reading

Behrend, E.N., Kemppainen, R.J. (2001) Diagnosis of canine hyperadrenocorticism. *Vet. Clin. North. Am.*, **31**, 985–1003.

Braddock, J.A., Church, D.B., Robertson, I.D., *et al.* (2004) Inefficacy of selegiline in treatment of canine pituitary-dependent hyperadrenocorticism. *Austr. Vet. J.*, **82**, 272–277.

Braddock, J.A., Church, D.B., Robertson, I.D., *et al.* (2003) Trilostane treatment in dogs with pituitary-dependent hyperadrenocorticism. *Austr. Vet. J.*, **81**, 600–607.

Feldman, E.C., Nelson, R.W. (2004) Canine hyperadrenocorticism (Cushing's syndrome), in *Feline and Canine Endocrinology and Reproduction*, 3rd edition (eds E.C.Feldman, R.W.Nelson), Saunders, Philadelphia, pp. 252–357.

Kintzer, P.P., Peterson, M.E. (1994) Mitotane treatment of cortisol secreting adrenocortical neoplasia: 32 cases (1980–1992). *J. Am. Vet. Med. Assoc.*, **205**, 54–61.

Kintzer, P.P., Peterson, M.E. (1991) Mitotane (o,p'-ddd) treatment of 200 dogs with pituitary-dependent hyperadenocorticism. *J. Vet. Intern. Med.*, **5**, 182–190.

Vaughn, M.A., Feldman, E.C., Hoar, B.R., Nelson, R.W. (2008) Evaluation of twice-daily, low-dose trilostane treatment administered orally in dogs with naturally occurring hyperadrenocorticism. *J. Am. Vet. Med. Assoc.*, **232**, 1321–1328.

Author: Ellen N. Behrend VMD, PhD, DACVIM

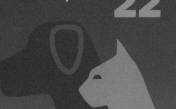
Feline Hyperadrenocorticism

DEFINITION

- Dysfunction of the hypothalamus–pituitary–adrenal axis resulting in an overproduction of cortisol.
- Pituitary-dependent hyperadrenocorticism (PDH) is the cause of HAC in 80–85% of feline cases; functional adrenal tumor (FAT) comprises the other 15–20%.
- Sequelae include: insulin-resistant DM, and fragile skin syndrome.
- Cases have been reported for over 30 years; however, this is a rare disease in cats, with less than 100 cases reported in peer-reviewed literature.

ETIOLOGY/PATHOPHYSIOLOGY

- PDH – over-secretion of ACTH due to expansion of corticotrophic cells found in the anterior lobe and/or pars intermedius of the pituitary.
- The pituitary becomes insensitive to negative feedback pathways and autonomous ACTH secretion occurs.
- The ZF and ZR of the adrenal gland rapidly produce cortisol in response to ACTH.
- Excessive ACTH stimulation results in bilateral adrenal hypertrophy and increased blood cortisol levels.
- The vast majority of PDH cases are adenomas, although rare adenocarcinomas have been reported.
- Less commonly, feline HAC is due to a FAT of the ZF and/or ZR, and is almost always a unilateral tumor. These tumors can be adenomas (50%) or adenocarcinomas (50%).
- Iatrogenic HAC has also been reported in the cat in association with chronic oral or injectable glucocorticoid administration.
- Ectopic secretion of ACTH from a neuroendocrine tumor (carcinoid) has been reported in humans, but not in cats.

Blackwell's Five-Minute Veterinary Consult Clinical Companion: Small Animal Endocrinology and Reproduction,
First Edition. Edited by Deborah S. Greco and Autumn P. Davidson. © 2017 John Wiley & Sons, Inc.
Published 2017 by John Wiley & Sons, Inc.
Companion Website: www.fiveminutevet.com/endocrinology

SIGNALMENT/HISTORY

- DSH cats and female cats may be over-represented. This remains unconfirmed due to the low incidence of disease.
- Unlike dogs, there is no size predisposition to PDH versus FAT. This may be due to the lack of a significant size difference in this species.
- This is primarily a disease of middle-aged to older cats.
- The median age at diagnosis is 10 years, with a range of 5 to 16 years.
- Insulin-resistant DM is commonly in the patient's history.
- In iatrogenic HAC, there is a history of chronic glucocorticoid administration.
- The cat typically presents for one or more of the following: muscle weakness, lack of ability to jump, lethargy, PU/PD, hair loss, tearing of the skin (even with routine grooming behavior) and dyspnea.

 ## CLINICAL FEATURES

- On physical examination the following may be seen: muscle wasting, atrophic skin with visible subcutaneous vessels (particularly on ventrum), pot-bellied appearance, seborrhea, comedones, hair loss, bruising, poor wound healing, fragile skin syndrome (often elicited with minimal restraint).
- Calcinotis cutis is not recognized in the cat.
- As the disease progresses, secondary insulin-resistant DM develops.
- DM is often diagnosed before the underlying HAC is recognized.

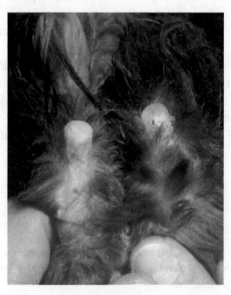

■ **Fig. 22.1.** Thin skin over the hocks of a cat with hyperadrenocorticism

- HAC diabetic cats often require large amounts of insulin and are poorly controlled.
- The renal tubules of the cat are not as responsive to excessive cortisol as the dog; therefore PU/PD is uncommon in a non-diabetic HAC cat.
- Cats are more resistant to cortisol-induced polyphagia, but become polyphagic with diabetes.
- Due to the immunosuppressive action of cortisol, secondary infections can occur.
- Iatrogenic HAC may present with curling of the ear pinnae.

 ## DIFFERENTIAL DIAGNOSIS

- Acromegaly, sex-hormone-producing functional adrenal tumor, pheochromocytoma.

 ## DIAGNOSTICS

Laboratory testing

- Early laboratory signs are usually mild, consisting only of variable increases in cholesterol and ALT.
- USG is usually normal. The feline kidney has a relatively low number of glucocorticoid receptors compared to the dog.
- ALP is not typically elevated due to the lack of a steroid isomer in the cat.
- Later in the disease, 90–100% of HAC cats develop DM and will present with increased blood glucose, increased fructosamine levels, and glucosuria.
- Diabetic monitoring in the HAC cat often reveals significant insulin resistance and poor control of the diabetic state.

Endocrine testing

- UCCR – If negative, this eliminates hyperadrenocorticism as a differential. If positive, further testing is required for diagnosis. The urine should be collected at home in a non-stressed environment. Cats typically have a higher UCCR than dogs, even in the absence of HAC.
- ACTH stimulation test – Not highly regarded as sensitive or specific in the cat for spontaneous HAC. This test should be used when iatrogenic HAC is suspected.
- Resting cortisol levels have been reported to be 67% sensitive and therefore can be used as part of an initial diagnostic evaluation to build suspicion of HAC
- LDDST – Lack of suppression (cortisol >1.5 µg/dl) at 8 hours is consistent with HAC. A higher dose of dexamethasone than the dog is required (0.1 mg/kg, IV).
- At Home LDDST using UCCR – Collect urine at 08:00 am on days 1 and 2 (can combine) for UCCR. After urine collection, administer 0.1 mg/kg oral dexamethasone in three doses, 6 hours apart. Collect a urine sample for UCCR at 08:00 am on Day 3. Client may mail samples to laboratory.
- HDDST – May be used to differentiate between PDH and FAT. A dose of 1 mg/kg is administered IV. PDH may suppress at 4 hours (<1.5 µg/dl) and escape at 8 hours (>1.5 µg/dl); however, a lack of suppression does not confirm FAT.

- An elevated endogenous ACTH is a very specific test for PDH. A negative result does not rule out PDH due to episodic secretion of ACTH in the cat. This test requires very special handling.

Imaging

- Radiographs are rarely helpful in diagnosis. Unless a mineralized adrenal tumor is present, even large tumors may be difficult to visualize.
- Abdominal ultrasound is a sensitive test. A skilled ultrasonographer should be utilized. Bilateral enlargement of the adrenal glands is supportive of PDH. Unilateral adrenal enlargement, especially with contralateral atrophy, is supportive of FAT; however, pheochromocytoma must also be considered.
- CT and MRI are sensitive and specific for pituitary tumors over 1 cm and also provide information on the effect of the tumor on surrounding tissue. This is mandatory before considering any surgical or radiation treatment for a pituitary tumor.

 THERAPEUTICS

PDH

- Mitotane is not recommended for the treatment of feline HAC.
- Trilostane: a synthetic steroid that inhibits β-hydroxysteroid dehydrogenase and decreases cortisol production. The initial dose is 30 mg/cat every 24 hours. An ACTH stimulation test should be performed 7–14 days after therapy is started. The pre-sample should be drawn 4 hours after trilostane is administered. A post-ACTH cortisol level of <2 mg/dl indicates that trilostane should be discontinued for 5–7 days and restarted at a 25–50% of the original dose. A level of 2.5–7.5 mg/dl indicates good control at the current dose. A level of >7.5 mg/dl indicates the dose should be increased by 25–50% and an ACTH stimulation should be performed two weeks later.
- Radiation therapy has achieved control of clinical signs and remission of insulin-resistant diabetes. Both, fractionated and surgical radiation techniques have been reported.
- Trans-sphenoidal hypophysectomy is the preferred treatment in humans. In animals, however, this technique is only performed a few surgeons in the world and does require very intensive postoperative care.

FAT

- Surgical removal of the adrenal tumor is the recommended.

Abbreviations

PDH   = Pituitary-dependent hyperadrenocorticism
HAC   = Hyperadrenocorticism
FAT   = Functional adrenal tumor

DM   = Diabetes mellitus
ACTH   = Adrenocorticotropic hormone
ZR   = Zona reticularis
ZF   = Zona fasiculata
PU/PD = Polyuria, polydipsia
USG   = Urine specific gravity
UCCR   = Urine cortisol creatinine test
LDDST = Low-dose dexamethasone suppression test
HDDST = High-dose dexamethasone suppression test

See Also

Diabetes mellitus
Acromegaly
Hypoadrenocorticism
Pheochromocytoma
Adrenal tumor

Suggested Reading

Feldman, E.C., Nelson, R.W. (1994) Comparative aspects of Cushing's syndrome in dogs and cats. *Endocrinol. Metab. Clin. North Am.*, **23**, 671–691.

Nelson, R.W., Feldman, E.C., Smith, M.C. (1988) Hyperadrenocorticism in cats: seven cases (1978–1987). *J. Am. Vet. Med. Assoc.*, **193**, 245–250.

Hoenig, M. (2002) Feline hypercortisolemia – where are we now? *J. Feline Med. Surg.*, **4**, 171–174.

Lien, Y.H., Huang, H.P., Chang, P.H. (2006) Iatrogenic hyperadrenocorticism in 12 cats. *J. Am. Anim. Hosp. Assoc.*, **42**, 414–423.

Elliott, D.A., Feldman, E.C., Koblik, P.D., Samii, V.F., Nelson, R.W. (2000) Prevalence of pituitary tumors among diabetic cats with insulin resistance. *J. Am. Vet. Med. Assoc.*, **216**, 1765–1768.

Mayer, M.N., Greco, D.S., LaRue, S.M. (2006) Outcomes of pituitary tumor irradiation in cats. *J. Vet. Intern. Med.*, **20**, 1151–1154.

Neiger, R., Witt, A.L., Noble, A., German, A.J. (2004) Trilostane therapy for treatment of pituitary-dependent hyperadrenocorticism in 5 cats. *J. Vet. Intern. Med.*, **18**, 160–164.

Author: Emily Cross DVM, DABVP (Canine/Feline)

chapter 23

Hyperglycemia

DEFINITION

- Transient or persistently increased serum glucose concentrations.

ETIOLOGY/PATHOPHYSIOLOGY

- Insulin resistance and pancreatic amyloidosis (type 2 DM in cats).
- Insulin resistance from endogenous hormones (growth hormone) or drugs (corticosteroids).
- Absolute or relative insulin deficiency (type 1 DM in dogs).
- Increased gluconeogenesis and increased glycogenolysis (epinephrine (adrenaline) release from stress, type 2 DM).

Systems Affected

- Endocrine/Metabolic – insulin resistance, hepatic glycogenolysis.
- Nervous – severe hyperglycemia may cause CNS dehydration from increasing serum osmolality. Hind limb weakness and plantigrade stance from diabetic neuropathy in cats.
- Ophthalmic – persistent hyperglycemia can cause cataracts in dogs.
- Renal/Urologic – osmotic diuresis from blood glucose exceeding the renal threshold (higher in the cat than dog) causes polyuria with secondary polydipsia.

SIGNALMENT/HISTORY

- Cats and dogs of any age or breed.

Blackwell's Five-Minute Veterinary Consult Clinical Companion: Small Animal Endocrinology and Reproduction, First Edition. Edited by Deborah S. Greco and Autumn P. Davidson. © 2017 John Wiley & Sons, Inc. Published 2017 by John Wiley & Sons, Inc.
Companion Website: www.fiveminutevet.com/endocrinology

CLINICAL FEATURES

General Comments

- Clinical signs vary and often reflect underlying disease.
- Some patients are asymptomatic, especially those with drug, stress-induced, and post-prandial hyperglycemia.

Historic Findings

- Variable by species and duration of hyperglycemia.
- May be normal.
- Dogs with diabetes: polydipsia, polyuria, depression, weight loss, obesity, polyphagia.
- Cats with diabetes: obesity, plantagrade stance, anorexia, vomiting, diarrhea, polydipsia/polyuria.
- CNS depression, coma – severe hyperglycemia with hyperosmolality.

Physical Examination Findings

- May be normal.
- Obesity in cats with type 2 DM.
- Plantigrade stance in cats.
- Cataracts in dogs.
- Emaciation in dogs with type 1 DM.
- Hepatomegaly resulting from diabetic hepatopathy.
- Chronic infections: respiratory, skin.
- Poor hair coat.

Causes

- Relative or absolute insulin deficiency – type 1 and type 2 DM.
- Insulin resistance – type 2 DM in cats, hyperadrenocorticism, pheochromocytoma, glucagonoma, hypersomatotropism, hyperthyroidism, high progesterone during diestrus (dogs), renal insufficiency, urinary tract infection.
- Physiologic—post-prandial fluctuation and stress (epinephrine (adrenaline)-induced) in cats.
- Drugs – thiazide diuretics, morphine, dextrose-containing fluids, progestins (e.g., megestrol acetate), growth hormone, glucocorticoids, and ACTH.
- Regulation problems in treated diabetics – high-carbohydrate diets (cats), insulin administration problems, insulin-induced hypoglycemic hyperglycemia (rare).
- Parenteral administration of nutritional solutions.
- Laboratory error.

Risk Factors

- Stress in cats.
- Concurrent disease – hyperadrenocorticism, acromegaly, and acute pancreatitis.
- Diabetogenic drugs – steroids, progestagens.
- Dextrose-containing fluids.

DIFFERENTIAL DIAGNOSIS

- Mild, transiently high blood glucose can be associated with stress.
- In patients with mild hyperglycemia and no history of polydipsia/polyuria, repeat blood glucose determination after 12-hour fast and perform serum fructosamine.

DIAGNOSTICS

Laboratory Findings

Drugs That May Alter Laboratory Results
- High blood glucose concentration – glucocorticoids, ACTH, dextrose-containing fluids, epinephrine, asparaginase, β-adrenergic agonists, and diazoxide.

Disorders That May Alter Laboratory Results
- Lipemia, hemolysis, and icterus may interfere with spectrophotometric assays.
- Delayed serum separation artificially lowers glucose concentration; must separate serum within 1 hour of collection to prevent cellular glucose use.
- Use of human glucometers – may read 25% below actual blood glucose value, repeat with monitor validated in dog or cat whole-blood.
- Blood glucose reagent strips require whole-blood.
- Measure glucose concentration in whole-blood within 30 minutes of collection.

Valid if Run in Human Laboratory?
- Yes.

CBC/Biochemistry/Urinalysis
- Hyperglycemia may be the only abnormal finding.
- CBC – may be normal; possible inflammatory leukogram in patients with sepsis.
- Urinalysis – may be normal; glucosuria, pyuria, bacteriuria, and ketonuria.
- Fasting hyperglycemia plus glucosuria suggests DM.
- Lipemia in patients with low lipoprotein lipase (miniature schnauzers), hyperadrenocorticism, acute pancreatitis, and postprandial blood sampling.

- High amylase and lipase activity suggests acute pancreatitis, especially in non-azotemic patients.
- Increased plasma lipase immunoreactivity in patients with acute pancreatitis.
- High liver enzyme activity may accompany fatty infiltration with diabetes.

Other Laboratory Tests

- Fructosamine – normal values rule-out diabetes as cause of hyperglycemia.
- ACTH stimulation or low-dose dexamethasone-suppression test to rule-out hyperadreno-corticism.

Imaging

- Not available.

Diagnostic Procedures

- Not available.

 THERAPEUTICS

- Insulin therapy (dogs and some cats), oral hypoglycemic agents (cats).
- Discontinue diabetogenic drugs.
- Dextrose-free fluids.

Drug(s) of Choice

- Insulin – regular (crystalline) insulin for diabetic ketoacidosis Lente insulin (dogs).
- Insulin glargine or PZI insulin in cats with DM.
- Oral hypoglycemics such as glipizide (cats with type 2 DM).

Contraindications

- Diabetogenic drugs (e.g., glucocorticoids).
- Dextrose-containing fluids.

Precautions

- Avoid rapid and aggressive insulin therapy that lowers blood glucose abruptly and causes hypoglycemia or cerebral edema.

Possible Interactions

- Not available.

Alternative Drug(s)

■ Acarbose 12.5 mg PO q.12 h; intestinal starch blocker.

Patient Monitoring

■ For return of clinical signs of diabetes such as polyuria, polydipsia, and polyphagia.
■ Blood glucose after discontinuing diabetogenic drugs.
■ Glycosylated hemoglobin and fructosamine on an outpatient basis to monitor long-term glucose control.

Possible Complications

■ High incidence of sepsis (and infection).
■ Severe hyperglycemia may be associated with CNS depression and coma because of hyperosmolarity.

 COMMENTS

Diet

■ High-protein, low-carbohydrate diet in cats with DM.
■ High-soluble fiber, low-fat diet in dogs with DM.

Associated Conditions

■ Hyperosmolarity.
■ Uremia may be associated with hyperglycemia.

Age-Related Factors

■ None

Zoonotic Potential

■ None

Pregnancy/Fertility/Breeding

■ Not available.

Synonyms

■ High blood sugar

See Also

Diabetes Mellitus without Complications – Cats
Diabetes Mellitus without Complications – Dogs
Hyperosmolarity

Abbreviations

ACTH = adrenocorticotropic hormone
CNS   = central nervous system
DM   = diabetes mellitus

Suggested Reading

Kaneko, J.J. (1989) Carbohydrate metabolism and its diseases, in *Clinical Biochemistry of Domestic Animals*, 4th edition (ed. J.J.Kaneko), Academic, San Diego, pp. 44–85.

Author: Deborah S. Greco DVM, PhD, DACVIM

chapter 24

Hyperkalemia

DEFINITION

- Serum potassium concentration >5.5 mEq/l (normal range: 3.5–5.5 mEq/l).

ETIOLOGY/PATHOPHYSIOLOGY

- Potassium is primarily an intracellular electrolyte (98% of total body potassium is intracellular); serum levels, however, may not accurately reflect total body concentrations.
- Potassium is predominantly responsible for the maintenance of intracellular fluid volume and is required for normal function of many enzymes.
- The resting cellular membrane potential is determined by the ratio of intracellular to extracellular potassium concentration, and maintained by the Na^+, K^+-ATPase pump. Conduction disturbances in susceptible tissues (cardiac, nerve, and muscle) are caused by rapid shifts in this ratio causing myoneural membrane hyperpolarization.

Systems Affected

- Neuromuscular – muscle weakness, including skeletal and muscles of respiration.
- Cardiac – electrocardiac changes and arrhythmias.
- Renal – hyposthenuria, nephropathy, and renal failure.
- Metabolic – acid-base balance (metabolic alkalosis); glucose homeostasis.

SIGNALMENT/HISTORY

Risk Factors

- Pseudohyperkalemia in certain East Asian dog breeds (e.g., Akitas, Shibas, Jindos, and Chinese shar-peis).

Blackwell's Five-Minute Veterinary Consult Clinical Companion: Small Animal Endocrinology and Reproduction, First Edition. Edited by Deborah S. Greco and Autumn P. Davidson. © 2017 John Wiley & Sons, Inc. Published 2017 by John Wiley & Sons, Inc.
Companion Website: www.fiveminutevet.com/endocrinology

CLINICAL FEATURES

Historic Findings

- Weakness.
- Collapse.
- Flaccid paralysis.
- Death.

Physical Examination Findings

- Arrhythmias, especially bradyarrhythmias.
- Weakness.
- Paralysis.

 DIFFERENTIAL DIAGNOSIS

- Hypoadrenocorticism.
- Fluid therapy with potassium supplementation.
- Parenteral nutrition.
- Administration of potassium-sparing diuretics.
- ACE inhibitors (e.g., enalapril, benazepril), disease.
- Acidosis.
- Trauma.
- Anuric or oliguric renal failure.
- Lower urinary tract blockage or rupture.
- Cystic calculi in male dogs.
- Thrombocytosis and leukemia.
- Pseudohyperkalemia.
- Phosphofructokinase deficiency.
- High potassium intake (KBr).
- Miscellaneous – third space (pleural effusion/ascites).
- Translocation of potassium – acidosis, reperfusion syndrome, thrombolysis in feline aortic thromboembolism, tumor lysis syndrome, muscle injury.
- Severe digitalis overdose, infusion of mannitol, and hyperglycemia causing hyperosmolality.

 DIAGNOSTICS

CBC/Biochemistry/Urinalysis

- Thrombocytosis ($>10^6$ cells/mm^3), leukocytosis ($>200\,000$ cells/mm^3), and abnormal (leukemic) leukocytes can cause release of large amounts of potassium into the serum if not separated quickly.

- INa:K ratio <20, consider hypoadrenocorticism.
- In patients with azotemia, consider hypoadrenocorticism, renal failure, and obstruction of the urinary tract.
- Presence of high creatine kinase, aspartate aminotransferase, and lactic dehydrogenase – consider muscle injury.
- With severe thrombocytosis or leukocytosis or if the patient is an East Asian dog breed – consider pseudohyperkalemia.

Other Laboratory Tests

- ACTH response test to rule out hypoadrenocorticism.

Imaging

- Radiographic contrast studies or ultrasound to rule out urinary tract rupture or obstruction.

Electrocardiogram

- Tall and spiked T waves.
- Wide QRS complexes.
- P-R intervals lengthen; the P waves become smaller and wider and, in animals with severe hyperkalemia, disappear (atrial standstill).
- Fusion of the QRS-T followed by ventricular fibrillation or asystole.
- ECG changes in animals with hyperkalemia vary and are diminished by hypernatremia, hypercalcemia, and alkalosis.

Pathological Findings

- Not available.

 # THERAPEUTICS

Drug(s) of Choice

- For patients with life-threatening hyperkalemia, administer calcium gluconate 10% (0.5–1 ml/kg slowly IV over 10 minutes) while monitoring the ECG.

Precautions/Interactions

- Kayexalate and sodium bicarbonate cause a sodium load that may lead to fluid retention in patients with cardiac or renal failure.
- Sodium bicarbonate lowers ionized calcium levels. Use cautiously in hypocalcemic patients.

Alternative Drugs

- Sodium bicarbonate: administer 1–2 mEq/kg slowly IV.
- Dextrose and regular insulin: 0.5 U/kg IV with 50% dextrose, 1 g/kg IV); dextrose can also be used without insulin.

Nursing Care

- Not available.

Diet

- Not available.

Surgical Considerations

- Not available.

 COMMENTS

Client Education

- Not available.

Patient Monitoring

- Recheck potassium following therapy and as dictated by underlying condition.
- ECG monitoring until arrhythmias resolve.
- ECG monitoring during IV calcium administration.

Prevention/Avoidance

- Avoid potassium-containing fluids and fluids that cause hyponatremia, acidosis, or hypocalcemia.
- Avoid drugs that contain potassium or interfere with potassium elimination (e.g., ACE inhibitors, trimethoprim antibiotics, and potassium-sparing diuretics).

Possible Complications

- Extreme elevations in serum potassium can be fatal.

Expected Course and Prognosis

- Depends on underlying disorder.

Synonyms

- Not available.

Abbreviations

ACE = angiotensin-converting enzyme
ACTH = adrenocorticotropic hormone
ECG = electrocardiogram/electrocardiography

Suggested Reading

Segev, G., Fascetti, A.J., Weeth, L.P., *et al.* (2010) Correction of hyperkalemia in dogs with chronic kidney disease consuming commercial renal therapeutic diets by a potassium-reduced home-prepared diet. *J. Vet. Intern. Med.*, **24** (3), 546–550.
Schaer, M. (2008) Therapeutic approach to chronic electrolyte emergencies. *Vet. Clin. North Am. Small Anim. Pract.*, **38** (3), 513–533.
Willard, M. (2008) Therapeutic approach to chronic electrolyte disorders. *Vet. Clin. North Am. Small Anim. Pract.*, **38** (3), 535–541.

Acknowledgment: The author and editors acknowledge the previous contribution of Frances W. K. Smith Jr. to *Blackwell's Five-Minute Veterinary Consult: Canine and Feline*, on which this topic is based.

Author: Deborah S. Greco DVM, PhD, DACVIM

chapter 25

Hyperlipidemia

DEFINITION

- Hyperlipidemia is the result of increased concentrations of lipids (fats) within the circulation. More specifically, hyperlipidemia refers to increased concentrations of triglycerides and/or cholesterol (hypertriglyceridemia, hypercholesterolemia) in a patient that has been fasted >12 hours.
- Lipemia occurs when the serum triglcyceride level exceeds 200 mg/dl, resulting in a turbid appearance to the serum or plasma.
- Lactescence occurs when the serum triglyceride level exceeds 1000 mg/dl, resulting in a milky appearance to the serum or plasma.
- Hyperlipidemia is common in dogs and can be primary in some breeds due to defective or ineffective lipid metabolism. The majority of cases of hyperlipidemia occur secondary to obesity, diet or an underlying disease process such as pancreatitis, hypothyroidism or diabetes mellitus.

ETIOLOGY/PATHOPHYSIOLOGY

Primary Hyperlipidemia

- Idiopathic hyperlipidemia of Miniature Schnauzers:
  - Primarily triglyceride defect.
  - First breed-related primary lipid disorder described in dogs.
  - The cause is unknown; absence of surface apoprotein C-II or mutation in the encoding gene are being evaluated.
  - Familial disorder.
  - Abnormal accumulation of VLDL or VLDL and chylomicrons.
- Idiopathic hypercholesterolemia:
  - Primary cholesterol defect.
  - Described in 15 breeds (UK); HDL1.

Blackwell's Five-Minute Veterinary Consult Clinical Companion: Small Animal Endocrinology and Reproduction,
First Edition. Edited by Deborah S. Greco and Autumn P. Davidson. © 2017 John Wiley & Sons, Inc.
Published 2017 by John Wiley & Sons, Inc.
Companion Website: www.fiveminutevet.com/endocrinology

- Family of rough-coated Collies (UK); HDL1, VLDL, LDL.
- Beagles, HDL1.
- Doberman Pinschers and Rottweilers; LDL.
- Hyperchylomicronemia in cats:
  - Familial, autosomal recessive.
  - Defect in lipoprotein lipase activity.

Secondary Hyperlipidemia

- Postprandial
  - Absorption of chylomicrons from the gastrointestinal tract occurs 30–60 minutes following ingestion of a meal.
  - May increase serum triglycerides for 3–10 hours.
- Obesity
  - Excessive hepatic synthesis of VLDS.
- Diabetes mellitus
  - Decreased LPL activity.
  - Increased hepatic synthesis of VLDL.
- Hypothyroidism
  - Increased triglycerides and cholesterol; HDL1, VLDL, LDL.
  - Decreased LPL activity.
  - Decreased lipolytic activity of catecholamines and other hormones.
  - Reduced hepatic degradation of cholesterol to bile acids.
- Hyperadrenocorticism
  - Naturally occurring and iatrogenic.
  - Elevated triglyceride and cholesterol.
  - Increased hepatic VLDL synthesis.
  - Decrease LPL activity.
- Hepatobiliary disease
  - Decreased excretion of cholesterol in the bile.
- Nephrotic syndrome
  - Decreased LDL activity.
  - Increased cholesterol synthesis secondary to low oncotic pressure.

Systems Affected

- Endocrine/Metabolic
- Gastrointestinal
- Nervous
- Ophthalmic
- Hepatobiliary

SIGNALMENT/HISTORY

Primary hyperlipidemia

- Dogs
    - Middle age >4 years of age.
    - Miniature Schnauzers, Beagles, Doberman Pinscher, Rottweiler.
- Cats
    - Young, 8–10 weeks, >8 months.
    - Himalayan, DSH, Persian, Siamese.

Secondary Hyperlipidemia

- Variable signalment and history bases on the underlying cause.

Risk Factors

- Genetic predisposition.
- Obesity.
- High-fat diet.
- Hypothyroidism.
- Hyperadrenocorticism.
- Diabetes mellitus.
- Hepatobiliary disease.
- Nephrotic syndrome.

Historic Findings

- Recent high-fat meal.
- Abdominal pain or distress.
- Seizures.
- Neuropathies.

CLINICAL FEATURES

- The most common clinical presentation in patients with hypertriglyceridemia waxing/waning vomiting, diarrhea and abdominal pain/discomfort.
- Severe hypertriglyceridemia (>1000 mg/dl)
    - Pancreatitis
    - Lipemia retinalis
    - Seizures

- Cutaneous xanthoma
  - □ Most common in cats
- Peripheral neuropathies
- Behavioral changes
- Severe hypercholesterolemia
  - Arcus lipoides corneae
  - Lipemia retinalis
  - Atherosclerosis

 DIFFERENTIAL DIAGNOSIS

- Postprandial
- Primary hyperlipidemia
- Obesity
- Pancreatitis
- Endocrine disorders
  - Hypothyroidism
  - Hyperadrenocorticism
  - Diabetes mellitus
- Hepatobiliary disease
  - Cholestasis
  - Mucocele
- Protein-losing nephropathy
  - Nephrotic syndrome
- Exogenous corticosteroid administration
- High-fat diet
- Lymphoma
- *Leishmania infantum*
- CHF secondary to DCM

 DIAGNOSTICS

Minimum Data Base

- If gross lipemia is present, samples should be promptly processed, centrifuged, and the serum separated. Lipemic serum in contact with red blood cells for a long period of time can result in hemolysis.

Complete Blood Count

- Typically normal.
- Nucleated RBC.
  - Hyperadrenocorticism.

- Mild normochromic, normocytic anemia.
  - Hypothyroidism.

Serum Biochemical Profile

- Elevated triglycerides
- Elevated cholesterol
- Hyperglycemia
  - Diabetes Mellitus
- Hypoalbuminemia
  - Nephrotic syndrome
- Increased ALP
  - Hyperadrenocorticism
  - Cholestatic disease
- Elevated serum lipase
  - Pancreatitis

Urinalysis

- Normal.
- Glycosuria.
  - Diabetes Mellitus.
- Hyposthenuria.
  - Hyperadrenocorticism.
- Proteinuria.
  - Nephrotic syndrome.
- The presence of hyperlipidemia can interfere with the results of other chemistry parameters, leading to falsely elevated total bilirubin, phosphorus, ALP, glucose, lipase and ALT; whereas TCO_2, cholesterol, BUN, and creatinine measurements may be falsely lowered.

Other Laboratory Tests

- Fasting Triglycerides
  - Consider submitting paired samples if triglycerides will be measured concurrently with other serum chemistry values. This allows one sample to be 'cleared' for more accurate analyte measurement.
- Endocrine Testing
  - Thyroid function testing (T4, FT4, TSH) to confirm hypothyroidism.
  - Adrenal axis testing (ACTH stimulation test or low-dose dexamethasone suppression test) to evaluate for hyperadrenocorticism.
- Chylomicron test
  - Obtain serum following a 12-hour fast.
  - Refrigerate serum for 12–14 hours; chylomicrons will rise to the surface to form a creamy layer.

- Lipoprotein electrophoresis
  - Separates LDL, VDL, HDL1 and HDL2.
  - Although measurement of HDL and LDL can be performed, the values have not been shown to be reliable in dogs and cats.
- LPL activity
  - Collect serum for triglycerides, cholesterol and lipoprotein electrophoresis prior to and 15 minutes following administration of heparin.
  - Administer heparin 90 IU/kg IV.
  - If there is no change in values before and after heparin administration, a defective LPL enzyme system should be suspected.

Pathological Findings

- Not available.

 ## THERAPEUTICS

- Identification and treatment of the secondary causes.
  - With appropriate recognition and therapy, hyperlipidemia should resolve.
- Dietary management is the mainstay of therapy of primary hyperlipidemia.
  - Fat-restricted diets; ideally they should contain <10% fat.
  - Hill's R/D.
  - Purina OM.
  - Royal Canin Low-Fat.

Drug(s)

- Diet should be the primary therapy, but if diet alone is not sufficient then additional medical management can be considered.
  - Gemfibrozil 7.5 mg PO q.12 h.
  - Fish oils linolenic acid (omega-3 polyunsaturated fat), 10–30 mg/kg PO q. 24 h.
  - Clofibrate and niacin are not currently recommended for use in dogs and cats.

 ## COMMENTS

- A 12-hour fast is required to evaluate for the presence of hyperlipidemia.
- Pancreatitis and seizures are potential complications of hyperlipidemia in the Miniature Schnauzer.
- In cats with hereditary chylomicronemia, xanthoma formation, lipemia retinalis, and neuropathies have been reported; peripheral neuropathies usually resolve 2–3 months after institution of a low-fat diet.

Expected Course and Prognosis

■ Ultimately depends on the underlying cause and response to therapy. Serum triglyceride levels should be maintained <500 mg/dl, to prevent acute pancreatitis.

Abbreviations

T4	= Levothyroxine, L-thyroxine, tetraiodothyronine
FT4	= Free T4
TSH	= Thyroid-stimulating hormone, thyrotropin
BUN	= Blood urea nitrogen
ALP	= Alkaline phosphatase
ALT	= Alanine aminotransferase
ACTH	= Adrenocorticotropic hormone
HDL	= High-density lipoprotein
LDL	= Low-density lipoprotein
VLDL	= Very-low-density lipoprotein
LPL	= Lipoprotein lipase
CHF	= Congestive heart failure
DCM	= Dilated cardiomyopathy

See Also

Diabetes Mellitus
Hypothyroidism
Hyperadrenocorticism
Hepatobiliary disease
Nephrotic syndrome
Pancreatitis
Obesity

Suggested Reading

Xenoulis, P.G., Steiner, J.M. (2010) Lipid metabolism and hyperlipidemia in dogs. *Vet. J.*, **183**, 12–21.

Elliot, D.A. (2005) Dietary and Medical Considerations in Hyperlipidemia, in *Textbook of Veterinary Internal Medicine* (eds S.J.Ettinger, E.C.Feldman), Elsevier Saunders, St Louis, MO, pp. 592–595.

Barrie, J., Watson, T. (1995) Hyperlipidemia, in *Kirk's Current Veterinary Therapy XII* (ed. J.D.Bonagura), Saunders, Philadelphia, pp. 430–434.

Ford, R. (1994) Canine hyperlipidemias, in *Textbook of Veterinary Internal Medicine* (eds S.J.Ettinger, E.C.Feldman), Elsevier Saunders, St Louis, MO, pp. 1414–1418.

Jones, B. (1994) Feline Hyperlipidemias, in *Textbook of Veterinary Internal Medicine* (eds S.J.Ettinger, E.C.Feldman), Elsevier Saunders, St Louis, MO, pp. 1410–1413.

Author: Julia Bates DVM, DACVIM

chapter 26

Hypernatremia

DEFINITION

- Serum sodium concentration >158 mEq/l in dogs or >165 mEq/l in cats.

PATHOPHYSIOLOGY

- Sodium is the most abundant cation in the extracellular fluid, so hypernatremia usually reflects hyperosmolality.
- Hypernatremia can be caused by excessive water loss, increased intake of sodium, or a combination of both.
- Common causes of hypernatremia include renal or gastrointestinal loss of water in excess of sodium loss and low water intake.

Systems Affected

- Endocrine/Metabolic
- Nervous

SIGNALMENT

- Dogs and cats

CLINICAL FEATURES

- Polydipsia.
- Disorientation.
- Coma.
- Seizures.
- Other findings depend on underlying cause.
- Severity of signs usually correlates to the degree of hypernatremia.

Blackwell's Five-Minute Veterinary Consult Clinical Companion: Small Animal Endocrinology and Reproduction,
First Edition. Edited by Deborah S. Greco and Autumn P. Davidson. © 2017 John Wiley & Sons, Inc.
Published 2017 by John Wiley & Sons, Inc.
Companion Website: www.fiveminutevet.com/endocrinology

Causes

- Total body sodium high – oral ingestion (rare); IV administration of NaCl during cardio-vascular resuscitation; hyperaldosteronism (rare); hyperadrenocorticism (may cause mild changes).
- Total body sodium normal plus water deficit – low water intake (e.g., no access to water and adipsia or hypodipsia); high urinary water loss (e.g., diabetes insipidus); high insensible water loss (e.g., panting and hyperthermia).
- Total body sodium low and hypotonic fluid loss (i.e., loss of fluid containing sodium without adequate water replacement) – urinary loss (e.g., diabetes mellitus, osmotic diuresis, and diuresis after acute urinary obstruction); gastrointestinal sodium loss (e.g., administration of osmotic cathartic, vomiting, and diarrhea).

DIAGNOSIS

 ## DIFFERENTIAL DIAGNOSIS

- Diabetes insipidus.
- Hyperosmolar non-ketotic syndrome.
- Hypertonic dehydration.
- Alterations in thirst reaction pathway – rare.
- Salt ingestion – rare.

Laboratory Findings

Drugs That May Alter Laboratory Results
- A wide variety of drugs interfere with renal capacity to concentrate urine, leading to water loss in excess of sodium and high serum sodium concentration; these drugs include lithium, demeclocycline, and amphotericin.

Disorders That May Alter Laboratory Results
- Lipemia or hyperproteinemia (>11 g/dl) can artifactually raise sodium concentration when the flame photometry method is used.

Valid if Run in a Human Laboratory?
- Yes.

CBC/Biochemistry/Urinalysis
- High serum sodium concentration.
- Diabetes insipidus – polyuria, low urinary specific gravity, and low urinary sodium concentration.

- Hyperosmolar non-ketotic syndrome – high blood glucose, low urine output, and high urinary specific gravity (usually >1.025).
- Hypertonic dehydration – low urinary sodium concentration and high urinary specific gravity (usually >1.030).

Other Laboratory Tests

- Modified water deprivation test to differentiate diabetes insipidus from other causes of polyuria and polydipsia; performed after results of CBC, biochemical analysis, urinalysis, and endocrine testing are evaluated to rule-out hyperadrenocorticism.
- After water restriction, patients with diabetes insipidus have little or no increase in urinary specific gravity or osmolality.
- After ADH or DDAVP administration, patients with nephrogenic diabetes insipidus have <10% increase in urinary specific gravity; those with central diabetes insipidus have a 10% to 800% increase.

Imaging

- CT scan or MRI in patients with diabetes insipidus to rule-out pituitary tumor.

TREATMENT

- After resolution of the hypernatremia, consider a sodium-restricted diet (especially in patients with nephrogenic diabetes insipidus).
- Water must be available at all times for patients with diabetes insipidus.

MEDICATION

Drug(s) of Choice

- If hypovolemia is severe – replace volume with isotonic saline (i.e., lactated Ringer's or normal saline) or isotonic fluids (i.e., 5% dextrose with half-normal saline).
- Hypernatremia – administer hypotonic fluids (e.g., 5% dextrose in water) to reduce serum sodium by 0.5 mEq/hour or by no more than 20 mEq/l/day; supplement with potassium and phosphate if needed.
- Central diabetes insipidus – DDAVP (one to two drops in subconjunctival sac q.12–24 h).
- Nephrogenic diabetes insipidus – hydrochlorthiazide (2–4 mg/kg PO q.12 h).

Contraindications

- Refer to manufacturer's literature.

Precautions

- Rapid correction of hypernatremia can cause pulmonary edema.
- Hypocalcemia may develop during correction of hypernatremia.

FOLLOW-UP

Patient Monitoring

- Acute setting – electrolytes, urine output, and body weight.
- Diabetes insipidus – water intake.

Possible Complications

- CNS thrombosis or hemorrhage.
- Hyperactivity.
- Seizures.
- Serum sodium >180 mEq/l often associated with residual CNS damage.
- Many patients recover, but possibility of neurologic damage is high.

 ## COMMENTS

Age-Related Factors

- None.

Zoonotic Potential

- None.

Synonyms

- None.

See Also

Diabetes Insipidus
Hyposthenuria

Abbreviations

ADH   = antidiuretic hormone
CNS   = central nervous system
CT   = computed tomography

DDAVP = brand name of desmopressin, a synthetic antidiuretic hormone preparation
MRI   = magnetic resonance imaging

Suggested Reading

DiBartola, S.P. (2005) *Fluid, Electrolyte, and Acid-base Disorders in Small Animal Practice*, 3rd edition, Saunders, Philadelphia.

Marks, S.L., Taboada, J. (1998) Hypernatremia and hypertonic syndromes. *Vet. Clin. North Am. Small Anim. Pract.*, **28** (3), 533–543.

Ross, D.B. (1989) *Clinical Physiology of Acid-base and Electrolyte Disorders*, 3rd edition, McGraw-Hill, New York.

Acknowledgment: The author and editors acknowledge the previous contribution of Rhett Nichols to *Blackwell's Five-Minute Veterinary Consult: Canine and Feline*, on which this topic is based.

Author: Melinda Fleming DVM

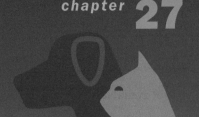

chapter 27

Diabetes Mellitus with Hyperosmolar Coma

DEFINITION

- Disease characterized by severe hyperglycemia, hyperosmolarity, severe dehydration, lack of urine or serum ketones, lack of or mild-to-moderate metabolic acidosis, and CNS depression.

ETIOLOGY/PATHOPHYSIOLOGY

- Insulin deficiency causes reduced use of glucose and excessive glucose production.
- The resultant high extracellular blood glucose concentration causes a hyperosmolar state with a reduced extracellular fluid volume.
- Intracellular dehydration, azotemia, and uremia develop, and intracellular dehydration becomes more pronounced as the glomerular filtration rate decreases; tissue hypoxia ensues.
- Azotemia, hyperglycemia, and hyperosmolarity worsen as a result of glucose retention and glucose-induced osmotic diuresis.
- Although ketonemia and ketonuria usually are not features of this syndrome, anorexia (especially when prolonged) may cause mild ketoacidosis in some patients, but increased lactic acid is a major contributor to the metabolic acidosis that may develop in these patients.

Systems Affected

- Renal/Urologic – prerenal and primary renal azotemia develop because of reduced extracellular fluid volume, reduced tissue perfusion, or diabetic glomerulonephropathy; urinary specific gravity is low because of osmotic diuresis, diabetic glomerulonephropathy, or concurrent renal insufficiency.
- Cardiovascular – hypotension because of low extracellular fluid volume, vascular collapse, and depressed myocardial contractility
- Nervous – depression, disorientation or mental confusion, seizures, and coma are caused by intracellular dehydration and hyperosmolarity; CNS dysfunction worsens as serum osmolarity rises.

Blackwell's Five-Minute Veterinary Consult Clinical Companion: Small Animal Endocrinology and Reproduction, First Edition. Edited by Deborah S. Greco and Autumn P. Davidson. © 2017 John Wiley & Sons, Inc. Published 2017 by John Wiley & Sons, Inc.
Companion Website: www.fiveminutevet.com/endocrinology

Genetics

- Not available.

Incidence/Prevalence

- Uncommon

 # SIGNALMENT/HISTORY

Species

- Dogs and cats.

Breed Predilection

- Not available.

Mean Age and Range

- Dogs – peak prevalence, 7–9 years of age.
- Cats – any age; most >6 years old.

Predominant Sex

- Dogs – female.
- Cats – neutered males.

 # CLINICAL FEATURES

Historic Findings

- Early signs – polydipsia, polyuria, polyphagia, and weight loss.
- Late signs – weakness, vomiting, anorexia, depression, stupor, and coma.

Physical Examination Findings

- Dehydration, hypothermia, prolonged capillary refill time, cataracts, lethargy, depression, seizures (severe hyperosmolarity), and stupor or coma (severe hyperosmolarity).

Causes

- Diabetes mellitus associated with severe hyperosmolarity, severe hyperglycemia, and severe dehydration.

Risk Factors

- Concurrent problems such as heart disease, renal insufficiency, pneumonia, acute pancreatitis, neoplasia and other severe diseases.
- Drugs – anticonvulsants, glucocorticoids, and thiazide diuretics may precipitate or aggravate this syndrome.

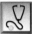 **DIFFERENTIAL DIAGNOSIS**

- Uncomplicated diabetes mellitus – mentally alert with fasting hyperglycemia and glucosuria.
- Ketoacidotic diabetes mellitus – fasting hyperglycemia with glucosuria, ketonuria, and metabolic acidosis.
- Extreme lethargy and depression with severe hyperosmolarity, severe hyperglycemia, severe dehydration without ketonemia and ketonuria usually differentiate diabetes mellitus non-ketotic hyperosmolar syndrome from uncomplicated and ketoacidotic diabetes mellitus.

 DIAGNOSTICS

CBC/Biochemistry/Urinalysis

- Severe hyperglycemia – usually >600 mg/dl.
- High BUN and creatinine concentration.
- Normokalemia (despite total body potassium depletion) or hypokalemia.
- Hyperkalemia is expected in patients with anuric or oliguric renal failure.
- Low TCO_2.
- High anion gap.
- Glucosuria.
- Low urinary specific gravity.

Other Laboratory Tests

- Severe hyperosmolarity – usually >350 mOsm/l.
- Estimated serum osmolarity may be calculated from serum chemistries as follows: 1.86(Na + K) + BUN/2.8 + glucose/18.
- High plasma lactate concentration may help confirm metabolic lactic acidosis in the absence of ketonemia and ketonuria.

Imaging

- Not available.

Diagnostic Procedures

- Not available.

Pathologic Findings

- Pancreatic islet cell atrophy

 # THERAPEUTICS

Appropriate Health Care

- A life-threatening medical emergency requiring inpatient treatment.

Nursing Care

- Fluid therapy is a major component of medical management.
- Replace one-half the fluid deficits in the first 12hours and the remainder during the next 24 hours.
- Administer normal saline (0.9%) IV if the patient is hypotensive or hyponatremic.
- Add potassium (20 mEq/l) to the initial fluids unless the patient has hyperkalemia.
- Switch to IV administration of 0.45% saline after restoration of normal blood pressure and urine output.
- Switch to 2.5–5% dextrose plus 0.45% saline when blood glucose <250 mg/dl, and continue until the patient is eating and drinking on its own.

Activity

- Not available.

Diet

- Low carbohydrate diet once patient is stablilzed.

Drugs Of Choice

- Administer regular insulin 2–4 hours after initiating IV fluid therapy.
- Regular insulin for patients <10 kg – initial dose is 2 U IM followed by 1 U IM hourly until blood glucose is <250 mg/dl.
- Regular insulin for patients >10 kg – initial dose is 0.25 U/kg IM followed by 0.1 U/kg IM, hourly until blood glucose is <250 mg/dl.
- Monitor blood glucose hourly; aim is to drop concentration by 50–100 mg/dl/h; adjust insulin dosage accordingly.

- Discontinue hourly IM regular insulin when blood glucose is <250 mg/dl; switch to regular insulin (0.5 U/kg) IM q.4–6 h or SC q.6–8 h if blood glucose concentration remains between 150 and 250 mg/dl.
- Alternatively, an IV constant-rate infusion of regular insulin may be used at a dosage of 1.1 U/kg/24 hours. Add 1.1 U/kg regular insulin to 250 ml 0.9% NaCl and administer at 10 ml/hour (0.045 U/kg/h) in a separate line. Discard the first 50 ml of the solution to compensate for insulin binding to the plastic tubing.
- Reduce the dosage/rate of the constant-rate infusion when the blood glucose is <250 mg/dl.
- Once the patient is stabilized (eating and drinking on its own without vomiting), discontinue fluids and regular insulin; NPH PZI, or Lente insulin can then be administered SC in a routine manner.
- Other concurrent diseases must be treated appropriately.

Contraindications

- Not available.

Precautions

- Avoid rapid reduction of serum osmolarity and glucose because the brain will become hyperosmolar compared with serum; fluid may then shift from extracellular to intracellular spaces, resulting in cerebral edema and worsening of neurologic status.

Possible Interactions

- Not available.

Alternative Drugs

- Once stable, oral hypoglycemics (e.g., glipizide, Glucotrol) may be tried; these agents are more likely to be efficacious in cats with type II (non-insulin-dependent diabetes mellitus) than in dogs.

Patient Monitoring

- Monitor blood glucose concentrations closely to avoid hypoglycemia and abrupt, precipitous decreases.
- Ideally, the blood glucose should drop 50–100 mg/dl/h until a concentration of 250 mg/dl is reached.
- Monitor blood glucose hourly before administering the next dose of regular insulin IM during initial stabilization.
- Monitor urine output for early detection of acute renal failure.

- Hydration status, ECG, CVP, serum electrolytes, BUN, and urine glucose every 2 hours during the initial stabilization period.
- Long-term glucose control by determining serum glycosylated hemoglobin and serum fructosamine concentrations.
- Watch for return of clinical signs such as polydipsia, polyuria, and polyphagia.

Prevention/Avoidance

- Avoid inappropriate insulin therapy.
- Avoid hypoglycemia, hypokalemia, and hyponatremia.

Possible Complications

- Irreversible coma and death are possible, especially in patients with renal insufficiency.
- Acute renal failure.

Expected Course and Prognosis

- Clinical signs and laboratory values may improve within the initial 24 hours of treatment, but these patients have a guarded prognosis.

 COMMENTS

Client Education

- Poor-to-guarded prognosis
- Intensive care and frequent monitoring are required during hospitalization.

Surgical Considerations

- Not available.

Associated Conditions

- Congestive heart failure, renal disease, infection, gastrointestinal hemorrhage, and other serious illnesses.

Synonyms

- Diabetic coma
- Hyperosmolar coma

See Also

Diabetes Mellitus Without Complication – Cats
Diabetes Mellitus Without Complication – Dogs
Diabetes with Ketoacidosis
Hyperosmolarity
Hyperglycemia

Abbreviations

BUN = blood urea nitrogen
CVP = central venous pressure
TCO_2 = total carbon dioxide

Suggested Reading

Brody, G.M. (1992) Diabetic ketoacidosis and hyperosmolar hyperglycemic nonketotic coma. *Top. Emerg. Med.*, **14**, 12–22.

Chastain, C.B., Nichols, C.E. (1981) Low dose intramuscular insulin therapy for diabetic ketoacidosis in dogs. *J. Am. Vet. Med. Assoc.*, **178**, 561–564.

MacIntire, D.K. (1995) Emergency therapy of diabetic crises: insulin overdose, diabetic ketoacidosis, and hyperosmolar coma. *Vet. Clin. North Am.*, **25**, 639–650.

Melendez, L.D. (1997) Diabetes mellitus, in *Veterinary Emergency Medicine Secrets* (ed. W. Wingfield), Hanley and Belfus, Philadelphia, pp. 253–258.

Koenig, A., Drobatz, K.J., Beale, A.B., King, L.G. (2004) Hyperglycemic, hyperosmolar syndrome in feline diabetics: 17 cases (1995–2001). *J. Vet. Emerg. Crit. Care*, **14** (1), 30–40.

Author: Margaret R. Kern DVM, DACVIM

chapter 28

Hyperparathyroidism

DEFINITION

- Hypersecretion of parathormone from the parathyroid glands resulting in hypercalcemia.

ETIOLOGY/PATHOPHYSIOLOGY

- Adenoma or less commonly hyperplasia or adenocarcinoma of the parathyroid glands.

Systems Affected

- Nervous
- Muscular
- Cardiac
- Gastrointestinal

SIGNALMENT/HISTORY

Risk Factors

- Older dogs and cats.
- Keeshound, Siberian husky and golden retriever.
- Siamese cats.

Historic Findings

- Lethargy.
- Weakness.
- Polydipsia and polyuria.
- Hematuria and stranguria.

Blackwell's Five-Minute Veterinary Consult Clinical Companion: Small Animal Endocrinology and Reproduction,
First Edition. Edited by Deborah S. Greco and Autumn P. Davidson. © 2017 John Wiley & Sons, Inc.
Published 2017 by John Wiley & Sons, Inc.
Companion Website: www.fiveminutevet.com/endocrinology

- Urolithiasis recurrent.
- Inappetance.
- Vomiting.
- Constipation.

 ## CLINICAL FEATURES

Physical Examination

- Listlessness.
- Muscle weakness.
- Cervical nodule (rarely palpable).
- Bradycardia (rare).

Clinical Pathology

- High total serum calcium.
- Low serum phosphorus.
- High plasma ionized calcium.

 ## DIFFERENTIAL DIAGNOSIS

- Hypercalcemia of malignancy
  - Lymphoma (LSA)
  - Apocrine gland tumor of the anal gland
  - Multiple myeloma
  - Squamous cell carcinoma (SCC)
  - Renal angiomyxoma
  - Thyroid carcinoma
  - Bone tumors
  - Thymoma
  - Mammary gland carcinoma/adenocarcinoma
  - Melanoma
  - Primary lung tumors
  - Chronic lymphocytic leukemia (CLL)
- Vitamin D toxicosis
- Renal disease
- Idiopathic hypercalcemia
- Hypoadrenocorticism
- Granulomatous disease
- Osteoporosis
- Multiple endocrine neoplasia (MEN) types 1 and 2

DIAGNOSTICS

Endocrine diagnostics

- PTH – high or inappropriately high.
- Ionized calcium – high.
- PTH-rp – low.

Imaging

- Ultrasound Fig. 28.1.
- Pertechnetate scan.

Pathological Findings

- Parathyroid adenoma.
- Less commonly, adenocarcinoma or hyperplasia (cats).

THERAPEUTICS

Drug(s) of Choice

- Emergency treatment of hypercalcemia
  - Saline fluids.
  - Lasix.
  - Bisphosphonates.

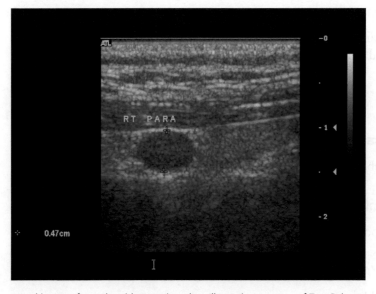

■ **Fig. 28.1.** Ultrasound image of parathyroid tumor in a dog. Illustration courtesy of Tom Baker.

Precautions/Interactions

■ Not available.

Alternative Drugs

■ Not available.

Appropriate Health Care

■ Not available.

Nursing Care

■ Postoperative monitoring for signs of hypocalcemia.

Diet

■ Good-quality diet.
■ Oral calcium postoperatively (see Hypoparathyroidism).
■ Oral Vitamin D2 or D3 (see Hypoparathyroidism).

Activity

■ Restricted postoperatively.

Surgical Considerations

■ Surgical parathyroidectomy.
■ Ultrasound guided heat ablation.

 COMMENTS

Client Education

■ Not available.

Patient Monitoring

■ 3–6 days postoperatively, monitor for signs of hypocalcemia.

Prevention/Avoidance

■ Not available.

Possible Complications

- Laryngeal nerve paralysis post surgical – especially if bilateral disease.

Expected Course and Prognosis

- Good prognosis with early diagnosis and treatment.

Synonyms

- None.

Abbreviations

PTH = Parathyroid hormone
LSA = Lymphosarcoma
SCC = Squamous cell carcinoma
CLL = Chronic lymphocytic leukemia

Suggested Reading

Greco, D.S. (2012) Endocrine causes of calcium disorders. *Top. Comp. Anim. Med.*, **27** (4), 150–145.

Author: Deborah S. Greco DVM, PhD, DACVIM

chapter 29

Hyperphosphatemia

DEFINITION

- Serum total phosphorus >5.5 mg/dl (dogs).
- Serum total phosphorus >6 mg/dl (cats).

ETIOLOGY/PATHOPHYSIOLOGY

- Control of phosphorus is complex and is influenced by the actions of PTH and vitamin D, and the interaction of these hormones with the gut, bone, kidneys, and parathyroid glands.
- High serum phosphorus results from excessive gastrointestinal absorption of phosphorus, excessive bone resorption of phosphorus, and reduced renal excretion of phosphorus.

Systems Affected

- Endocrine
- Metabolic
- Renal

SIGNALMENT/HISTORY

- Dogs and cats.
- Any age, but commonly young, growing animals or old animals with renal insufficiency.

CLINICAL FEATURES

Historic Findings

- Depends on the underlying cause of hyperphosphatemia.
- No specific signs directly attributable to hyperphosphatemia.
- Acute hyperphosphatemia causes hypocalcemic tetany and/or vascular collapse.

Blackwell's Five-Minute Veterinary Consult Clinical Companion: Small Animal Endocrinology and Reproduction, First Edition. Edited by Deborah S. Greco and Autumn P. Davidson. © 2017 John Wiley & Sons, Inc. Published 2017 by John Wiley & Sons, Inc.
Companion Website: www.fiveminutevet.com/endocrinology

Physical Examination Findings

- Chronic hyperphosphatemia causes calcification of soft tissues, resulting in chronic renal failure and tumoral calcinosis.

Causes

- Reduced glomerular filtration rate.
- Prerenal azotemia.
- Renal azotemia.
- Post-renal azotemia.
- Hyperphosphatemia secondary to excessive bone resorption or muscle breakdown.
- Young growing dogs.
- Hypoparathyroidism.
- Hypersomatotropism.
- Hyperphosphatemia caused by excessive gastrointestinal absorption of phosphorus.
- Osteolysis.
- Disuse osteoporosis.
- Osseous neoplasia.
- Hyperthyroidism.
- Phosphorus-containing enemas.
- Vitamin D toxicosis.
- Phosphorus dietary supplementation.
- Nutritional secondary hyperparathyroidism.

Risk Factors

- Renal disease.
- Use of phosphorus-containing enemas in small animals such as cats.

 DIFFERENTIAL DIAGNOSIS

Differential Diagnosis

- Hypoparathyroidism – also characterized by clinical signs of hypocalcemia such as seizures and tetany.
- Prerenal azotemia as a cause of hyperphosphatemia – associated with disease states that result in low cardiac output such as congestive heart failure, dehydration, hypoadrenocorticism, and shock.
- Renal insufficiency, either acute or chronic renal failure – attended by azotemia and abnormal findings on urinalysis (low urinary specific gravity).
- Young, growing animals – can have serum phosphorus concentrations twice those of adults.
- Vitamin D intoxication – history of vitamin D supplementation or ingestion of rodenticides (e.g., Rampage).

- Nutritional secondary hyperparathyroidism – history of dietary calcium–phosphorus imbalance.
- Hyperthyroidism in cats – clinical signs of weight loss, polyphagia, and polydipsia and polyuria.
- Hypersomatotropism – attended by a history of progesterone administration in dogs and insulin-resistant diabetes mellitus in cats.
- Non-azotemia tumoral calcinosis – observed in human beings as an autosomal dominant disorder; rare cause of hyperphosphatemia associated with large bone lesions.
- Jasmine toxicity – history of plant ingestion.
- Factitious.

DIAGNOSTICS

Laboratory Findings

Drugs That May Alter Laboratory Results
- Phosphorus-containing enemas.
- Intravenous potassium phosphate.
- Anabolic steroids.
- Furosemide.
- Hydrochlorothiazide.
- Minocycline.

Disorders That May Alter Laboratory Results
- Hemolysis and lipemia can falsely raise phosphorus concentrations.
- Collection in citrate, oxalate, or EDTA.

Valid If Run in Human Laboratory?
- Yes.

CBC/Biochemistry/Urinalysis
- Serum phosphorus >6 mg/dl.
- Low serum calcium in patients with primary hypoparathyroidism.
- High serum calcium in patients with vitamin D intoxication.
- Azotemia and isosthenuria help define degree of renal impairment.
- Hyperkalemia and hyponatremia suggest hypoadrenocorticism.

Other Laboratory Tests
- Serum PTH measurement – intact molecule and two-site assay methods have the greatest specificity; high-normal or high concentrations suggest primary hyperparathyroidism; low concentrations suggest neoplasia.

- Thyroxine concentrations – indicated in cats with hyperphosphatemia and clinical signs consistent with hyperthyroidism.
- Insulin-like growth factor 1 concentrations – indicated in dogs or cats with unexplained hyperphosphatemia and clinical signs consistent with acromegaly; IGF-1 concentrations are elevated in animals with hypersomatotropism.
- Vitamin D assays are not readily available.
- ACTH stimulation testing to confirm hypoadrenocorticism.

Imaging

- Abdominal radiography to assess renal size and symmetry.
- Renal ultrasonography to detect soft-tissue mineralization.
- Thyroid scan to rule out hyperthyroidism.
- Radiography of long bones to detect osteoporosis or neoplasia.

Diagnostic Procedures

- Renal biopsy

 # THERAPEUTICS

- Inpatient, because of the deleterious effects of hyperphosphatemia and the need for fluid therapy; consider severe hyperphosphatemia a medical emergency.
- Restrict dietary phosphorus.
- Normal saline is the fluid of choice.

Drug(s) of Choice

Acute Hyperphosphatemia
- Dextrose (1 g/kg IV) and insulin (0.5 U/kg IV).
- Avoid phosphorus-containing fluids.

Chronic Hyperphosphatemia
- Oral administration of phosphate binders (e.g., aluminum hydroxide or aluminum carbonate, 30–100 mg/kg/day PO with meals).

Contraindications

- Not available.

Precautions

- Not available.

Possible Interactions

- Not available.

Alternative Drug(s)

- Not available.

Patient Monitoring

- Monitor serum calcium every 12 hours.
- Renal function tests – urine output must be monitored, particularly if oliguric renal failure is suspected, in which case urine output should be measured carefully; oliguria cannot be determined unless the patient is fully hydrated.
- Hydration status – indicators of overhydration include increased body weight, increased central venous pressure, and edema (pulmonary or subcutaneous).

Possible Complications

- Hypophosphatemia resulting in hemolysis.
- Soft-tissue mineralization.

 # COMMENTS

Associated Conditions

- Hypocalcemia.

Age-Related Factors

- Mild elevations in phosphorus may be normal in growing animals.

Zoonotic Potential

- None.

Pregnancy/Fertility/Breeding

- Not available.

See Also

Hypoparathyroidism

Abbreviations

ACTH = adrenocorticotropic hormone
EDTA = ethylene diamine tetra-acetic acid
IGF-1 = insulin-like growth factor 1
PTH   = parathyroid hormone

Suggested Reading

Aurbach, G.D., Marx, S.J., Spiegel, A.M. (1985) Parathyroid hormone, calcitonin, and the calciferols, in *Williams Textbook of Endocrinology*, 7th edition (eds J.D. Wilson, D.W. Foster DW), Saunders, Philadelphia, pp. 1208–1209.
Willard, M.D., Tvedten, H., Turnwald, G.H. (1989) *Clinical Diagnosis by Laboratory Methods*. Saunders, Philadelphia.

Author: Deborah S. Greco DVM, PhD, DACVIM

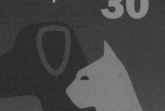

Hypersomatotropism and Acromegaly in the Dog

chapter 30

DEFINITION

- Hypersomatotropism (HS) is defined as the pathological overproduction of growth hormone (GH).and GH-induced insulin-like growth factor-1 (IGF-1), causing several pathological changes known as the clinical syndrome of acromegaly.

ETIOLOGY/PATHOPHYSIOLOGY

- Acromegaly in the dog is usually caused by chronic GH secretion from hyperplasia of mammary tissue resulting from endogenous (diestrus) or exogenous progestins.
- Rarely, pituitary adenomas, similar to the cause in humans and cats, may be the cause of acromegaly in the dog.

Systems Affected

- Endocrine/Metabolic
  - HS induces insulin resistance and subsequent pancreatic beta-cell dysfunction and failure, resulting in diabetes mellitus.
  - Diabetes mellitus which may be reversible if the HS is treated definitively.
  - Weight gain.
  - Total protein concentrations have been shown to be significantly elevated.
- Reproductive
  - Mammary enlargement due to hyperplasia; mammary tumors.
  - Diestrus.
- Musculoskeletal
  - The anabolic effects of excess GH and IGF-1 can induce a range of changes including broad facial features, big (clubbed) paws, arthropathies (in extreme, longstanding cases joint collapse) and protrusion of lower jaw (prognathia inferior).

Blackwell's Five-Minute Veterinary Consult Clinical Companion: Small Animal Endocrinology and Reproduction, First Edition. Edited by Deborah S. Greco and Autumn P. Davidson. © 2017 John Wiley & Sons, Inc. Published 2017 by John Wiley & Sons, Inc.
Companion Website: www.fiveminutevet.com/endocrinology

- **Respiratory**
  - Anabolic effects can also induce soft tissue thickening in the upper airway which commonly leads to respiratory stridor.
- **Nervous**
  - The poorly controlled diabetes can result in a state of lethargy.
  - Mentation changes may also more rarely be associated with the expansion of the slow-growing pituitary adenoma (rare).

 # SIGNALMENT/HISTORY

- Intact female dogs

Risk Factors

- Treatment with exogenous progestins (e.g., ovaban, proligestone).

Historic Findings

- Dogs are usually presented with signs referable to diabetes mellitus, i.e., polydipsia, polyuria and polyphagia.
- Weight gain is common despite the uncontrolled diabetes.
- In many cases the diabetes mellitus proves difficult to control even with high doses of insulin.

 # CLINICAL FEATURES

Physical examination

- Broad facial features.
- Prognathia inferior (protrusion of lower jaw).
- Clubbed (big) paws.
- Cranial abdominal organomegaly.
- Mammary tumor or hyperplasia.
- Respiratory stridor.
- Lethargy.
- Overall large stature.

 # DIFFERENTIAL DIAGNOSIS

- Polydipsia/polyuria
  - Hyperadrenocorticism
  - Gestational diabetes
  - Diabetes insipidus

- Weight gain
  - Hypothyroidism
- Stridor
  - Laryngeal paralysis

 ## DIAGNOSTICS

- History of progestin therapy for estrus suppression
- Intact bitch with clinical signs consistent with acromegaly.
- Serum total IGF-1 is the initial screening test of choice (72–165 ng/ml).
- Elevated serum GH (0.5–3 ng/ml).
- Rule out hyperadrenocorticism (LDDS, ACTH stim) and hypothyroidism (TT4, FT4, eTSH).

Pathological Findings

- Mammary hyperplasia, diestrus uterus/ovaries.
- The main finding that dogs with HS caused by a pituitary tumor containing acidophils (GH producing cells in pars distalis of the anterior pituitary).

 ## THERAPEUTICS

Drug(s)

- Discontinue exogenous progestins.

Surgery

- Ovariohysterectomy if endogenous progestins are involved.
- Hypophysectomy if pituitary adenoma.
- A trans-sphenoidal approach is currently preferred.

Radiotherapy

- In a proportion of cases radiation therapy is able to reduce the size of pituitary adenoma as well as reduce the excess hormone secretion.
- Radiation does not usually normalize GH and IGF-1 concentrations in contrast to hypophysectomy.

 ## COMMENTS

Expected Course and Prognosis

- Excellent after OHE or discontinuation of exogenous progestins.
- If diagnosed and treated early, diabetic remission will be achieved in most patients.

Abbreviations

TT4 = Total thyroxine
FT4 = Free thyroxine
TSH = Thyroid stimulating hormone
HS = hypersomatotropism
GH = growth hormone
IGF-1 = Insulin-like growth factor 1

See Also

Feline Hypersomatotropism

Suggested Reading

Eigenmann, J.E., Venker-van Haagen, A.J. (1981) Progestagen-induced and spontaneous canine acromegaly due to reversible growth hormone overproduction: Clinical picture and pathogenesis. *J. Am. Anim. Hosp. Assoc.*, **17**, 813–822.

Eigenmann, J.E., Eigenmann, R.Y., Rijnberk, A., *et al.* (1983) Progesterone-controlled growth hormone overproduction and naturally occurring canine diabetes and acromegaly. *Acta Endocrinol. (Copenh.)*, **104**, 167–176.

Selman, P.J., Mol, J.A., Rutteman, G.R., *et al.* (1994) Progestin-induced growth hormone excess in the dog originates in the mammary gland. *Endocrinology*, **134**, 287–292.

Mol, J.A., van Garderen, E., Selman, P.J., *et al.* (1995) Growth hormone mRNA in mammary gland tumors of dogs and cats. *J. Clin. Invest.*, **95**, 2028–2034.

Mol, J.A., Lantinga-van Leeuwen, I., van Garderen, E., *et al.* (2000) Progestin-induced mammary growth hormone (GH) production. *Adv. Exp. Med. Biol.*, **480**, 71–76.

Rijnberk, A., Mol, J.A. (1997) Progestin-induced hypersecretion of growth hormone: an introductory review. *J. Reprod. Fertil. Suppl.*, **51**, 335–338.

van Garderen, E., de Wit, M., Voorhout, W.F., *et al.* (1997) Expression of growth hormone in canine mammary tissue and mammary tumors. Evidence for a potential autocrine/paracrine stimulatory loop. *Am. J. Pathol.*, **150**, 1037–1047.

Murai, A., Nishii, N., Morita, T., *et al.* (2012) GH-producing mammary tumors in two dogs with acromegaly. *J. Vet. Med. Sci.*, **74**, 771–774.

Author: Deborah S. Greco DVM, PhD, DACVIM

chapter 31

Hypersomatotropism and Acromegaly in the Cat

DEFINITION

- Hypersomatotropism (HS) is defined as the pathological overproduction of growth hormone (GH).
- In the cat, HS is caused by either a pituitary tumor or pituitary hyperplasia.
- Chronic exposure to the catabolic and anabolic effects of excess GH, as well as the anabolic effects of GH-induced insulin-like growth factor-1 (IGF-1), ultimately induces several pathological changes known as the clinical syndrome of acromegaly.

ETIOLOGY/PATHOPHYSIOLOGY

- HS in the cat is usually caused by a functional adenoma or, more rarely, carcinoma or hyperplasia of the pars distalis of the pituitary producing excess GH.
- The excess GH has a host of anabolic and catabolic effects and also induces IGF-1 production, mainly by the liver, which is mainly anabolic in nature.
- The combined effects of both GH and IGF-1 eventually lead to the clinical syndrome of acromegaly.
- Initially, however, cats will not have apparent physical changes and clinical signs associated with the induction of diabetes mellitus are often the first and only presenting complaints patients are presented with.
- Although HS was previously thought to be rare, it has recently been estimated that up to one in three or four diabetic cats in fact have HS-induced diabetes mellitus. It is therefore possible that currently many cats with HS are misdiagnosed as regular diabetics and therefore miss out on appropriate treatment and prognostication.
- The diabetes mellitus in cats with HS is caused by the insulin resistance induced by excess GH, which ultimately also leads to beta-cell dysfunction and failure.
- In the long-run, the excess GH and IGF-1 will cause classical changes to occur in the physique of cats, including broad facial features, protrusion of the lower jaw (prognathia inferior), big (clubbed) paws, hepatomegaly and renomegaly.

Blackwell's Five-Minute Veterinary Consult Clinical Companion: Small Animal Endocrinology and Reproduction, First Edition. Edited by Deborah S. Greco and Autumn P. Davidson. © 2017 John Wiley & Sons, Inc. Published 2017 by John Wiley & Sons, Inc. Companion Website: www.fiveminutevet.com/endocrinology

- Any diabetic with poor glycemic control yet weight gain instead of weight loss should be suspected of suffering from HS.
- It could also be argued that in light of its prevalence and impact on treatment and prognosis, all diabetic cats should be screened for HS.

SYSTEMS AFFECTED

- Endocrine/Metabolic
  - HS induces insulin resistance and subsequent pancreatic beta-cell dysfunction and failure, resulting in diabetes mellitus.
  - Diabetes mellitus is often the first disease to be diagnosed, whereas other consequences of HS (discussed below) are usually only witnessed after a longer-standing history of HS.
  - The diabetes is, at least initially, reversible in nature if the HS is treated definitively.
  - Weight gain occurs frequently, which should ring alarm bells about the possible presence of HS in any poorly controlled diabetic cat, which normally present with weight loss.
  - Total protein concentrations have been shown to be significantly elevated in cats with HS compared to regular diabetic cats.
- Musculoskeletal
  - The anabolic effects of excess GH and IGF-1 can induce a range of changes including broad facial features, big (clubbed) paws, arthropathies (in extreme, longstanding cases joint collapse) and protrusion of lower jaw (prognathia inferior).
  - The insulin resistance often causes the resulting diabetes to be poorly controlled despite insulin therapy which can result in diabetic neuropathy displayed by a plantigrade stance of the hind limbs.
- Cardiovascular
  - The anabolic effects of excess GH and IGF-1 are thought to be responsible for a higher prevalence of cardiomyopathies and possible resulting heart failure.
  - Controversy exists over whether hypertension is more common among cats with HS.
  - Nevertheless, cats with HS are usually middle-aged to older and therefore should be checked for hypertension regularly and ideally also associated retinal changes.
- Respiratory
  - Anabolic effects can also induce soft-tissue thickening in the upper airway which commonly leads to respiratory stridor (frequently reported by owners as snoring) and, rarely, airway collapse in longstanding cases.
  - HS-associated cardiac changes can result in congestive heart failure and thus tachynea and dyspnea.
- Nervous
  - The poorly controlled diabetes can result in a state of lethargy.
  - Mentation changes may also more rarely be associated with the expansion of the slow growing pituitary adenoma.
  - The latter can also result in seizures and blindness.

- Gastrointestinal
  - Many cats with HS show polyphagia, which can be more extreme than in regular diabetics.
  - The polyphagia can result in large stools.
- Hepatobiliary-pancreas
  - Cranial abdominal organomegaly, including hepatomegaly is frequently noticed.
  - Elevation of hepatic enzymes occurs and is thought to be secondary to the induced diabetes mellitus.
  - HS is suspected to be associated with a high rate of pancreatic changes, including pancreatic nodular hyperplasia.
- Renal/urologic
  - Renomegaly is common in longstanding cases.
  - Renal dysfunction occurs among cats with HS, although it remains to be proven if its frequency is significantly higher than in the general geriatric cat population.
  - Urinary tract infections should be regularly excluded, given their assumed higher prevalence among diabetic cats.
- Ophthalmic
  - Retinal changes might occur due to age-associated hypertension (although hypertension has previously been suggested to occur more frequently in cats with HS).
  - Vision might ultimately be lost due to a large pituitary mass impinging on the optic chiasm.

 ## SIGNALMENT/HISTORY

- Most cats have been described to be middle-aged to older male neutered domestic short-haired cats. However, a range of breeds have been shown to be affected by this endocrinopathy.
- The youngest cats described thus far was 6 years of age.
- The median age of cats with HS is 11 years.
- A genetic basis has not yet been discovered.

Risk Factors

- Unknown.

Historic Findings

- Cats are usually presented with signs referable to diabetes mellitus, i.e., polydipsia, polyuria and polyphagia.
- The polyphagia in some cases is extreme.
- Weight gain is common despite the uncontrolled diabetes.
- In many cases the diabetes mellitus proves difficult to control even with high doses of insulin.
- Cats might display diabetic neuropathy and a resulting plantigrade stance.

- Only rarely will owners report physical changes to have occurred, even when they seem apparent to the clinician.
- The latter emphasizes the subtle nature of such changes and/or gradual onset, as well as owners' difficulties in spotting such changes.
- Rare cases present with central nervous system signs (seizures, depression), blindness or respiratory problems (due to soft-tissue thickening of the airways or congestive heart failure).

 ## CLINICAL FEATURES

- Interestingly, only 24% of clinicians suspected the presence of HS in diabetic cats found to have a serum IGF-1 >1000 ng/ml (an indicator strongly suggesting HS; see below).
- This suggests the likely presence of a subtle phenotype in a majority of cases in the first phases of the disease.
- Physical examination might be indistinguishable from any other diabetic cat.
- In longer-standing cases findings might include:
  - Broad facial features (Figs 31.1 and 31.2).
  - Prognathia inferior (protrusion of lower jaw).
  - Clubbed (big) paws.
  - Cranial abdominal organomegaly.

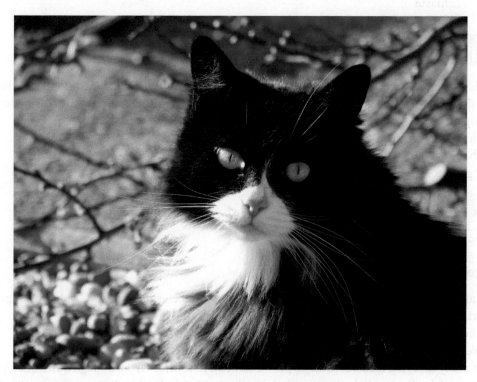

■ **Fig. 31.1.** Facial features of a cat prior to the onset of HS-induced acromegaly.

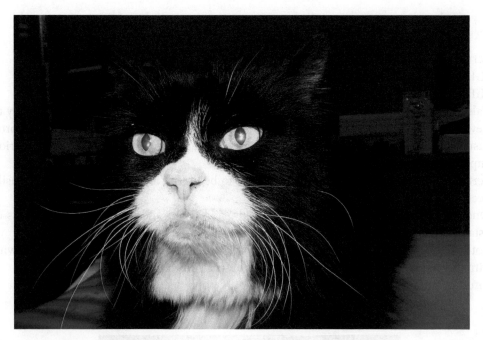

■ **Fig. 31.2.** Facial features of the cat in Fig. 31.1 after the onset of HS-induced acromegaly.

- Heart murmur.
- Respiratory stridor.
- Plantigrade stance hind limbs.
- Lethargy.
- Overall large stature.

 ## DIFFERENTIAL DIAGNOSIS

- Since HS is associated with diabetes mellitus, any other disease causing secondary diabetes mellitus as well as primary diabetes mellitus are relevant differential diagnoses.
- Secondary diabetes mellitus associated with hyperadrenocorticism is a particularly important differential diagnosis since it is also associated with insulin-resistant diabetes mellitus and (most commonly) a pituitary tumor.
- However, the insulin resistance associated with HS tends to be more extreme than in hyperadrenocorticism.
- Cases with hyperadrenocorticism might also show other typical signs including coat color changes, fragile skin syndrome, bruising and muscle loss.
- Hyperadrenocorticism more commonly presents with a 'catabolic picture' including weight loss rather than the predominantly 'anabolic picture' including weight gain, seen with HS.
- A low-dose dexamethasone suppression test (using 0.1 mg/kg dexamethasone) can be helpful to differentiate cases, although false positives can be seen in any ill or stressed cat (including those suffering from HS).

DIAGNOSTICS

- Serum total IGF-1 is for many the initial screening test of choice.
- IGF-1 is induced by GH and mainly produced in the liver.
- IGF-1 reflects the GH secretion over the past 24 hours.
- False-positive and false-negative IGF-1 results can be seen though, the latter especially in newly diagnosed diabetics since IGF-1 production is dependent on the presence of portal insulin. IGF-1 might therefore prove low prior to or early into the insulin treatment period (up to 8 weeks after starting insulin).
- Serum and plasma GH have also been shown to be useful, although assays are not easily accessible.
- Once a suspicion of HS has been established using IGF-1 and/or GH, the next step is to establish whether there is a pituitary abnormality.
- Both CT and MRI are useful for this purpose, although microadenomas and cases with pituitary hyperplasia might show normal brain imaging (Fig. 31.3).
- Pituitary imaging also enables the planning of hypophysectomy and radiotherapy.

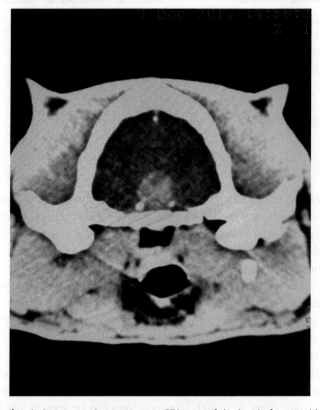

■ **Fig. 31.3.** Presence of a pituitary tumor in a transverse CT-image of the head of a cat with HS. The tumor is the contrast-enhancing protrusion beyond the rim of the sella turcica at the base of the skull.

Pathological Findings

- The main finding that cats with HS have in common constitutes a pituitary adenoma of the acidophils (GH-producing cells in pars distalis of the anterior pituitary).
- Rarely, acidophilic hyperplasia or an acidophilic carcinoma is found. Additionally, in long-standing cases GH- and IGF-1-induced changes can be observed, including hypertrophy of the myocardium.

 # THERAPEUTICS

- Ideally, the HS is treated definitively by removing the pituitary tumor (hypophysectomy). Alternatively, the tumor can be reduced in size and function by radiation therapy or inhibited by drugs. A conservative approach consists of only treating the resulting diabetes mellitus.

Surgery

- Hypophysectomy is considered the treatment of choice in human hypersomatotropism.
- It has also proven to be the only consistently effective and reliable method to cure HS in cats.
- An experienced neurosurgeon and appropriate pre-, peri-, and postoperative care are essential for success.
- A trans-sphenoidal approach is currently preferred (incising the soft palate).
- In the long-run, cats need to be supplemented with thyroid hormone and a glucocorticoids; synthetic ADH (DDAVP) supplementation can often be ceased with 6–8 weeks postoperatively.
- When performed early in the disease process, diabetic remission is a realistic outcome and often occurs within 2 months after the procedure.

Drug(s)

- Somatostatins and dopamine agonists have been used to try to inhibit GH secretion by the pituitary, mostly unsuccessfully.
- Recently, a novel somatostatin analog Pasireotide® (Novartis, Basel, Switzerland) has been shown to be effective at achieving this, although further research is required to evaluate the use of this drug, including dosing regimens, in the long run.

Radiotherapy

- In a proportion of cases radiation therapy is able to reduce the size of pituitary adenoma as well as reduce the excess hormone secretion.
- Some cats even achieve diabetic remission.
- Several important disadvantages are associated with this treatment option, including: high costs, need for multiple anesthetics, and especially, the variable and unpredictable response.

- Radiation does not usually normalize GH and IGF-1 concentrations, in contrast to hypophysectomy.

Palliative treatment

- When definitive treatment is not possible, the focus should lie on gaining more control of the diabetes mellitus and treating possible comorbidities.
- Eventually, most cats tend to need high dosages of insulin and/or combinations of short-acting and long-acting insulin types to ensure an adequate quality of life for both pet and owner.
- Nevertheless, a minority achieve an adequate quality of life.
- Regular veterinary assessment is recommended.
- Iatrogenic hypoglycemia is a major concern given the pulsatile nature of GH secretion (and therefore associated insulin resistance).
- Home monitoring of blood glucose concentrations can prove very useful to avoid under- and especially overdosage.

 COMMENTS

- A diagnosis of HS in a diabetic cat has great implications on treatment and prognosis.
- Given the newly uncovered prevalence of HS among diabetic cats, screening diabetic cats for HS using IGF-1 can prove a wise investment.
- Since false-negatives can occur in the first 6–8 weeks of insulin treatment, clinicians can either choose to measure IGF-1 after 8 weeks of treatment or check immediately. Measurements should be repeated if the value proves low at the initial check.

Expected Course and Prognosis

- If diagnosed and treated effectively early, diabetic remission will be achieved in most patients and ensure a normal quality of life with good life expectancy.
- Even if diabetic remission does not occur, effective HS treatment can ensure more stable glycemia with more conservative insulin dosages.
- Given the slow-growing nature of most tumors and the relatively shorter life expectancy of cats (versus humans), most cats will enjoy a normal life expectancy when treated successfully with hypophysectomy.
- A proportion of cats treated successfully with radiotherapy will show a relapse of the disease months to years after treatment. Some will not be treated effectively with radiotherapy in the first place.
- Continuous quality of life assessment is crucial to ensure the patient is managed in the most appropriate way, especially if the HS is not being treated definitively.
- When non-definitive treatment is applied, HS-induced acromegalic changes will eventually lead to the demise of the patient, which might include congestive heart failure, upper-airway occlusion and suspected GH- and IGF-1-induced neoplasia.

■ In many cases, quality of life changes related to uncontrolled diabetes mellitus will lead to a decision of euthanasia in the long-run if the HS is not being treated directly.

Abbreviations

HS   = hypersomatotropism
GH   = growth hormone
IGF-1 = Insulin-like growth factor 1

See Also

Diabetes Mellitus without Complication – Cats

Suggested Reading

Berg, R.I., Nelson, R.W., Feldman, E.C., *et al.* (2007) Serum insulin-like growth factor-I concentration in cats with diabetes mellitus and acromegaly. *J. Vet. Intern. Med.*, **21** (5), 892–898.

Niessen, S.J., Khalid, M., Petrie, G., *et al.* (2007) Validation and application of an ovine radioimmunoassay for the diagnosis of feline acromegaly. *Veterinary Record*, **160**, 902–907.

Niessen, S.J., Petrie, G., Gaudiano, F., *et al.* (2007) Feline acromegaly: an underdiagnosed endocrinopathy? *J. Vet. Intern. Med.*, **21** (5), 899–905.

Niessen, S.J. (2010) Feline acromegaly: an essential differential diagnosis for the difficult diabetic. *J. Feline Med. Surg.*, **12** (1), 15–23.

Niessen, S.J., Forcada, Y., Jensen, K., *et al.* (2011) Routine screening of diabetic cats for acromegaly: overdue or overkill? *J. Vet. Intern. Med.*, **25**,1489–1490.

Niessen, S.J., Church, D.B., Forcada, Y. (2013) Hypersomatotropism, Acromegaly, and Hyperadrenocorticism and Feline Diabetes Mellitus. *Vet. Clin. North Am. Small Anim.*, **43** (2), 319–350.

Author: Stijn J. Niessen DVM, PhD, DECVIM

chapter 32

Hyperthyroidism

DEFINITION

- Hyperthyroidism (thyrotoxicosis) is a multisystemic disorder resulting from excessive circulating concentrations of the active thyroid hormones triiodothyronine (T3) and thyroxine (T4).
- Most common endocrine disease of cats, affecting 10% of all cats older than 10 years of age. The incidence of hyperthyroidism appears to be increasing in this species.
- Most cats have benign lesions of their thyroid gland (adenomatous hyperplasia or adenoma) that are responsible for the hyperthyroid state.
- Rare disease in dogs. In contrast to cats, spontaneous hyperthyroidism generally occurs in dogs with thyroid carcinoma. More often, hyperthyroidism develops in dogs that are over-supplemented with exogenous thyroid hormone.

ETIOLOGY/PATHOPHYSIOLOGY

- Benign adenomatous hyperplasia (adenoma) of one (30%) or both (70%) thyroid lobes is the most common pathological abnormality associated with hyperthyroidism in cats, occurring in 96–98% of cases.
- Thyroid carcinoma is a rare cause of hyperthyroidism in cats, accounting for approximately 2–4% of cats.
- Extremely uncommon in dogs, it is most commonly seen in some dogs with thyroid carcinoma (most dogs with thyroid gland neoplasia are euthyroid) and in dogs given excessive doses of exogenous thyroid hormone.

Systems Affected

- Metabolic – metabolic rate, weight loss despite increase in appetite.
- Musculoskeletal – cachexia, muscle wasting.
- Cardiovascular – tachycardia, cardiac murmurs, myocardial hypertrophy and hypertension.
- Respiratory – tachypnea, dyspnea.

Blackwell's Five-Minute Veterinary Consult Clinical Companion: Small Animal Endocrinology and Reproduction, First Edition. Edited by Deborah S. Greco and Autumn P. Davidson. © 2017 John Wiley & Sons, Inc. Published 2017 by John Wiley & Sons, Inc.
Companion Website: www.fiveminutevet.com/endocrinology

- Gastrointestinal – vomiting, diarrhea, decreased gastrointestinal transit time, and malabsorption in some animals.
- Hepatobiliary – high liver function tests.
- Renal/urologic – high GFR may mask underlying chronic renal failure, possible hyperfiltration injury, and decreased urine-concentrating ability.
- Nervous – nervousness, restlessness, or aggressive behavior.
- Behavioral – psychogenic alopecia, miliary dermatitis.

 # SIGNALMENT/HISTORY

- Hyperthyroidism most commonly occurs in middle-aged to older cats with a median age of 12–13 years.
- Only 5% of hyperthyroid cats are less than 10 years of age.
- There is no obvious breed susceptibility. Two genetically related breeds (Siamese and Himalayan) and purebred cats have been reported to be at decreased risk of developing hyperthyroidism.
- Male and female cats are affected equally.

Risk Factors

- To date, the underlying etiology responsible for the thyroid changes remains obscure and is probably multifactorial. Advancing age certainly increases the risk of developing this disease.
- In addition, studies have indicated the following environmental and nutritional risk factors, which may play a role in the pathogenesis of this disorder:
  - Diet composed entirely or primarily of canned cat food.
  - Certain varieties of canned cat good (fish, liver, or giblet flavor).
  - Cans with plastic linings and pop-top lids may pose a greater risk than sachets or cans that require a can opener to open them. This is potentially due to the release of chemicals such as bisphenol-A and bisphenol-F from the lacquer linings of the pop-top cans.
  - Diets containing either excess or deficient amounts of iodine have been implicated.
  - Regular use of insecticidal products (flea products) on the cat or fly sprays within the household.
  - Exposure to herbicides and fertilizers.
  - Exposure to flame-retardant chemicals contaminants including polybrominated diphenyl ethers (PBDEs). Excessive PBDEs have been identified in household dust from contaminated carpet padding, polyurethane foams, furniture and mattresses.

Historic Findings

- Weight loss – Loss of body weight is the most commonly recognized sign of hyperthyroidism in cats. Hyperthyroidism is so common that it should always be considered in cats that have lost weight, whether supporting signs such as tachycardia are present or not.

- Polyphagia – The weight loss seen in cats with hyperthyroidism is often associated with an increased appetite. However, some cats maintain a normal appetite, or even develop a reduced appetite.
- Gastrointestinal signs – not uncommon in cats with hyperthyroidism. Vomiting may be associated with rapid overeating; diarrhea is most likely due to intestinal hypermotility, although malabsorption may also play a role.
- Hyperactivity – Nervousness, restlessness, or aggressive behavior may be apparent in some hyperthyroid cats. These signs may be more obvious when attempts are made to restrain the cat and are, therefore, often more noticeable to veterinarians than to owners themselves.
- Anxiety and restlessness – Night-time yowling, aimless pacing, or easily interrupted sleep patterns sometimes develop. This presumably reflects a state of confusion, anxiety and nervousness in these cats.
- Skin changes – Cutaneous signs that often develop in hyperthyroid cats include a dull or matted hair coat. Some hyperthyroid cats can groom obsessively, resulting in alopecia of the ventral abdomen or caudal thighs.
- Polyuria and polydipsia – Increased thirst or urination, or both, occur in about half of hyperthyroid cats and can be severe in some cats. Various mechanisms may be responsible, including concurrent primary renal dysfunction, renal medullary washout because of increased renal blood flow, and primary polydipsia because of a hypothalamic disturbance.

 CLINICAL FEATURES

Physical Examination Findings

- Large thyroid gland – 70% of cats have bilateral thyroid nodules.
- Poor body condition – weight loss, muscle wasting.
- Unkempt appearance – cachexia, hair matting.
- Heart murmur – hyperthyroid cardiac murmurs are associated with dynamic right and left ventricular outflow obstruction rather than primary mitral or tricuspid regurgitation. Hyperthyroidism is probably the single most important factor for the development of murmurs in older cats.
- Tachycardia – A powerful apex beat and rapid heart rate (>240 beats per minute) are relatively common, found in about half of hyperthyroid cats.
- Gallop rhythms and other arrhythmias, such as ectopic atrial and ventricular arrhythmias can occasionally be detected.
- Hypertension – Mild to moderate hypertension can be observed, but when present this may simply reflect the reduced tolerance of hyperthyroid cats to stressful situations such as the veterinary examination ('white-coat' phenomenon).

 DIFFERENTIAL DIAGNOSIS

- Because the clinical signs of hyperthyroidism in cats can be so variable and generally affect many body systems, a number of differential diagnoses must be considered in cats having a possible diagnosis of hyperthyroidism. These diseases include the following:

- Diabetes mellitus.
- Chronic kidney disease.
- Hepatic disease.
- Gastrointestinal disease.
- Neoplasia.
- Primary cardiac disease (cardiomyopathy).
- Cardiac disease secondary of other conditions (e.g., hypertension, acromegaly, etc.).
- Anxiety-related misbehavior.

DIAGNOSTICS

- In addition to the characteristic physical examination findings, a routine laboratory work-up, including a complete blood count, serum chemistry analysis, and complete urinalysis, are recommended in the work-up of all cats with suspected hyperthyroidism. Often, this database simply lends support to the diagnosis, but these screening tests are most useful if concurrent disorders are present and an accurate prognosis is required. Specific thyroid function tests, especially a total serum T4 determination, are necessary to confirm a diagnosis.

Palpation of the Thyroid Nodule

- All cats with hyperthyroidism have a thyroid nodule affecting one or both lobes, since all of these cats have underlying thyroid pathology leading to their disease (e.g., thyroid adenomatous hyperplasia, adenoma, or carcinoma). Therefore, a palpable cervical thyroid nodule (goiter) is present in most, if not all, cats with hyperthyroidism, and the presence of a goiter plays a key role in diagnosis of these cats. Thyroid gland palpation is an important noninvasive and inexpensive diagnostic tool, and should be a standard part of the physical examination of all cats, but especially in those older than 10 years of age, when hyperthyroidism becomes more prevalent.
- There are two general techniques used to palpate the thyroid gland in cats, both of which can and should be used to perform thyroid palpation. In my experience, it is not uncommon to miss a thyroid nodule with one technique but pick up a nodule with the second technique on the same examination.
  - With the classic palpation technique: the cat is restrained in a sitting position and the front legs held still. The neck of the cat is extended, and the clinician's thumb and index finger are placed on each side of the trachea and swept downwards from the larynx to the sternal manubrium. Palpation of a mobile subcutaneous nodule or a 'blip' that slips under the fingertips determines the presence of a goiter.
  - With the alternative technique, the clinician is positioned directly behind the standing cat. The head of the cat is raised and turned (45°) alternatively to the right or left, away from the side that is assessed (i.e., to palpate the right

thyroid lobe, turn the cat's head to the left). The tip of the clinician's index finger is placed in the groove formed by the trachea and sternothyroid muscle just below the larynx and then moved downwards in the groove to the thoracic inlet). If the thyroid lobe is enlarged, a characteristic 'blip' is felt as the index finger passes the goiter.

Hematology (Complete Blood Count)

- Hematological findings are usually non-specific and mostly not clinically important.
  - Mild erythrocytosis is fairly common.
  - Less commonly, leukocytosis, lymphopenia, and eosinopenia – all represent a stress response associated with hyperthyroid state.
  - Anemia, when present, is almost never caused by the hyperthyroid state and a search for another cause should be undertaken.

Serum Chemistry Profile

- Serum biochemistry abnormalities are common in cats with hyperthyroidism.
  - Mild to marked increases in the serum activities of many liver enzymes, including alanine aminotransferase (ALT) and alkaline phosphatase (ALP) are the most common and striking biochemical abnormalities of feline hyperthyroidism. These high liver enzyme abnormalities are more common in cats with severe hyperthyroidism, and return to normal upon successful treatment of hyperthyroidism.
  - Before treatment, mild to moderate increases in serum concentrations of urea and creatinine may be found in just over 20% of hyperthyroid cats. Such a prevalence of concurrent renal dysfunction or chronic kidney disease (CKD) is not unexpected in a group of older or aged cats.
  - These abnormalities, particularly the high urea concentration, may be exacerbated by the increased protein intake and protein catabolism of hyperthyroidism.
  - On the other hand, in hyperthyroid cats without concurrent CKD or azotemia, circulating creatinine concentrations are lowered, which may be related in part to a loss of muscle mass.
  - However, this lowering of serum creatinine (and urea in some cats) is primarily the result of the increase in glomerular filtration rate (GFR) that occurs in hyperthyroid cats. These effects have implications in assessing the presence of primary renal dysfunction in hyperthyroid cats (see below).

Complete Urinalysis

- Urinalysis is generally unremarkable but is useful in differentiating other diseases with similar clinical signs such as diabetes mellitus.
  - The urine specific gravity is variable, but concurrent (masked) renal disease should be considered in all cats that have values <1.040. Cats with concurrent CKD can occasionally have values >1.040, but most cats have less-concentrated urine.

- Mild proteinuria is commonly observed and may reflect glomerular hypertension and hyperfiltration or differences in tubular handling of protein. Proteinuria found on routine urinalysis should be confirmed by measuring the urine protein-to-creatinine ratio.
  - □ Normal cats have a UPC ratio of less than 0.2, where many hyperthyroid cats have borderline high (0.2-0.4) or overt proteinuria (>0.4).
  - □ Such proteinuria resolves upon successful treatment of hyperthyroidism.

Chest Radiography

- Thoracic radiography is useful in assessing the severity of cardiac disease.
  - Mild to severe cardiac enlargement is evident in about half of hyperthyroid cats.
  - In the vast majority of cats, this is a secondary type of cardiomegaly and is reversible with correction of the hyperthyroid state.
  - With severe hyperthyroidism, cats may develop congestive heart failure, as evidenced by pleural effusion and pulmonary edema on thoracic radiography.
  - Dogs generally do not develop clinical heart disease, but thoracic radiography should always be performed to look for pulmonary metastasis from a thyroid carcinoma (most hyperthyroid dogs have thyroid cancer).

Chest and Abdominal Ultrasonography

- Echocardiography may be useful in assessing the severity of cardiac disease.
  - The most common echocardiographic findings in hyperthyroid cats include left ventricular hypertrophy, left atrial and ventricular dilation, and interventricular septum hypertrophy.
    - □ Most of these changes are subtle and are of little clinical relevance.
    - □ Increased fractional shortening (reflecting increased cardiac contractility) common and invariably normalizes upon successful treatment of the hyperthyroidism.
  - Abdominal ultrasound may be useful to explore underlying renal disease and rule out other causes of weight loss (liver or gastrointestinal disease).

Thyroid Scintigraphy (Thyroid Imaging)

- Thyroid scintigraphy provides valuable information regarding both thyroid anatomy and physiology and can play an integral role in the diagnosis, staging, and management of thyroid disease in cats.
  - Thyroid gland scintigraphy can be used to confirm hyperthyroidism, which is very useful in cats in which a thyroid nodule cannot be palpated.
    - □ Thyroid scintigraphy is considered the 'gold standard' for diagnosing mild hyperthyroidism in cats.
    - □ With thyroid imaging (scintigraphy), hyperthyroid cats usually exhibit increased thyroidal uptake of radioisotope: radioactive iodine (123-I or 131-I) or technetium-99M as pertechnetate (99m-TcO$_4^-$).

□ Percentage uptake or increased thyroid:salivary ratio may be calculated, and both are strongly correlated with circulating thyroid hormone concentration and provide a sensitive means of diagnosing hyperthyroidism.
- Thyroid imaging also helps determine the location of abnormal thyroid tissue.
  □ In addition to visualization of functional cervical thyroid nodules, thyroid scintigraphy will detect ectopic thyroid tissue, which can be located anywhere from the base of the tongue to the heart.
  □ Thyroid imaging can locate large tumors that gravity has pulled into the thoracic cavity, which cannot be palpated on physical examination.
- Thyroid scintigraphy also provides valuable information in the diagnosis and evaluation of hyperthyroid cats with thyroid carcinoma.
- However, apart from expense and the difficulties in dealing with radioisotopes, few veterinarians have access to the nuclear medicine equipment needed to obtain thyroid images or perform thyroid uptake determinations.

Thyroid Function Tests

- Confirming the diagnosis of hyperthyroidism requires use of one or more thyroid function tests to demonstrate increased production of circulating thyroid hormones or suppressed pituitary thyroid-stimulating hormone secretion. High circulating thyroid hormone concentrations (T4 and T3) are the biochemical hallmarks of hyperthyroidism, and are extremely specific for its diagnosis. Methods for their measurement are readily accessible, relatively cheap, and do not involve specific sampling requirements.
- Serum total T4 concentration – measures for protein-bound and free (unbound) T4; a high resting concentration confirms the diagnosis of hyperthyroidism.
  - Serum total T4 is preferable as a screening test for hyperthyroidism, with a test sensitivity of over 90%. However, approximately 10% of all hyperthyroid cats have serum total T4 concentration within the reference range limits. Such T4 values are usually within the mid- to high-end of the reference range. Thus, while a high total T4 value is indicative of hyperthyroidism, finding a single reference range T4 value does not preclude such a diagnosis.
  - In early or mildly affected cases, serum total T4 concentrations can fluctuate in and out of the reference range. Such fluctuation occurs in all hyperthyroid cats, but the degree of fluctuation is of little diagnostic significance in cats with markedly elevated T4 concentrations.
  - Severe non-thyroidal illness is capable of suppressing serum total T4 concentrations to below the reference range in euthyroid cats. Similarly, marginally elevated serum total T4 concentrations may be suppressed to the mid- to high-end of the reference range in cats with mild hyperthyroidism and concurrent moderate to severe non-thyroidal disease.
  - In early or mildly hyperthyroid cats (with no concurrent illnesses), serum total T4 concentrations will eventually increase into the diagnostic thyrotoxic range upon retesting a few weeks later.

- Concurrent hyperthyroidism should always be suspected in severely ill cats with mid- to high-reference range serum total T4 concentrations.
- Serum total T3 concentration – less useful than T4 as a diagnostic test, since over 30% of hyperthyroid cats will have a normal circulating T3 concentration.
  - The majority of hyperthyroid cats with normal T3 concentrations are early or mildly affected.
  - Measurement of total T3 alone (without a total T4) is not recommended for investigation of hyperthyroidism in cats.
- Free T4 (FT4) concentration – a more sensitive diagnostic test than total T4 in cats with hyperthyroidism. May be used to help diagnose mild or early hyperthyroidism in cats, which may have normal resting serum TT4 concentrations.
  - Up to 98% of hyperthyroid cats will have a high free T4 value, compared to 90% of cats with high total T4 values.
  - Free T4 cannot, however, be used as a routine screening test since non-thyroidal disease can cause falsely high free T4 values in up to 12% of non-hyperthyroid cats. These cats generally have corresponding total T4 values in the lower half or below the reference range.
  - Caution is, therefore, advised in using serum free T4 measurements as the sole diagnostic test for hyperthyroidism. It is more reliable if interpreted with a corresponding total T4 value. High-normal total and free T4 concentrations are consistent with hyperthyroidism, whereas a low total T4 together with a high free T4 is usually associated with non-thyroidal illness.
- Serum canine thyroid-stimulating hormone (cTSH) concentration – a species-specific feline TSH assay has not yet been developed; however, assays for measuring cTSH are widely available and may provide some diagnostic information in cats with suspected hyperthyroidism.
  - Serum TSH levels should be low in early stages of hyperthyroidism before the circulating T4 or T3 concentrations are elevated.
  - About 95% of hyperthyroid cats will almost always have a low TSH value, at or below the limit of detection of the assay.
  - The best use for the current TSH measurements is to help exclude hyperthyroidism, i.e., by finding a mid- to high-normal value rather than a suppressed value.
  - However, since 5% of hyperthyroid cats will have detectable serum TSH concentration (>0.03 ng/ml), one can never completely exclude that diagnosis on the basis of this test.
  - As a diagnostic test for feline hyperthyroidism, serum TSH should never be run alone, but should be measured in tandem with T4 (and free T4) concentrations.
- Dynamic thyroid function testing – in cats with suspected hyperthyroidism but normal serum T4 concentrations, dynamic thyroid function testing (e.g., T4 suppression test or the TRH stimulation test) can be used to help in diagnosis.
  - However, in the majority of hyperthyroid cats found to have a normal T4 concentration, identification of concurrent disease, repeat total T4 values, or simultaneous measurement of free T4 concentrations allows confirmation of the diagnosis. Further diagnostic tests are rarely required.

- Nowadays, such dynamic tests should only be considered in cats with clinical signs suggestive of hyperthyroidism when repeated total T4 concentration remains within reference range, or free T4 analysis and thyroid imaging is unavailable or diagnostically unhelpful.

Pathologic Findings

- Histopathological examination of thyroid tissue helps confirm the diagnosis of adenomatous hyperplasia (thyroid adenoma), which is the typical finding in cats with hyperthyroidism. In dogs, thyroid biopsy is essential in differentiating thyroid adenoma from carcinoma, the most common pathologic finding in dogs with hyperthyroidism).

 # THERAPEUTICS

- Hyperthyroidism can be treated in three ways: medical management with methimazole or carbimazole, surgical thyroidectomy, and radioactive iodine (131-I). Each form of treatment has advantages and disadvantages that should be considered when formulating a treatment plan for the individual hyperthyroid cat. The major advantages and disadvantages of the main forms of therapy are outlined in Table 32.1.

Treatment Considerations: Concurrent Non-Thyroidal Conditions and Cost of Therapy

- Chronic kidney disease (CKD):
  - CKD is very common in older cats so it is not surprising that CKD is commonly found concurrent with hyperthyroidism. The increased GFR and reduced muscle mass induced by hyperthyroidism can mask underlying CKD.
  - Because it is not always possible to predict which hyperthyroid cats have underlying CKD, a treatment trial with methimazole or carbimazole should be considered in all cats in which CKD is suspected.
  - Immediate permanent therapy (131-I or surgical thyroidectomy) without a methimazole/carbimazole trial is appropriate for relatively young cats with completely normal serum urea and creatinine concentration, and urine specific gravity >1.040.
  - The serum T4 and renal parameters should be re-checked after 30 days of methimazole/carbimazole administration. If renal parameters remain normal after euthyroidism is restored, it is safe to proceed with permanent therapy such as thyroidectomy or radioactive iodine.
  - Mild to moderate kidney disease should not preclude the permanent treatment of hyperthyroidism. Recent research provides evidence that hyperthyroidism may contribute to the development or progression of CKD in cats, suggesting that leaving a hyperthyroid cat untreated (or poorly regulated with methimazole) may be detrimental to long-term kidney function. Treating and curing hyperthyroidism may help to both reverse renal damage and preserve the remaining kidney function.

TABLE 32.1. Advantages and disadvantages of treatment modalities for cats with hyperthyroidism.

Advantage/ disadvantage	Methimazole or carbimazole	Low-iodine diet	Surgical thyroidectomy	Radioiodine
Availability of treatment	Readily available	Readily available	Skilled surgeon needed	Radiation license needed
Ease of treatment	Intermediate	Simple§	Most difficult	Simple
Hospitalization time	None	None	1–7 days	3–7 days
Anesthesia required	No	No	Yes	No
Time until euthyroid	1–3 weeks	4–12 weeks	1 day	5–90 days
Persistent hyperthyroidism	Low (dose-related)	High (cat refuses to solely eat diet)	Rare (usually ectopic tissue)	Low (dose-related)
Reversible or permanent	Reversible	Reversible	Permanent	Permanent
Cures disease	No	No	Yes	Yes
Relapse/ recurrence	High	High	Intermediate	Low
Lifelong treatment	Yes	Yes	No	No
Cost	Variable	Variable	Intermediate to high	Generally highest
Complications				
Hypoparathyroidism	Never	Never	Common	Never
Permanent hypothyroidism	Never	Never	Common	Common
Anorexia, vomiting	Common	May refuse food	No	No
Hematologic effects	Rare†	Never	Never	Extremely rare
Neurologic damage	Never	Never	Rare*	Never
Muscle wasting	No	Yes	No	No
Progression to thyroid carcinoma	Yes	Yes	No	No

§Treatment will only be successful if cat only eats the iodine deficient diet. No other food or treats can be given.
†Thrombocytopenia, agranulocytosis, or development of positive serum ANA.
*Vocal cord paralysis or Horner's syndrome.

- Thyrotoxic heart disease:
  - Cardiac disease associated with hyperthyroidism is mild and reversible in most cats with hyperthyroidism. Murmurs and tachycardia are common but often do not result in clinical signs.
  - On the occasions when cats show more severe cardiac changes, such as congestive heart failure or aortic thromboembolism, these should be stabilized before a cat undergoes thyroidectomy or radioiodine therapy.
- Secondary hypertension:
  - High blood pressure develops in approximately 10–15% of untreated hyperthyroid cats. However, hypertension is generally mild to moderate in severity, and reversible upon induction of euthyroidism.

- Conversely, some cats that are normotensive at time of diagnosis of hyperthyroidism will become hypertensive after becoming euthyroid. Most of these cats, however, have some degree of concurrent renal disease.
- If hypertension is severe or persists after treatment of hyperthyroidism, these cats should be managed with amlodipine.
- Hepatic disease:
  - Liver disease may be suspected in cats with untreated hyperthyroidism because of their high liver enzymes (serum ALT and alkaline phosphatase). At the time of diagnosis it is not always possible to know if increased liver enzymes are due to hepatic disease unrelated to hyperthyroidism, or merely a manifestation of hyperthyroidism.
  - If underlying primary liver disease is expected, especially if the cat is showing signs of apathetic hyperthyroidism (e.g., anorexia, depression, etc.), a treatment trial with methimazole or carbimazole should be considered.
- Client circumstances:
  - Cost of therapy is a major consideration for many cat owners.
  - The initial cost of medical or nutritional therapy is far less than surgical thyroidectomy or radioiodine. However, the cost of ongoing monitoring can exceed that of thyroidectomy or 131-I therapy over a period of many months to years.

Medical Therapy

- Chronic management with antithyroid drugs is a practical treatment option for many cats and has many advantages over other treatments.
  - Medical management requires no special facilities and is readily available.
  - Anesthesia is avoided, as are the surgical complications associated with thyroidectomy (Table 32.1).
- However, medical management also has its disadvantages.
  - This form of treatment is not curative, is highly dependent on owner and cat compliance, and requires regular biochemical monitoring to ensure the efficacy of treatment.
  - Most importantly, the thyroid tumor continues to grow and, after many months, may transform from adenoma to thyroid carcinoma in some cats.
- Indications:
  - Long-term medical management best reserved for cats of advanced age or for those with concurrent diseases, and for when owners refuse either surgery or radioactive iodine.
  - In addition to long-term treatment, medical management is also necessary prior to surgical thyroidectomy to decrease the metabolic and cardiac complications associated with hyperthyroidism.
  - Short-term medical management is often recommended as trial therapy prior to 131-I therapy to determine the effect of restoring euthyroidism on renal function.
- Methimazole and carbimazole are antithyroid drugs used in cats.
  - Methimazole is specifically licensed for treatment of feline hyperthyroidism both in Europe and USA as 2.5 mg and 5 mg tablets (Felimazole®; Dechra Veterinary Products). For most hyperthyroid cats, a starting dose of 1.25–2.5 mg methimazole administered once- to twice-daily is recommended.

- Carbimazole is available for human use in many European countries and Japan. It exerts its antithyroid effect through immediate conversion to methimazole when administered orally. For most hyperthyroid cats, a starting dose of regular carbimazole of 5 mg twice-daily is effective is restoring euthyroidism.
- Carbimazole, as a novel once-daily controlled-release formulation (10 or 15 mg tablets) was recently licensed for cats in Europe (Vidalta®; Intervet Schering Plough). Administration of this drug with food significantly enhances its absorption. The starting dose for controlled release carbimazole is 15 mg administered once-daily. In cats with mild hyperthyroidism (total T4 concentration <100 nmol/l), a 10 mg once-daily treatment is recommended.
- Carbimazole and methimazole can be reformulated in a pluronic lecithin organogel (PLO) for transdermal administration. Both antithyroid drugs are generally effective in cats when administered at a dose of 2.5 mg twice-daily transdermally. The gel is applied in a thin layer to the non-haired portion of the pinnae.
  - ☐ Transdermal administration is associated with fewer gastrointestinal side effects than the oral route, but some cats resent manipulation of their ears and crusting can occur between doses leading to erythema.
  - ☐ Such custom formulation increases expense of therapy and the stability of the product is not guaranteed.
- Monitoring of cats on antithyroid drugs is extremely important.
  - Initially, cats should be reassessed after 2–3 weeks and a serum total T4 concentration measured. If euthyroidism has not been achieved, the dose of methimazole or carbimazole can be altered in 2.5- to 5-mg increments, reassessing the cat again in 2–3 weeks. Lack of owner or cat compliance should first be eliminated as a reason for a failure of therapy.
  - When monitoring, the time of serum T4 sampling in relation to administration of the antithyroid drug is not important.
  - The goal of medical therapy is to maintain total T4 concentrations within the middle third of the reference range.
  - For long-term management (once euthyroidism has been achieved), the daily antithyroid drug dosage is adjusted to the lowest possible dose that effectively maintains euthyroidism. Once the dosage has stabilized, the cat should be monitored every 3–6 months and as needed clinically.
  - Because antithyroid medications have no effect on the underlying lesion, the thyroid nodules continue to grow larger and larger over time. This may necessitate an increased daily dose with time.
- Adverse effects associated with antithyroid drugs
  - Most clinical adverse reactions occur within the first 3 months of therapy.
  - Mild clinical side effects of vomiting, anorexia, or depression occur in approximately 10–15% of cats, usually within the first 3 weeks of therapy. In most cats, these reactions are transient and do not require permanent drug withdrawal.
  - Early in the course of therapy, mild and transient hematological abnormalities, including lymphocytosis, eosinophilia or leucopenia, develop in up to 15% of cats, without any apparent clinical effect. More serious hematological

complications occur in less than 5% of cats and include agranulocytosis and thrombocytopenia.
- Self-induced excoriations of the head and neck occasionally develop, usually within the first 6 weeks of therapy.
- Hepatopathy characterized by marked increases in liver enzymes and bilirubin concentration occurs in less than 2% of cats. Withdrawal of the medication and symptomatic therapy is required.
- Other rarely reported side effects include a bleeding tendency without thrombocytopenia, prolongation of clotting times, and acquired myasthenia gravis.
- All of the adverse effects are reversible upon discontinuation of the medication.

Nutritional Therapy (Iodine-Deficient Diet)

- Recent studies have indicated that use of a diet with severely restricted iodine levels (Hill's Prescription Diet y/d Feline –Thyroid Health) can result in normalization of T4 levels in hyperthyroid cats and provide a further option for medical management of this disease.
- The basis for using this diet is that iodine is an essential component of both T4 and T3; without sufficient iodine, the thyroid cannot produce excess thyroid hormones. This is an iodine-deficient diet, containing levels below the minimum daily requirement for adult cats.
  - Time to become euthyroid on diet:
    - By 4 weeks, about 70% of hyperthyroid cats exclusively eating y/d will be euthyroid.
    - By 8 weeks, about 90% of cats will be euthyroid.
    - By 12 weeks, almost all cats should have normal T4 values.
    - This therapy appears to be more effective in cats with only moderate elevations of T4 than cats with severe hyperthyroidism.
  - Indications for nutritional management:
    - A major indication for the use of this y/d diet for management of feline hyperthyroidism is in cats that are not candidates for definitive treatment of the underlying thyroid tumor(s) with surgery or radioiodine, which remains the treatments of choice.
    - Nutritional management with y/d food (canned rather than the dry y/d) could be considered in cats whose owners are not able to give oral medication or in cats that develop side effects from methimazole/carbimazole.
  - Despite some advantages, nutritional management has many disadvantages:
    - First, feeding this diet cannot cure hyperthyroidism. Rather, feeding y/d just offers control (withholding fuel for thyroid tumor). The thyroid tumor remains and will continue to grow larger. In cats with longstanding hyperthyroidism, transformation of adenoma to thyroid carcinoma can occur unless definitive treatment (surgery or radioiodine treatment) is used to cure the disease.
    - The cats fed this diet must not eat any other cat diet, table food, or treats because even tiny amounts of iodine may lead to failure of this diet to effectively control hyperthyroidism.
    - If the diet is stopped, relapse will develop; the cat must eat only this diet for the rest of its lifetime.

□ The long-term consequences of this iodine deficient diet are not known, especially in normal cats in households that are also fed this diet. For this reason, y/d should not be the only diet fed to normal cats, which can be an issue for owners with multiple cats in the same household.

□ The composition (protein/fat/carbohydrate breakdown) of y/d reveals that it is a high-carbohydrate, relatively low-protein diet. Feeding y/d for long periods is less than an 'ideal' diet for an obligate carnivore, especially in an older hyperthyroid cat with severe muscle wasting (see Table 32.1).

Surgical Thyroidectomy Therapy

- Thyroidectomy is a highly curative treatment for hyperthyroidism. However, thyroidectomy can be associated with significant morbidity and mortality, especially in cats with severe hyperthyroidism (Table 32.1).

- Ideally, the cat would be managed preoperatively with antithyroid drugs. After methimazole or carbimazole treatment has maintained euthyroidism for 1–3 weeks, anesthetic and surgical complications will be greatly minimized. The last dose of methimazole or carbimazole should be given on the morning of surgery.

- In cats that cannot tolerate antithyroid drug treatment, alternate preoperative preparation with β-adrenoceptor blocking drugs (e.g., propranolol or atenolol) should be used.

- Surgical therapy entails either unilateral or bilateral thyroidectomy. Because most cats have involvement of both thyroid lobes, bilateral thyroidectomy is indicated in most cats.

- The two major techniques for bilateral thyroidectomy include the intracapsular and extracapsular methods. The aim of both techniques is to remove the adenomatous thyroid tissue while preserving parathyroid function.

  • The major problem with the intracapsular technique for thyroidectomy is that it can be difficult to remove the entire thyroid capsule (and, therefore, all abnormal thyroid tissue) while concurrently preserving parathyroid function. Small remnants of thyroid tissue that remain attached to the capsule may regenerate and produce recurrent hyperthyroidism.

  • The main advantage of the extracapsular technique is that the incidence of relapse is much less than that of the intracapsular technique because the entire thyroid capsule is removed together with the thyroid lobe.

- Many potential complications are associated with thyroidectomy, including hypoparathyroidism, laryngeal nerve damage (most commonly associated with voice change), and Horner's syndrome (Table 32.1).

  • The most serious complication is hypocalcemia, which develops after the parathyroid glands are injured or inadvertently removed. Since only one parathyroid gland is required for maintenance of normocalcemia, hypoparathyroidism develops only in cats treated with bilateral thyroidectomy.

  • If the surgeon recognizes that all parathyroid glands have been inadvertently removed, they can autotransplant parathyroid tissue into a muscular pouch in the neck where revascularization and return of function may occur.

- After bilateral thyroidectomy, it is important to monitor serum calcium concentration daily until it has stabilized within the normal range.
- In most cats with iatrogenic hypoparathyroidism, clinical signs associated with hypocalcemia will develop within 1–3 days of surgery.
- Although mild hypocalcemia (6.5–7.5 mg/dl; 1.6–1.9 mmol/l) is common during this immediate postoperative period, laboratory evidence of hypocalcemia alone does not require treatment. However, if accompanying signs of muscle tremors, tetany, or convulsions develop, therapy with vitamin D and calcium is strongly indicated.
- Although hypoparathyroidism may be permanent in some cats, spontaneous recovery of parathyroid function may occur weeks to months after surgery.
■ Temporary hypothyroidism develops in most cats after unilateral or bilateral thyroidectomy, with serum T4 concentrations falling to subnormal levels for 2–3 months. However, clinical signs of hypothyroidism are rare, and L-T4 supplementation is rarely required (Table 32.1).
  - If signs of postoperative hypothyroidism do develop (e.g., severe lethargy), L-T4 (0.1–0.2 mg/day) can be given, but this supplementation can generally be stopped after 2–3 months.
  - Serum T4 concentrations almost always spontaneously return to reference range limits within a few weeks to months in cats treated with thyroidectomy.
■ Because of the potential for recurrence of hyperthyroidism, all cats should have serum T4 concentration monitored once or twice a year (Table 32.1).
  - If hyperthyroidism recurs after bilateral thyroidectomy, treatment with either antithyroid drugs or radioiodine is favored over reoperation; the incidence of surgical complications (especially hypoparathyroidism) is considerably higher in subsequent operations.

Radioactive iodine therapy

■ Radioactive iodine (radioiodine; 131-I) provides a simple, effective, and safe treatment for cats with hyperthyroidism and is regarded by most veterinarians to be the treatment of choice for cats with hyperthyroidism.
  - Advantages of radioiodine treatment over the other treatment methods:
    □ 131-I treatment avoids the inconvenience of daily oral administration of antithyroid drugs, as well as the side effects commonly associated with these drugs.
    □ Eliminates the risks and perioperative complications associated with anesthesia and surgical thyroidectomy (Table 32.1).
    □ A single administration of radioiodine restores euthyroidism in most (95%) hyperthyroid cats. The therapy is simple and relatively stress-free for most cats.
  - Downsides of radioiodine treatment:
    □ Its use requires special radioactive licensing and hospitalization facilities, and extensive compliance with local and state radiation safety laws.
    □ The major drawback for most owners is that their cat must be kept hospitalized for a period (3–10 days in most treatment centers; but up to a month in some places), and visiting is not allowed.

- The principle behind this treatment is that thyrocytes concentrate iodine but do not differentiate between stable and radioactive iodine.
  - □ In cats with hyperthyroidism, radioiodine is concentrated primarily in the hyperplastic or neoplastic thyroid cells, where it irradiates and destroys the hyperfunctioning tissue.
  - □ In hyperthyroid cats, any normal thyroid tissue tends to be protected from the effects of radioiodine, because the uninvolved thyroid tissue is suppressed and receives only a small dose of radiation.
- The goal of treatment is to administer a dose of radioiodine that will restore euthyroidism while avoiding iatrogenic hypothyroidism. Unfortunately, there is no definitive method to determine the best dose of 131-I for cats.
  - □ Fixed doses are not recommended as they can provide too-low a 131-I dose and not cure the disease. More commonly, fixed dose methods give too-high a 131-I dose, resulting in hypothyroidism.
  - □ More precise, variable 131-I doses can be estimated by use of a scoring system that takes into consideration the severity of clinical signs, the size of the cat's thyroid gland, and the serum T4 concentration.
  - □ Yet more precision can be gained with thyroid imaging (scintigraphy), since it can also be used to estimate thyroid tumor volume and identify ectopic (intrathoracic) thyroid tissue.
- Most hyperthyroid cats treated with radioactive iodine are cured by a single dose. Approximately 5% of cats, however, fail to respond completely and remain hyperthyroid after treatment with radioiodine.
  - □ In cats that remain hyperthyroid 3 months after initial 131-I treatment, retreatment is generally recommended because virtually all cats with persistent hyperthyroidism after the first treatment can be cured by a second treatment.
- A proportion of cats treated with radioiodine will develop permanent hypothyroidism, with clinical signs developing 3–6 months after treatment.
  - □ Clinical signs associated with iatrogenic hypothyroidism are generally very mild, but may include lethargy, non-pruritic seborrhea sicca, matting of hair, and marked weight gain; bilateral symmetric alopecia does not develop.
  - □ Diagnosis of hypothyroidism is based on clinical signs, subnormal serum total T4 and free T4 concentrations, high serum cTSH values, and the response to replacement L-T4 therapy).
  - □ Life-long L-T4 supplementation is needed (i.e., 0.1–0.2 mg L-thyroxine per day).
- In cats with thyroid carcinoma (incidence <2–4% of all hyperthyroid cats), radioiodine offers the best chance for successful cure of the tumor because it concentrates in all hyperactive thyroid cells, i.e., carcinomatous tissue, as well as metastasis.
  - □ Thyroid carcinomas are more resistant to the effect of 131-I than thyroid adenomas (adenomatous hyperplasia), and the size of thyroid carcinomas is usually much larger.
  - □ Therefore, extremely high doses of radioiodine (30 mCi; 1110 mBq) are almost always needed for the destruction of all malignant tissue.

- ☐ A combination of surgical debulking followed by high-dose 131-I is also useful in treating cats with thyroid carcinoma.
- ☐ Longer periods of hospitalization will be required with use of such high-dose 131-I administration because of the prolonged radioiodine excretion.

 COMMENTS

Expected Course and Prognosis

- With correct treatment, the prognosis of most cats with uncomplicated hyperthyroidism is good to excellent.
  - The specific prognosis for each individual cat depends on the cat's age and condition at the time of diagnosis, duration of the disease, and the presence of concurrent diseases (e.g., CKD).
  - Like most other diseases, hyperthyroidism is best diagnosed and treated in its early rather than the advanced stages. The prognosis also depends on the treatment type, as well as the cat's response to treatment.
  - Cats with pre-existing renal disease have a poorer prognosis. Renal failure is the most common cause of death in hyperthyroid cats.
  - Recurrence of hyperthyroidism is possible with all treatments, and is most commonly associated with poor owner compliance with medical management; re-growth of hyperthyroid tissue is possible but uncommon after surgical thyroidectomy or radioiodine treatment.
- In hyperthyroid dogs with thyroid carcinoma, the prognosis is generally guarded to poor.
  - Methimazole or carbimazaole can be used to lower serum T4 concentration and control signs of hyperthyroidism, but antithyroid drugs do nothing to stop tumor growth or metastasis
  - Treatment with radioiodine, surgery, or both is usually followed by recurrence of disease; adjuvant chemotherapy is of questionable benefit.

Abbreviations

ALP = alkaline phosphatase
AST = aspartate transaminase
BUN = blood urea nitrogen
CBC = complete blood count
FT4 = free thyroxine
GFR = glomerular filtration rate
LDH = lactate dehydrogenase
T3   = triiodothyronine
T4   = thyroxine
TRH = thyrotropin-releasing hormone
TSH = thyroid-stimulating hormone
TT4 = total thyroxine

See Also

Cardiomyopathy, Hypertrophic – Cats
Congestive Heart Failure, Left-sided
Hypertension, Systemic
Hypoparathyroidism

Suggested Reading

Birchard, S.J. (2006) Thyroidectomy in the cat. *Clin. Tech. Small Anim. Pract.*, **21**, 29–33.

Frenais, R., Rosenberg, D., Burgaud, S., *et al.* (2009) Clinical efficacy and safety of a once-daily formulation of carbimazole in cats with hyperthyroidism. *J. Small Anim. Pract.*, **50**, 510–515.

Melendez, L.M., Yamka, R.M., Forrester, S.D., *et al.* (2011) Titration of dietary iodine for reducing serum thyroxine concentrations in newly diagnosed hyperthyroid cats. *J. Vet. Intern. Med.*, **25**, 683.

Peterson, M.E., Melian, C., Nichols, R. (2001) Measurement of serum concentrations of free thyroxine, total thyroxine, and total triiodothyronine in cats with hyperthyroidism and cats with nonthyroidal disease. *J. Am. Vet. Med. Assoc.*, **218**, 529–536.

Peterson, M. (2012) Hyperthyroidism in cats: What's causing this epidemic of thyroid disease and can we prevent it? *J. Feline Med. Surg.*, **14**, 804–818.

Peterson, M.E., Broome, M.R. (2013) Radioiodine for feline hyperthyroidism, in *Kirk's Current Veterinary Therapy*, *Volume XV* (eds J.D. Bonagura, D.C. Twedt), Saunders Elsevier, Philadelphia. in press.

Peterson, M.E. (2013) More than just T4: diagnostic testing for hyperthyroidism in cats:. *J. Feline Med. Surg.*, **15** (9), 765–777.

Peterson, M.E., Broome, M.R. (2012) Hyperthyroid cats on long-term medical treatment show a progressive increase in the prevalence of large thyroid tumors, intrathoracic thyroid masses, and suspected thyroid carcinoma. *J. Vet. Intern. Med.*, **26**, 1523.

Syme, H.M. (2007) Cardiovascular and renal manifestations of hyperthyroidism. *Vet. Clin. North Am. Small Anim. Pract.*, **37**, 723–743.

Trepanier, L.A. (2007) Pharmacologic management of feline hyperthyroidism. *Vet. Clin. North Am. Small Anim. Pract.*, **37**, 775–788.

Wakeling, J. (2010) Use of thyroid stimulating hormone (TSH) in cats. *Can. Vet. J.*, **51** (1), 33–34.

Williams, T.L., Peak, K.J., Brodbelt, D., *et al.* (2010) Survival and the development of azotemia after treatment of hyperthyroid cats. *J. Vet. Intern. Med.*, **24** (4), 863–869.

Yu, S., Wedekind, K.J., Burris, P.A., *et al.* (2011) Controlled level of dietary iodine normalizes serum total thyroxine in cats with naturally occurring hyperthyroidism. *J. Vet. Intern. Med.*, **25**, 683.

Author: Mark E. Peterson DVM, Dip. ACVIM

chapter 33

Canine Hypoadrenocorticism (Addison's Disease)

DEFINITION

- Hypoadrenocorticism is an endocrine disorder resulting from a deficient production of glucocorticoids and/or mineralocorticoids. Primary hypoadrenocorticism is due to destruction of the adrenal cortices, typically resulting in glucocorticoid and mineralocorticoid deficiency.
- Addison's disease refers to a deficiency of both glucocorticoids and mineralocorticoids resulting from idiopathic (immune-mediated) primary hypoadrenocorticism.
- The term atypical hypoadrenocorticism has been applied to the subset of dogs with primary hypoadrenocorticism that present with normal electrolytes. Recent work, however, has demonstrated that most of these dogs are mineralocorticoid deficient and thereby may not be so atypical.
- Secondary hypoadrenocorticism is results from pituitary ACTH insufficiency, resulting in inadequate glucocorticoid production by the adrenal cortices.

ETIOLOGY/PATHOPHYSIOLOGY

- Mineralocorticoid (aldosterone) deficiency results in a diminished ability to excrete potassium and retain sodium, disrupting sodium and potassium balance in the body.
- Sodium deficiency leads to diminished effective circulating volume. This then contributes to pathophysiologic changes and clinical abnormalities including prerenal azotemia, hypotension, dehydration, weakness, and depression.
- Hyperkalemia can contribute to clinical abnormalities including weakness, lethargy and anorexia. In combination with other electrolyte and metabolic derangements, it may result in myocardial toxicity as evidenced by bradycardia and various arrhythmias.
- Glucocorticoid (cortisol) deficiency contributes to the occurrence of anorexia, vomiting, diarrhea, melena, lethargy, and weight loss. Due to its role in glucose homeostasis hypocortisolemia predisposes to hypoglycemia. In addition, free water excretion is impaired.

Blackwell's Five-Minute Veterinary Consult Clinical Companion: Small Animal Endocrinology and Reproduction,
First Edition. Edited by Deborah S. Greco and Autumn P. Davidson. © 2017 John Wiley & Sons, Inc.
Published 2017 by John Wiley & Sons, Inc.
Companion Website: www.fiveminutevet.com/endocrinology

Systems Affected

- Gastrointestinal
- Musculoskeletal
- Cardiovascular
- Renal/urologic
- Skin

Genetics

- A genetic basis has been determined in Standard Poodles, Bearded Collies, Nova Scotia duck tolling retrievers, West Highland white terriers, Great Danes and Leonbergers.

Incidence/Prevalence

- No exact figures available; considered uncommon to rare in dogs and very rare in cats.

 SIGNALMENT/HISTORY

Species

- Dog and cat.

Breed Predilections

- Great Danes, Rottweilers, Portuguese Water dogs, Standard Poodles, Bearded Collies, Leonbergers, West Highland White terriers, Novia Scotia Duck Tolling Retreivers and Wheaten terriers have increased relative risk. Golden Retrievers and Chihuahuas have decreased relative risk.
- No predilection in cats.

Mean Age and Range

- Dogs – range, <1 to >12 years; median 4 years; most are young to middle-aged.
- Cats – range 1–9 years; most are middle-aged.

Predominant Sex

- Female dogs are at an increased relative risk; no predilection in cats.

CLINICAL FEATURES

General Comments

- Signs vary from mild and few in some patients with chronic hypoadrenocorticism to severe and life-threatening in an acute Addisonian crisis. Multiple organ systems may be involved; type and extent of involvement varies from case to case.

Historic Findings

- Dogs – lethargy, anorexia, vomiting, weakness, weight loss, diarrhea, waxing/waning course, diarrhea, previous response to therapy, shaking, PU/PD, melena.
- Cats – lethargy, anorexia, weight loss, vomiting, waxing/waning course, previous response to therapy, PU/PD.

Physical Examination Findings

- Dogs – depression, weakness, dehydration, collapse, hypothermia, slow CRT, melena, weak pulse, bradycardia, painful abdomen, hair loss.
- Cats – dehydration, weakness, hypothermia, slow CRT, depression, weak pulse, bradycardia, collapse.

Causes

- Primary hypoadrenocorticism – idiopathic (immune-mediated), mitotane overdose, trilostane overdose, granulomatous disease, metastatic tumors, fungal disease, coagulopathy.
- Secondary hypoadrenocorticism – iatrogenic following withdrawal of long-term glucocorticoid administration, isolated ACTH deficiency, panhypopituitarism, pituitary or hypothalamic lesions.

Risk Factors

- Not available.

 DIFFERENTIAL DIAGNOSIS

- Signs are nonspecific and are seen in other, more common medical disorders, particularly gastrointestinal and renal diseases.
- Although no signs are pathognomonic, a waxing and waning course and previous response to nonspecific medical intervention ('fluids and steroids') should alert the clinician to consider the diagnosis.

DIAGNOSTICS

CBC/Biochemistry/Urinalysis

- Hematologic abnormalities may include anemia, eosinophilia, and lymphocytosis.
- The absence of a stress (glucocorticoid influence) leukogram in a patient that has been ill for a few days should prompt consideration of hypoadrenocorticism.
- Serum biochemical findings may include hyperkalemia, azotemia, hyponatremia, hypochloremia, decreased total CO_2, hyperphosphatemia, hypercalcemia, increased ALT, increased serum alkaline phosphatase, and hypoglycemia.
- Urinalysis often reveals impaired urine-concentrating ability and in some cases isothenuria. Some patients with isothenuria are also azotemic, potentially causing confusion with primary renal disease.
- Some patients with hypoadrenocorticism exhibit normal electrolyte levels (so-called atypical hypoadrenocorticism).

Other Laboratory Tests

- Definitive diagnosis is by demonstration of undetectable-to-low baseline serum cortisol concentrations that fail to increase appropriately following ACTH administration. We prefer to determine cortisol concentrations before and 1 hour after administration of synthetic ACTH IV (5 µg/kg in dogs, 0.125 mg in cats). Alternatively, ACTH gel can be given IM (2 U/kg in dogs, 10 U in cats). ACTH gel (usually 40 U/ml) is available from several compounding pharmacies. Based on a recent study performed in normal dogs, it was recommended that serum cortisol concentrations be determined at both 1 and 2 hours post-ACTH administration when using a compounded ACTH gel.
- In hypovolemic dehydrated animals, use synthetic ACTH IV or delay testing until after initial fluid administration is completed and tissue perfusion restored.
- If IV synthetic ACTH is used, the ACTH stimulation test can be performed during initial stabilization and treatment if dexamethasone is used since it does not cross react with the cortisol assay.
- If prednisone, prednisolone, or hydrocortisone have been administered, these treatments must be discontinued, and the ACTH stimulation test performed at least 24 hours after changing the glucocorticoid to dexamethasone.
- A recent study showed that a resting cortisol concentration above 2 µg/dl would make hypoadrenocorticism very unlikely in a dog that had not recently received glucocorticoids. Please note that this cut-off is a guideline and may vary a little based on the methodology of the cortisol assay used, as well as from laboratory to laboratory using the same methodology. Also, a low resting cortisol does NOT confirm hypoadrenocorticism; an ACTH stimulation test is required. Determine the plasma ACTH concentration in patients with normal electrolyte levels to differentiate primary from secondary hypoadrenocorticism; it is essential to collect a sample before initiating therapy, especially glucocorticoids.

Carefully follow sample handling instructions from the laboratory being used. Plasma ACTH concentrations are high with primary hypoadrenocorticism and undetectable-to-low with secondary hypoadrenocorticism.
- ACTH/cortisol ratios

Imaging

- Radiographs may reveal microcardia, narrowed vena cava or descending aorta, hypoperfused lung fields, less commonly microhepatica, and very rarely megaesophagus. Abdominal ultrasound may reveal small adrenal glands.

Diagnostic Procedures

- Not available.

Pathologic Findings

- Gross examination – atrophy of the adrenal glands.
- Microscopically – lymphocytic-plasmacytic adrenalitis and/or adrenocortical atrophy. Other abnormalities may be present depending on etiology (neoplasia, fungal disease, etc.)

 # THERAPEUTICS

Appropriate Health Care

- An acute Addisonian crisis is a medical emergency requiring intensive therapy and 24-hour observation and care. The diagnostic work-up is performed while initial treatment and stabilization are ongoing. Feline patients often respond slower than canine ones.
- The intensity of treatment for patients with chronic hypoadrenocorticism depends on the severity of clinical signs; usually initial stabilization and therapy are conducted on an inpatient basis.

Nursing Care

- Treat acute Addisonian crisis with rapid correction of hypovolemia and restoration of volume status using isotonic fluids (preferably 0.9% NaCl).
- Monitor hydration status, blood pressure, urine output, temperature and heart rate and rhythm.

Activity

- Avoid unnecessary stress and exertion during an Addisonian crisis.

Diet

- No need to alter.

COMMENTS

Client Education

- Life-long glucocorticoid and/or mineralocorticoid replacement therapy is required.
- Increased dosages of glucocorticoid (above maintenance requirements) are required during periods of stress such as travel, boarding, hospitalization, and surgery.

Surgical Considerations

- Not available.

Medications

Drug(s) of Choice

- Chronic primary hypoadrenocorticism – Most patients will need daily glucocorticoid replacement (prednisone, 0.1–0.2 mg/kg/day), as well as mineralocorticoid replacement (DOCP, Percorten®; 2.2 mg/kg IM or SC typically given monthly, and adjusted as needed on the basis of serial electrolyte determinations). The initial monthly DOCP dose for an average-size cat is 12.5 mg. Though not preferred, an alternative means of administering glucocorticoid replacement to cats is Depo-Medrol® (10 mg IM monthly).
- Alternatively, an oral mineralocorticoid replacement can be used (fludrocortisone acetate, Florinef®, 10–20 µg/kg/day divided BID, adjusted by 0.05- to 0.1-mg increments on the basis of serial electrolyte determinations). Fludrocortisone acetate has some glucocorticoid activity and the maintenance dose of prednisone required may be lower than that of dogs receiving DOCP. A few dogs develop PU/PD and/or polyphagia on fludrocortisone acetate.
- In an Addisonian crisis, parenteral administration of a rapidly acting glucocorticoid such as dexamethasone sodium phosphate or prednisolone sodium succinate is indicated; dexamethasone sodium phosphate is preferred because prednisolone cross-reacts with cortisol assays. Dexamethasone sodium phosphate is given at a dose of 2–4 mg/kg IV; this dose can be repeated in 2 to 6 hours if necessary. Glucocorticoid is gradually tapered as the condition improves. If prednisone, prednisolone, or hydrocortisone have been given, ACTH stimulation testing will need to be delayed until the glucocorticoid has been switched to dexamethasone for at least 24 hours.
- Fluid therapy with 0.9% NaCl as needed based on the patient's hydration, volume status and blood pressure. In an Addisonian crisis, fluids are typically initiated at a rate of 60–80 ml/kg/hour for the first 1–2 hours, then tapered based on the clinical status and discontinued when appropriate. If severe hyponatremia is noted on preliminary labwork, correct no quicker than 10–12 mEq/l per day over the first 48 hours of therapy.
- If necessary, a colloid also can be given to help treat hypotension and hypovolemia.
- Treat hypoglycemia if present with IV dextrose.
- Sodium bicarbonate therapy is rarely needed; reserve for severe acidosis.

- Treat hyperkalemic myocardial toxicity with an intravenous insulin and glucose protocol. Alternatively, use intravenous calcium chloride or calcium gluconate (cardioprotective only). Patients with confirmed secondary hypoadrenocorticism require only glucocorticoid supplementation (prednisone 0.1–0.2 mg/kg/day).

Contraindications

- Not available.

Precautions

- Not available.

Possible Interactions

- Not available.

Alternative Drug(s)

- See Hyperkalemia topic for specific recommendations for emergency management of severe hyperkalemia.
- See Hyponatremia topic for specific recommendations for emergency management of severe hyponatremia.

Patient Monitoring

- Depending on their clinical presentation, patients hospitalized for treatment of hypoadrenocorticism may require intensive monitoring and frequent laboratory evaluations. Monitor clinical status, urine output, CBCs, blood chemistries and ECGs as needed. Blood glucose and electrolytes may need to be evaluated several times daily during initial therapy. Determine blood gas status when necessary.
- After the first two injections of DOCP, ideally measure electrolyte levels at 2, 3, and 4 weeks to determine the duration of effect; thereafter, check electrolyte levels at the time of injection for the next 3–6 months (and adjust the dosage of DOCP if necessary) and then every 6 months.
- DOCP is usually required at monthly intervals; rare patients need injections as often as every 2 or 3 weeks. On the other hand, an occasional dog will require DOCP as infrequently as every 6 weeks. Less than 5% of dogs require a dose of DOCP higher than 2.2 mg/kg per injection.
- The large majority of dogs with hypoadrenocorticism will be well controlled on a maintenance DOCP dose of 2.2 mg/kg per injection every month. If necessary, the DOCP dosage can be sequentially decreased based on electrolyte determinations, as some dogs can be controlled on a monthly dosage that is significantly less than 2.2 mg/kg. Alternatively, the interval between injections can be increased while monitoring electrolyte concentrations.

- Adjust the daily dose of fludrocortisone by 0.05- to 0.1-mg increments as needed, based on serial electrolyte determinations; following initiation of therapy, check electrolyte levels weekly until they stabilize in the normal range; thereafter, check electrolyte concentrations monthly for the first 3–6 months and then every 3–12 months.
- In many dogs given fludrocortisone, the daily dose required to control the disorder increases incrementally, usually during the first 6–24 months of therapy; in most dogs, the final fludrocortisone dosage needed is 20–30 µg/kg/day; very few can be controlled on 10 µg/kg/day or less. In patients that were initially azotemic, monitor creatinine concentrations as needed following discharge from the hospital.

Prevention/Avoidance

- Continue hormonal replacement therapy for the lifetime of the patient.
- Increase the dosage of replacement glucocorticoid during periods of stress such as travel, boarding, hospitalization, and surgery.

Possible Complications

- PU/PD may occur from prednisone administration, necessitating decreasing or discontinuing the drug or trying an alternative glucocorticoid.
- PU/PD may occur from fludrocortisone administration, necessitating a change to DOCP therapy.
- Side effects from DOCP are very uncommon; rarely, weight gain is seen and very rarely, PU/PD.

Expected Course and Prognosis

- Except for patients with primary hypoadrenocorticism caused by granulomatous or metastatic disease and secondary hypoadrenocorticism caused by a pituitary mass, the vast majority of patients carry a good to excellent prognosis with proper stabilization, treatment, and monitoring.

 COMMENTS

Associated Conditions

- Concurrent endocrine gland failure occurs in up to 5% of dogs—hypothyroidism, diabetes mellitus, and/or hypoparathyroidism.

Age-Related Factors

- Not available.

Zoonotic Potential

- None.

Pregnancy/Fertility/Breeding

- Not available.

Synonyms

- Addison's disease (primary hypoadrenocorticism).

See Also

Hyperkalemia
Hyponatremia

Abbreviation

PU/PD = polyuria/polydipsia

Suggested Reading

Church, D.B. (2012) Canine hypoadrenocorticism, in *BSAVA Manual of Canine and Feline Endocrinology*, 4th edition (eds C.T. Mooney, M.E. Peterson), British Small Animal Veterinary Association, Quedgeley, Gloucester.

Greco, D.S., Peterson, M.E. (1989) Feline hypoadrenocorticism, in *Current Veterinary Therapy X* (ed. R.W. Kirk), Saunders, Philadelphia, pp. 1042–1045.

Kemppainen, R.J., Behrend, E.N., Busch, K.A. (2005) Use of compounded adrenocorticotropic hormone (ACTH) for adrenal function testing in dogs. *J. Am. Anim. Hosp. Assoc.*, **41**, 368.

Kintzer, P.P., Peterson, M.E. (2014) Canine hypoadrenocorticism, in *Current Veterinary Therapy XV* (eds J.D. Bonagura, D.C. Twedt), Elsevier, Philadelphia.

Lennon, E.M., *et al.* (2007) Use of basal serum or plasma cortisol concentrations to rule out a diagnosis of hypoadrenocorticism in dogs: 123 cases (2000–2005). *J. Am. Vet. Med. Assoc.*, **231**, 413.

Peterson, M.E., Kintzer, P.P., Kass, P.H. (1996) Pretreatment clinical and laboratory findings in dogs with hypoadrenocorticism: 225 cases (1979–1993). *J. Am. Vet. Med. Assoc.*, **208**, 85–91.

Author: Peter P. Kintzer DVM, DACVIM

chapter 34

Feline Hypoadrenocorticism

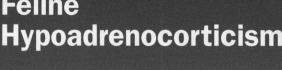

DEFINITION

- Low circulating levels of cortisol and/or mineralocorticoids resulting in clinical signs of deficiency.

ETIOLOGY/PATHOPHYSIOLOGY

- Primary hypoadrenocorticism
  - Immune-mediated destruction of the adrenal cortex.
  - Lymphomatous infiltration of the adrenal glands.
- Secondary hypoadrenocorticism from hypopituitarism

Systems Affected

- Endocrine/Metabolic.
- Gastrointestinal.
- Renal.
- Cardiovascular.

SIGNALMENT/HISTORY

- Young to middle-aged cats of any breed

Risk Factors

- None.

Historic Findings

- Lethargy.
- Anorexia.

Blackwell's Five-Minute Veterinary Consult Clinical Companion: Small Animal Endocrinology and Reproduction, First Edition. Edited by Deborah S. Greco and Autumn P. Davidson. © 2017 John Wiley & Sons, Inc. Published 2017 by John Wiley & Sons, Inc. Companion Website: www.fiveminutevet.com/endocrinology

- Weight loss.
- Vomiting.
- Polydipsia.
- Polyuria.

CLINICAL FEATURES

- The most common clinical presentation is a waxing/waning vomiting, diarrhea and abdominal pain/discomfort.
- Slow capillary refill.
- Weight loss.
- Weakness.
- Dehydration.
- Bradycardia.
- Weak pulse.

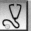

DIFFERENTIAL DIAGNOSIS

- Acute or chronic renal failure
- Inflammatory bowel disease
- Hyperthyroidism

DIAGNOSTICS

Minimum Data Base

Complete Blood Count
- Mild normochromic, normocytic anemia.
- Eosinophilia.
- Lymphocytosis.

Serum Biochemical Profile

- Hyperkalemia.
- Hyponatremia.
- Hypochloremia.
- Na/K ratio < 20.
- Azotemia.
- Hypercalcemia.
- Hyperphosphatemia.

Urinalysis

- Normal.

Other Laboratory Tests

- Protocols for dynamic adrenal function testing in cats.
  - Cosyntropin – 0.5 U/kg aqueous corticotropin IV or IM, serum samples at 0, 30, and 60 minutes (cat).
  - ACTH gel – 2.2 U/kg corticotropin gel IM, serum samples at 0, 1, and 2 hours (cat).
  - Normals: Pre: 1–4 µg/dl (28–110 mmol/l). Post ACTH: <20 µg/dl (550 mmol/l).
  - Endogenous ACTH – Single plasma sample (may be collected prior to screening test and frozen for later analysis). Collect in EDTA Vacutainer (with aprotinin), centrifuge and store in plastic, ship at 4°C (or frozen if not collected in aprotinin).
  - Normals: 20–80 pg/ml (4.4–8.8 pmol/l).
  - ACTH stimulation test:
    - □ Low baseline cortisol usually <2 µg/dl.
    - □ No response (increase in serum cortisol) to exogenous ACTH after 30 minutes or 1 hour.
  - Endogenous ACTH:
    - □ High with primary hypoadrenocorticism.
    - □ Low with secondary (pituitary failure) hypoadrenocorticism.

Pathological Findings

- Lymphocytic, plasmacytic infiltration of adrenal tissue.
- Lymphomatous infiltration of adrenal tissue.

 # THERAPEUTICS

Drug(s)

- Deoxycorticosterone pivalate 12.5 mg IM q. 30 days.
- Methylpredinisolone acetate (DepoMedrol®) 10 mg IM q. 30 days.

 # COMMENTS

Expected Course and Prognosis

- Cats may take 3–5 days to respond to emergency therapy for hypoadrenocorticism
- Excellent with proper therapy.

Abbreviations

ACTH = Adrenocorticotropic hormone

See Also

Addison's disease

Suggested Reading

Peterson, M.E., Greco, D.S., Orth, D.R. (1989) Hypoadrenocorticism in ten cats. *J. Vet. Intern. Med.*, **3**, 55–58.
Parnell, N.K., Powell, L.L., Hohenhaus, A.E., Patnaik, A.K., Peterson, M.E. (1999) Hypoadrenocorticism as the primary manifestation of lymphoma in two cats. *J. Am. Vet. Med. Assoc.*, **214**, 8, 1208–1211.

Author: Deborah S. Greco DVM, PhD, DACVIM

chapter 35

Hypoglycemia

DEFINITION

- Blood glucose <60 mg/dl (3 mmol/l).

ETIOLOGY/PATHOPHYSIOLOGY

- Decreased glucose production from glycogenolysis or gluconeogenesis – Liver disease, PSS, hypoadrenocorticism, hypothyroidism, hyposomatotropism, puppy hypoglycemia, hunting dog hypoglycemia, glycogen storage disease.
- Increased glucose utilization – insulin overdose, insulinoma, leiomyoma/sarcoma, hemangiosarcoma, sepsis, xylitol toxicity.

Iatrogenic

- Insulin administration.
- Oral hypoglycemic agents.

Systems Affected

- Neurologic.
- Neuromuscular.
- Gastrointestinal.
- Metabolic.
- Endocrine.

SIGNALMENT/HISTORY

- Acute collapse
- Muscle tremors
- Seizures

Blackwell's Five-Minute Veterinary Consult Clinical Companion: Small Animal Endocrinology and Reproduction, First Edition. Edited by Deborah S. Greco and Autumn P. Davidson. © 2017 John Wiley & Sons, Inc. Published 2017 by John Wiley & Sons, Inc. Companion Website: www.fiveminutevet.com/endocrinology

- Agitation
- Coma
- Anorexia
- Hunger

 CLINICAL FEATURES

- Seizure or coma
- Muscle tremors/shivering
- Weakness
- Disorientation

 DIFFERENTIAL DIAGNOSIS

- Spurious:
    - Lab error – Not separating clot from serum.
    - Inaccurate POC glucometers.
    - Polycythemia.
- Insulinoma.
- Leiomyoma/leiomyosarcoma.
- Hemangiosarcoma.
- Hepatocellular carcinoma.
- Neonatal, juvenile hypoglycemia.
- Hunting dog hypoglycemia.
- Liver failure – cirrhosis.
- Portosystemic shunts.
- Hypoadrenocorticism.
- Hypothyroidism.
- Growth hormone deficiency.
- Insulin administration.
- Xylitol toxicity.
- Glycogen storage disease.
- Sepsis.

 DIAGNOSTICS

- Care should be taken to rule out iatrogenic or spurious causes of hypoglycemia including use of a portable glucose monitoring device (results can be 25% below the actual value), old test strips, and delayed separation of serum from red blood cells.
- Whipple's triad may be used to support a diagnosis of insulinoma. Whipple's triad is composed of: (i) symptoms which occur after feeding or exercise; (ii) serum glucose <50 mg/dl at the time of symptoms; and (iii) symptoms relieved by the administration of glucose.

- Fructosamine – chronic hypoglycemia will result in low or below normal serum fructosamine.
- Serum insulin should be measured when serum glucose <60 mg/dl. Only insulin assays which have been validated for use in the dog and cat should be used for the diagnosis of insulinoma.
  - In order to document hyperinsulinemia, an animal should be fed a normal meal early in the day, and then fasted.
  - Glucose should be monitored at hourly intervals until the glucose is <60 mg/dl (<3 mmol/l); a blood sample should then be obtained for insulin and glucose measurements.
  - The animal is then fed small high-protein meals (1/4-can) hourly over the next several hours. An insulin concentration >20 µU/ml when the serum glucose is <60 mg/dl is diagnostic for insulinoma.
- An insulinoma is probable if serum insulin is in the normal range (5–20 µU/ml) when serum glucose is <60 mg/dl (<3 mmol/l).
- In cases where the insulin concentration is suspect but not diagnostic for insulinoma, an amended insulin:glucose ratio (AIGR) may be used. An AIGR >30 is diagnostic for an insulinoma.

$$AIGR = \frac{\text{serum insulin (µU/ml)} \times 100}{\text{serum glucose (mg/dl)} - 30}$$

Imaging

- Ultrasound of the pancreas may document a large pancreatic beta cell mass and/or metastasis to regional lymph nodes or liver.
- Scintigraphic imaging of the pancreas has also been described for the diagnosis of insulinoma in animals.

 THERAPEUTICS

Drug(s) of Choice

- Dextrose 50% bolus, diluted 1:4.
- D5W drip.

Precautions/Interactions

- Perivascular injection of dextrose can cause phlebitis.
- Dilute 50% dextrose.

Alternative Drugs

- Glucagon 5–10 ng/kg/minute.

COMMENTS

Appropriate Health Care

Nursing Care

- Frequent and well-timed feeding is essential in juvenile/hunting dog hypoglycemia.

Diet

- Dogs – diet rich in complex and simple carbohydrates.
- Cats – high-protein diet as cats replenish glycogen via gluconeogenesis.

Activity

- Hunting dog hypoglycemia – time feeding around exercise.

Surgical considerations

- See Insulinoma.

Suggested Reading

Feldman, E.C., Nelson, R.W. (1996) Beta-cell neoplasia: Insulinoma, in *Canine and Feline Endocrinology and Reproduction* (eds E.C. Feldman, R.W. Nelson), WB Saunders, Philadelphia, p. 422.

Schrauwen, E., Van Ham, L., Desmidt, M., *et al.* (1996) Peripheral polyneuropathy associated with insulinoma in the dog: Clinical, pathological, and electrodiagnostic features. *Prog. Vet. Neurol.*, 7, 16.

Simpson, K.W., Cook, A. (1998) Hypoglycaemia, in *BSAVA Manual of Small Animal Endocrinology* (eds A.G. Torrance, C.T. Mooney), British Small Animal Veterinary Association, Shurdington, Cheltenham, p. 141.

Thompson, J.C., Jones, B.R., Hickson, P.C. (1995) The amended insulin-to-glucose ratio and diagnosis of insulinoma in dogs. *N. Z. Vet. J.*, 43, 240.

Author: Deborah S. Greco DVM, PhD, DACVIM

chapter 36

Hypokalemia

DEFINITION

- Serum potassium concentration <3.5 mEq/l (normal range: 3.5–5.5 mEq/l).

ETIOLOGY/PATHOPHYSIOLOGY

- Potassium is primarily an intracellular electrolyte (98% of total body potassium is intracellular); serum levels, however, may not accurately reflect total body concentrations.
- Potassium is predominantly responsible for the maintenance of intracellular fluid volume and is required for the normal function of many enzymes.
- The resting cellular membrane potential is determined by the ratio of intracellular to extracellular potassium concentration, and is maintained by the Na+, K+-ATPase pump. Conduction disturbances in susceptible tissues (cardiac, nerve, and muscle) are caused by rapid shifts in this ratio causing myoneural membrane hyperpolarization.
- Hypokalemia can be caused by decreased intake, loss (via the gastrointestinal tract or kidneys), or translocation of potassium from the extracellular to the intracellular fluid space.

Systems Affected

- Neuromuscular – muscle weakness, including skeletal and muscles of respiration.
- Cardiac – electrocardiac changes and arrhythmias.
- Renal – hyposthenuria, nephropathy, and renal failure.
- Metabolic – acid–base balance (metabolic alkalosis); glucose homeostasis.

SIGNALMENT/HISTORY

- Dogs and cats with predispositions to increased potassium loss, translocation of potassium, or decreased intake of potassium.
- Young Burmese cats with recurrent hypokalemic periodic paralysis episodes.

Blackwell's Five-Minute Veterinary Consult Clinical Companion: Small Animal Endocrinology and Reproduction, First Edition. Edited by Deborah S. Greco and Autumn P. Davidson. © 2017 John Wiley & Sons, Inc. Published 2017 by John Wiley & Sons, Inc.
Companion Website: www.fiveminutevet.com/endocrinology

CLINICAL FEATURES

- Generalized muscle weakness or paralysis.
- Muscle cramps.
- Lethargy and confusion.
- Vomiting.
- Anorexia.
- Carbohydrate intolerance and weight loss.
- Polyuria.
- Polydipsia.
- Decreased bowel motility (humans; maybe dogs and cats).
- Hyposthenuria.
- Ventroflexion of the neck (cats and dogs).
- Respiratory muscle failure.

Causes

Decreased Intake

- Anorexia or starvation.
- Administration of potassium-deficient or potassium-free intravenous fluids.
- Bentonite clay ingestion (e.g., clumping cat litter).

Gastrointestinal Loss

- Vomiting.
- Diarrhea.
- Both upper and lower gastrointestinal obstruction; especially pyloric outflow obstruction.

Urinary Loss

- Chronic renal disease.
- Renal tubular acidosis.
- Hypokalemic nephropathy.
- Post-obstructive diuresis.
- Dialysis (hemodialysis or peritoneal).
- Intravenous fluid diuresis.
- Mineralocorticoid excess.
- Hypochloremia.
- Drugs (loop diuretics, amphotericin B, penicillins, rattlesnake envenomation).

Translocation (Extracellular to Intracellular Fluid)

- Glucose administration.
- Insulin administration.
- Sodium bicarbonate administration.

- Catecholamines.
- Alkalemia.
- β2-adrenergic agonist overdose (e.g., albuterol).
- Hypokalemic periodic paralysis (Burmese cats).
- Rattlesnake envenomation (mechanism unknown).

Risk Factors

- Acidifying diets with negligible potassium.
- Diuresis or dialysis with potassium-deficient fluids.
- Chronic illness (sustained anorexia and muscle wasting).

 ## DIFFERENTIAL DIAGNOSIS

- PU/PD, hyperglycemia, and glucosuria – rule-out diabetes mellitus.
- PU/PD, azotemia, and isosthenuria – rule-out chronic renal failure and nephropathy.
- Vomiting, metabolic alkalosis, and hypochloremia – rule-out upper gastrointestinal tract obstruction.
- Metabolic acidosis with urine pH >6.5 – rule-out renal tubular acidosis.
- Urethral obstruction – rule-out post-obstructive diuresis.
- Young Burmese cat with episodic muscle weakness – rule-out hypokalemic periodic paralysis.

 ## DIAGNOSTICS

Laboratory Findings

- **Drugs That May Alter Laboratory Results**
  - Falsely elevated potassium measurement can be caused by excessive K_3EDTA relative to the blood sample, as found in 'purple-stoppered' blood tube for hematology; this is not a problem with 'red-stoppered' tubes for serum.
- **Disorders That May Alter Laboratory Results**
  - None.
- **Valid if Run in Human Laboratory?**
  - Yes.

CBC/Biochemistry/Urinalysis

- Hyperglycemia, glucosuria, ± ketonuria, ± ketoacidosis in patients with diabetes mellitus.
- Normocytic, normochromic, non-regenerative anemia in patients with chronic renal failure.
- Elevated BUN and creatinine, with isosthenuria in patients with chronic renal failure or hypokalemic nephropathy.

- Low total CO_2 or HCO_3^- in patients with renal tubular acidosis (RTA) or renal failure.
- Normal anion gap metabolic acidosis in RTA.
- Urine pH >6.5 in patients with distal tubular acidosis.
- High total CO_2 or HCO_3^- in patients with metabolic alkalosis.

Other Laboratory Tests

- Increased aldosterone and decreased renin in patients with primary hyperaldosteronism.
- Elevated urinary fractional excretion of potassium in patients with chronic renal failure or hypokalemic nephropathy.
- ACTH stimulation tests are used to diagnose adrenal gland disorders.

Imaging

- Radiography, ultrasonography are helpful to diagnose gastrointestinal tract obstructions (mass or foreign bodies), pancreatitis, chronic renal failure work-up, adrenal gland diseases (hyperadrenocorticism, hyperaldosteronism, and adrenal tumors).
- Upper gastrointestinal tract barium study to additionally diagnose gastrointestinal obstructions (anatomic or functional).
- Computed tomography or magnetic resonance imaging to further diagnose adrenal gland diseases.

Other Diagnostic Procedures

- Endoscopy to diagnose upper gastrointestinal tract disorders.

 ## THERAPEUTICS

- Mild hypokalemia (3.0–3.5 mEq/l) can be treated by oral supplementation.
- Moderate hypokalemia (2.5–3.0 mEq/l) is best treated by inpatient administration of oral ± intravenous supplementation and carefully monitored.
- Severe hypokalemia (<2.5 mEq/l) should be hospitalized for intensive intravenous potassium supplementation. Patients – especially cats – should be carefully monitored for cardiac arrhythmias and impaired ventilation.

Medications

Drug(s) of Choice
- Oral supplementation with potassium gluconate (e.g., Tumil-K) is effective in mildly affected patients. The initial dosage is 1/4 teaspoon (2 mEq) per 4.5 kg body weight in food twice daily.
- With severe life-threatening hypokalemia (serum potassium <2.0 mEq/l), potassium chloride can be administered at a rate of 1.0–1.5 mEq/kg/hour, with ECG monitoring.

Table 36.1. Potassium supplementation for hypokalemia using a sliding scale

Patient K⁺ concentration (mEq/l)	KCl/l (mEq)
3.5–4.5	20
3.0–3.5	30
2.5–3.0	40
2.0–2.5	60
< 2.0	80

Note: Do not exceed an intravenous supplementation rate or 0.5 mEq/kg/hour unless continually monitoring and on the verge of ventilator muscle failure.

- Parenteral supplementation is required in anorectic or vomiting patients, or in patients with moderate-to-severe hypokalemia (<3.0 mEq/l). Potassium chloride is added to intravenous fluids according to data in Table 36.1, best delivered via an infusion pump or with a pediatric fluid administration set (60 drops/ml/minute). Monitor and taper accordingly.

Contraindications

- Glucose supplementation.
- Insulin administration.
- Sodium bicarbonate administration.
- Untreated hypoadrenocorticism.
- Hyperkalemia.
- Renal failure or severe renal impairment.
- Acute dehydration.
- Severe hemolytic reactions.
- Impaired gastrointestinal motility.

Precautions

- Administer with caution, avoid oversupplementation, monitor frequently.

Possible Interactions

- Concurrent potassium supplementation with ACE inhibitors (e.g., enalapril), potassium-sparing diuretics (e.g., spironolactone), prostaglandin inhibitors (e.g., nonsteroidal anti-inflammatory drugs), beta-blockers (e.g., atenolol), or cardiac glycosides (e.g., digoxin) can cause adverse effects.

Alternative Drug(s)

- Potassium phosphate can be used in patients with concurrent hypophosphatemia.

Patient Monitoring

- Check serum potassium every 6–24 hours based on severity of hypokalemia.

Possible Complications

- Electrolyte disturbances and arrhythmias. It is essential to close the IV fluid outflow valve and thoroughly mix the fluid contents while adding potassium chloride solution to the parenteral fluid bag.

 COMMENTS

Associated Conditions

- Hypokalemic nephropathy.
- Hypophosphatemia.
- Hypomagnesemia.
- Metabolic alkalosis.

Age-Related Factors

- None.

Zoonotic Potential

- None.

Pregnancy/Fertility/Breeding

- Not available.

See Also

Alkalosis, Metabolic
Diarrhea
Hypochloremia
Renal Failure, Chronic
Renal Tubular Acidosis
Vomiting, Chronic

Abbreviations

ACE = angiotensin-converting enzyme
ACTH = adrenocorticotropic hormone
ATPase = adenosine triphosphate

CO_2 = carbon dioxide
HCO_3^- = bicarbonate
K^+ = potassium
Na^+ = sodium
PU/PD = polyuria/polydipsia

Suggested Reading

Boag, A.K., Coe, R.J., Martinez, T.A., *et al.* (2005) Acid-base and electrolyte abnormalities in dogs with gastrointestinal foreign bodies. *J. Vet. Intern. Med.*, **19**, 816–821.

DiBartola, S.P., Autran de Morais, H. (2102) Disorders of potassium: Hypokalemia and hyperkalemia, in *Fluid Therapy in Small Animal Practice*, 4th edition (ed. S.P. DiBartola), Saunders, Philadelphia, pp. 92–120.

Nager, A.L. (2011) Fluid and electrolyte therapy in infants and children, in *Emergency Medicine – A Comprehensive Study Guide*, 7th edition (ed. J.E.Tintinalli), McGraw-Hill, New York, pp. 971–976.

Greenlee, M., Wingo, C.S., McDonough, A.A., *et al.* (2009 Narrative review: evolving concepts in potassium homeostasis and hypokalemia. *Ann. Intern. Med.*, **150**, 619–625.

Author: Michael Schaer DVM, DACVIM, DACVECC

chapter 37

Hyponatremia

DEFINITION

- Serum sodium concentration below the lower limit of the reference range.

ETIOLOGY/PATHOPHYSIOLOGY

- Sodium is the most abundant cation in the extracellular fluid. Hyponatremia usually, but not always, reflects hypoosmolality and is typically associated with a decreased total body sodium content. Either solute loss or water retention can theoretically cause hyponatremia. Most solute loss occurs in isoosmotic solutions (e.g., vomit and diarrhea) and, as a result, water retention in relation to solute is the underlying cause in almost all patients with hyponatremia. In general, hyponatremia occurs only when a defect in renal water excretion is present.

Systems Affected

- Nervous – severe neurologic dysfunction is not usually seen until serum sodium concentration falls below 110–115 mEq/l. Clinical signs may be more related to the rate of decline in serum sodium concentration than the actual nadir. Dogs with chronic hyponatremia often have mild, if any, clinical signs.
- Overly rapid correction of hyponatremia can also cause neurologic damage.

SIGNALMENT/HISTORY

Species

- Dogs and cats

Blackwell's Five-Minute Veterinary Consult Clinical Companion: Small Animal Endocrinology and Reproduction, First Edition. Edited by Deborah S. Greco and Autumn P. Davidson. © 2017 John Wiley & Sons, Inc. Published 2017 by John Wiley & Sons, Inc. Companion Website: www.fiveminutevet.com/endocrinology

CLINICAL FEATURES

- Lethargy
- Weakness
- Confusion
- Nausea/vomiting
- Seizures
- Obtundation
- Coma
- Other findings depend on the underlying cause.

Causes

- Hyperlipemia
- Hyperproteinemia

Hyperosmolar Hyponatremia

- Hyperglycemia
- Mannitol infusion

Hypoosmolar Hyponatremia

- **Normovolemic**
  - Primary polydipsia
  - Hypothyroid myxedema coma
  - Hypotonic fluid infusion
  - SIADH
- **Hypervolemic**
  - Congestive heart failure
  - Hepatic cirrhosis
  - Nephrotic syndrome
  - Severe renal failure
- **Hypovolemic**
  - Gastrointestinal losses
  - Renal failure
  - Third space losses
  - Cutaneous losses
  - Diuresis
  - Hypoadrenocorticism

DIFFERENTIAL DIAGNOSIS

- Hypoadrenocorticism.
- Severe GI disease.
- Hypothyroidism.
- Metabolic or respiratory acidosis (DKA).
- Congestive heart failure.
- Primary polydipsia.

DIAGNOSTICS

Laboratory Findings

- **Drugs That May Alter Laboratory Results**
  - Mannitol can cause pseudohyponatremia.
  - Diuretic administration can cause hyponatremia.
- **Disorders That May Alter Laboratory Results**
  - Hyperlipidemia, hyperglycemia, and hyperproteinemia can cause pseudohyponatremia.
- **Valid if Run in a Human Laboratory?**
  - Yes.

CBC/Biochemistry/Urinalysis

- Low serum sodium concentration.
- Other abnormalities may point to the underlying cause.

Other Laboratory Tests

- Plasma osmolality is usually low; if plasma osmolality is normal or high, exclude hyperlipidemia, hyperglycemia, hyperproteinemia, and mannitol administration.
- Urine osmolality <100–150 mosmol/kg indicates primary polydipsia or reset osmostat. Urine osmolality >150–200 mosmol/kg indicates impaired renal water excretion.
- Urinary sodium concentration <15–20 mEq/l indicates low effective circulating volume, pure cortisol deficiency, primary polydipsia with high urine output. Urinary sodium concentration >20–25 mEq/l indicates syndrome of inappropriate ADH secretion, adrenal insufficiency, renal failure, reset osmostat, diuretic administration, or vomiting with marked bicarbonate loss.

THERAPEUTICS

- Inpatient versus outpatient treatment depends on severity of hyponatremia, associated neurologic dysfunction, and the underlying disorder.

Medications

Drug(s) of Choice

- Treatment consists of addressing the underlying cause and increasing the serum sodium concentration if necessary. Overly rapid normalization of the hyponatremia can have potentially severe neurologic sequela and may be more detrimental than the hyponatremia itself. Therefore, isotonic saline is the fluid of choice in the large majority of cases. More aggressive correction of the serum sodium concentration with hypertonic saline is rarely necessary.
- Hypervolemic (edematous) patients are typically managed with diuretics and salt restriction. Isotonic saline and furosemide may be useful in more affected patients.
- Hypovolemic patients are managed by replacing the volume deficit with isotonic saline.
- The use of hypertonic saline may be considered in selected patients with severe symptomatic hyponatremia. The sodium deficit is estimated by 0.5 × lean BW (kg) × (120 – serum sodium concentration). The serum sodium concentration is corrected by 10–12 mEq/l/day (0.5 mEq/l/h) or less. Once the serum sodium concentration reaches 120–125 mEq/l, discontinue hypertonic saline and continue to slowly normalize the serum sodium concentration using isotonic saline or water restriction, as dictated by the underlying cause of the hyponatremia.
- Other therapeutic interventions are dictated by the underlying cause of the hyponatremia.

Precautions

- Overly rapid correction of hyponatremia can result in neurologic damage (demyelination); avoid increasing serum sodium concentration by more than 10–12 mEq/l/day (0.5 mEq/l/h).

Patient Monitoring

- Serial serum sodium determinations to avoid overly rapid correction of the serum sodium concentration and to assure appropriate response to NaCl and other indicated therapies.
- Monitor hydration status.
- Monitor other serum electrolyte concentrations as indicated by the patient's clinical condition and underlying disorder.

Prevention/Avoidance

- Depends on the underlying disorder.

Possible Complications

- Depends on the underlying disorder.

Expected Course And Prognosis

- Depends on the underlying disorder.

 COMMENTS

Client Education

- Depends on the underlying disorder.

Associated Conditions

- Other electrolyte and acid–base abnormalities are often associated with the clinical disorders that cause hyponatremia.

See Also

Cirrhosis and Fibrosis of the Liver
Congestive Heart Failure, left-sided
Hyperglycemia
Hyperlipemia
Hypoadrenocorticism (Addison's disease)
Myxedema and Myxedema coma
Nephrotic syndrome
Polyuria and Polydipsia
Renal Failure, chronic

Abbreviations

ADH   = antidiuretic hormone
DKA   = diabetic ketoacidosis
SIADH = syndrome of inappropriate ADH secretion

Suggested Reading

Cluitmans, F.H., Meinders, A.E. (1990) Management of severe hyponatremia: Rapid or slow correction? *Am. J. Med.*, **88**, 161.

Author: Melinda Fleming DVM

chapter 38

Hypoparathyroidism

DEFINITION

- Clinical signs of hypocalcemia caused by an absolute or relative deficiency of parathyroid hormone.

ETIOLOGY/PATHOPHYSIOLOGY

- Immune-mediated destruction of the parathyroid glands.
- Secondary to thyroidectomy (feline).

Systems Affected

- Neuromuscular
- Nervous
- Cardiovascular
- Ophthalmic
- Respiratory
- Renal
- Cardiovascular

SIGNALMENT/HISTORY

Risk Factors

- Surgical thyroidectomy.

Species

- Dogs, cats:
  - Toy poodle
  - Miniature schnauzer

Blackwell's Five-Minute Veterinary Consult Clinical Companion: Small Animal Endocrinology and Reproduction, First Edition. Edited by Deborah S. Greco and Autumn P. Davidson. © 2017 John Wiley & Sons, Inc. Published 2017 by John Wiley & Sons, Inc.
Companion Website: www.fiveminutevet.com/endocrinology

- German shepherd dog
- Labrador retriever
- Scottish terrier
- Mixed-breed cats

- Age
  - Dogs – young to middle-aged.
  - Cats – secondary to thyroidectomy: older cats (>10 years).
  - Spontaneous: young to middle-aged.
- Slight female predilection.

Historic Findings

- Dogs
  - Seizures.
  - Tense, splinted abdomen.
  - Ataxia/stiff gait.
  - PU/PD.
  - Vomiting.
  - Anorexia.
- Cats
  - Lethargy.
  - Anorexia.
  - Depression.

 CLINICAL FEATURES

Dogs

- Facial rubbing.
- Muscle trembling, twitching, and fasciculations.
- Growling.
- Panting.
- Posterior lenticular cataracts.
- Weakness.
- Fever.

Cats

- Seizures.
- Muscle trembling, twitching.
- Panting.
- Posterior lenticular cataracts.
- Bradycardia.
- Fever.
- Hypothermia.

DIFFERENTIAL DIAGNOSIS

Muscle tremors

- Puerperal tetany (eclampsia).
- Hypercalcemia.
- Toxins (tetanus, strychnine).

Muscle weakness

- Hypoadrenocorticism.
- Hypoglycemia.
- Anemia.
- Hypothyroidism.
- Myasthenia gravis.
- Polyradiculoneuropathy.
- Tick paralysis.
- Botulism.
- Organophosphate toxicity.
- Congestive heart failure.

Seizures

- Hypoglycemia.
- Hepatic encephalopathy.
- Syncope.
- Epilepsy.
- Neoplasia.
- Inflammatory.
- Infectious.
- Toxic.

 # DIAGNOSTICS

CBC/Biochemistry/Urinalysis

- Complete blood count normal.
- Urinalysis usually normal.
- Hypocalcemia (usually <6.5 mg/dl) and normal or mild to moderate hyperphosphatemia.
- Corrected Ca = [Ca (mg/dl) – albumin (g/dl)] + 3.5 or Corrected Ca = [Ca (mg/dl) – {0.4 × total protein (g/dl)}] + 3.3.

- Hypocalcemia caused by hypoalbuminemia in cats cannot be corrected by these formulas, although hypoalbuminemia causes reduced serum calcium in cats.
- CRF reduces serum calcium and raises serum phosphorus, but is easily distinguished from hypoparathyroidism by the presence of azotemia.

Other Laboratory Tests

- Serum PTH determination – demonstrates undetectable or very low concentration of PTH.
- Other causes of hypocalcemia (e.g., renal failure) have a normal-to-high concentration of PTH.

Imaging

- Radiography and ultrasonography are normal.

Diagnostic Procedures

- ECG changes seen in patients with hypocalcemia include prolongation of the ST and QT segments; sinus bradycardia and wide T waves or T wave alternans is occasionally seen.
- Cervical exploration reveals absence or atrophy of the parathyroid glands.

Pathologic Findings

- Dogs – normal tissue with mature lymphocytes, plasma cells, and fibrous connective tissue along with chief cell degeneration.
- Cats – parathyroid gland atrophy.

 THERAPEUTICS

Drug(s) of Choice

- Acute treatment – IV calcium chloride or gluconate (see Table 38.1):
    - 5–15 mg of calcium/kg over 10–30 minutes.
    - 10% diluted calcium gluconate (diluted with an equal volume of saline prior to injection) SC q. 4–6 hours.
- Chronic treatment:
    - Vitamin D3 – calcitriol (1,25-dihydroxycholecalciferol) (see Table 38.2).
    - 0.03–0.06 µg/kg/day.
    - 0.25 and 0.5 µg capsules, 1.0 µg/ml oral solution.
    - 1 µgram/ml injectable.

Precautions/Interactions

- Do not mix calcium solution with LRS.

TABLE 38.1. Calcium preparations.

Preparation	Dose of elemental calcium	Available calcium	Size available (needs to be converted to elemental calcium)
Calcium carbonate	Canine: 1–4 g/day	40%	Tablets: 500, 600, 650, 1250, 1500 mg Chewable tablets: 400, 420, 500, 750, 850, 1000, 1250 mg
	Feline: 0.5–1 g/day		Capsules: 1250 mg Oral suspension: 250 mg/ml
Calcium gluconate	Canine: 1–4 g/day Feline: 0.5–1 g/day	10%	Tablets: 500, 650, 975 mg Chewable tablets: 500 mg Capsules: 500, 700 mg Powder for suspension: 70 mg/ml
Calcium lactate	Canine: 1–4 g/day Feline: 0.5–1 g/day	13%	Tablets: 650, 770 mg Capsules: 500 mg
Calcium acetate	Canine: 1–4 g/day Feline: 0.5–1 g/day	25%	Tablets, gelcaps, and capsules: 667 mg
Calcium citrate	Canine: 1–4 g/day Feline: 0.5–1 g/day	21%	Tablets: 950, 1150 mg Effervescent tablets: 2380 mg Capsules: 850, 1070 mg Powder for oral suspension: 725 mg/ml
Calcium glubionate	Canine: 1–4 g/day Feline: 0.5–1 g/day	30%	Syrup: 360 mg/ml

TABLE 38.2. Vitamin D preparations.

Preparation	Dose	Maximal effect	Size
1,25-Dihydroxycholecalciferol (active vitamin D_3, calcitriol)	0.03–0.06 µg/kg/day	1–4 days	0.25 and 0.5 µg capsules, 1.0 µg/ml oral solution, and 1 and 2 µg/ml injectable
Dihydrotachysterol	Initial: 0.02–0.03 mg/kg/day Maintenance: 0.01–0.02 mg/kg/24–48 hours	1–7 days	Currently unavailable; formerly available as 0.125 mg, 0.2 mg, 0.4 mg tablets and 0.2 mg/ml syrup
Ergocalciferol (vitamin D_2)	Initial: 4000–6000 U/kg/day Maintenance: 1000–2000 U/kg/day-week	5–21 days	25 000 and 50 000 U capsules and 8000 U/ml syrup

Alternative Drugs

- Vitamin D2 (ergocalciferol): Initial 4000–6000 U/kg/day; maintenance: 1000–2000 U/kg/day.
- Calcium carbonate: 1–4 g/day.

Nursing Care

- Monitor ECG and calcium during initial treatment.

Diet

- Balanced commercial diet.

Activity

- Not available.

Surgical Considerations

- Not available.

 # COMMENTS

Client Education

- Naturally occurring primary hypoparathyroid will require lifelong therapy and monitoring.
- Most cases of iatrogenic hypoparathyroidism (e.g., thyroidectomy) will recover and only require transient management and monitoring.

Patient Monitoring

- ECG while administering IV calcium.
- Serum total or ionized calcium during SC calcium therapy – discontinue once oral medications have normalized serum calcium (>8 mg/dl).
- Once weekly calcium until normalized on calcitriol therapy.
- Adjustments in vitamin D and oral calcium administration can be expected during the course of management, especially during the initial 2–6 months.
- Cats with hypoparathyroidism secondary to thyroidectomy usually require only transient treatment because they typically regain normal parathyroid function within 4–6 months, often within 2–3 weeks.

Prevention/Avoidance

- Overdosage of calcitriol – will resolve in 48 hours after discontinuation.
- Overdosage of ergocalciferol – may take several weeks.

Possible Complications

- Hypercalcemia from vitamin D overdose.

Expected Course and Prognosis

- Excellent prognosis with vitamin D3 therapy.

Synonyms

- None

Abbreviations

Ca   = calcium
ECG   = electrocardiogram
PTH   = parathyroid hormone
PU/PD = polyuria and polydipsia

Suggested Reading

Bruyette, D.S., Feldman, E.C. (1988) Primary hypoparathyroidism in the dog. Report of 15 cases and review of 13 previously reported cases. *J. Vet. Intern. Med.*, **2**, 7–14.

Greco, D.S. (2012) Endocrine causes of hypercalcemia and hypocalcemia. *Top. Comp. Anim. Med.*, **27** (4), 150–155.

Henderson, A.K., Mahony, O. (2005) Hypoparathyroidism: pathophysiology and diagnosis. *Compend. Contin. Educ. Pract. Vet.*, **27** (4), 270–279.

Henderson, A.K., Mahony, O. (2005) Hypoparathyroidism: treatment. *Compend. Contin. Educ. Pract. Vet.*, **27** (4), 280–287.

Peterson, M.E., James, K.M., Wallace, M., *et al.* (1991) Idiopathic hypoparathyroidism in five cats. *J. Vet. Intern. Med.*, **5**, 47–51.

Author: Deborah S. Greco DVM, PhD, DACVIM

chapter 39

Hypophosphatemia

DEFINITION

- Serum phosphorus concentration <2.5 mg/dl.

ETIOLOGY/PATHOPHYSIOLOGY

- Control of phosphorus is influenced by the actions and interactions of PTH and vitamin D with the gastrointestinal tract, bone, kidneys, and parathyroid glands.
- Decreased serum phosphorus concentrations can be caused by the translocation of phosphorus from the extracellular fluid in cells, decreased renal reabsorption, or decreased intestinal absorption of phosphorus.
- Low serum phosphorus can lead to ATP depletion, which affects cells with high ATP-energy demands (skeletal muscle, cardiac muscle, nerve tissues, and RBCs.
- Many important enzyme systems are dependent on adequate phosphorus levels, including glycolysis, ammoniagenesis, 1-hydroxylation of 25-(OH)-cholecalciferol, and 2,3-diphosphoglycerate, which are essential for energy production, acid excretion, calcium balance, and tissue oxygenation, respectively.
- Phosphorus is required for maintenance of cell membrane integrity by playing an essential role in the production of ATP, guanosine triphosphate, cyclic AMP, and phosphocreatinine.
- Diabetic (ketotic and non-ketotic) patients at increased risk due to depleted phosphorus stores, lost muscle mass, and urinary losses. Insulin administration yields ATP from glycolysis, causing the translocation of phosphorus.

Systems Affected

- Hemic/Lymphatic/Immune – hemolysis, impaired oxygen delivery to tissues, impaired leukocyte and platelet function.
- Neurologic – impaired glucose uptake leads to encephalopathy, seizures, and coma.

Blackwell's Five-Minute Veterinary Consult Clinical Companion: Small Animal Endocrinology and Reproduction, First Edition. Edited by Deborah S. Greco and Autumn P. Davidson. © 2017 John Wiley & Sons, Inc. Published 2017 by John Wiley & Sons, Inc.
Companion Website: www.fiveminutevet.com/endocrinology

- Musculoskeletal – rhabdomyolysis, weakness, pain, ventilator failure, and gastrointestinal ileus.
- Cardiac – impaired contractility.

SIGNALMENT/HISTORY

- Older dogs and cats.
- Diabetic patients.

CLINICAL FEATURES

Historic Findings

- Usually consistent with the primary condition responsible for the hypophosphatemia; however, evidence of severe hypophosphatemia (e.g., hemolysis) is usually not observed unless serum phosphorus concentrations decrease to 1.0 mg/dl, or less.

Physical Examination Findings

- Hemolytic anemia causes pallor, tachypnea, dyspnea, and/or red-discolored urine.
- Skeletal and respiratory muscle weakness.
- Mental dullness.

Causes

- Maldistribution (translocation) – treatment of diabetes ketoacidosis, insulin administration or carbohydrate load, total parenteral nutrition or nutritional recovery, hyperventilation or respiratory alkalosis.
- Reduced renal reabsorption (increased renal loss) – primary hyperparathyroidism, renal tubular disorders (e.g., Fanconi syndrome), proximal tubule diuretics (e.g., carbonic anhydrase inhibitors), eclampsia (hypocalcemic tetany), hyperadrenocorticism, sodium bicarbonate administration.
- Reduced intestinal absorption (decreased intake) – phosphorus-deficient diets, vitamin D deficiency, malabsorption disorders, phosphate binders.
- Laboratory error – hemolysis, icterus, osmotic diuretic (e.g., mannitol) administration.

Risk Factors

- Phosphorus-deficient diets or parenteral nutrition (refeeding syndrome).
- Diabetes mellitus.
- Prolonged anorexia, malnutrition, or starvation.
- Primary hyperparathyroidism.

DIFFERENTIAL DIAGNOSIS

- Concurrent hyperglycemia, glucosuria, ketonuria, and high anion gap metabolic acidosis – rule-out diabetic ketoacidosis.
- Concurrent glucosuria, normoglycemia, isosthenuria ± azotemia – rule-out renal tubular defects.
- Concurrent hypercalcemia and proteinuria – rule-out primary hyperparathyroidism.
- Concurrent hypocalcemia – rule-out hypocalcemic tetany.
- Concurrent high serum alkaline phosphatase – rule-out hyperadrenocorticism.
- Concurrent panhypoproteinemia – rule-out intestinal malabsorption.

 # DIAGNOSTICS

Laboratory Findings

- **Drugs That May Alter Laboratory Results**
  - Osmotic diuretics (e.g., mannitol) may falsely lower serum phosphorus concentrations.
- **Disorders That May Alter Laboratory Results**
  - Hemolysis and icterus may falsely lower serum phosphorus concentrations.
- **Valid If Run In Human Laboratory?**
  - Yes.

CBC/Biochemistry/Urinalysis

- Serum phosphorus less than 2.5 mg/dl.
- Hyperglycemia, glucosuria, ketonuria, and high anion gap metabolic acidosis with diabetic ketoacidosis.
- Glucosuria, normoglycemia, isosthenuria, or azotemia with renal tubular defect.
- Hypercalcemia with primary hyperparathyroidism.
- Hypocalcemia with hypocalcemic tetany.
- High serum alkaline phosphatase, proteinuria with hyperadrenocorticism.
- Panhypoproteinemia with intestinal malabsorption.

Other Laboratory Tests

- Serum fructosamine – to diagnose or rule-out diabetes mellitus.
- Parathyroid hormone assay – to diagnose or rule-out hyperparathyroidism.
- PTH-rp for hypercalcemia of malignancy.
- Vitamin D metabolite measurement – to diagnose or rule-out vitamin D deficiency.

Imaging

- Radiography may reveal urolithiasis in cases of primary hyperparathyroidism or poor bone quality/pathologic fractures with disorders of vitamin D metabolism.
- Ultrasonography (cervical) may reveal parathyroid mass.

Other Diagnostic Procedures

- Surgical exploration of the cervical area may reveal a parathyroid mass.
- Urine anion gap can reveal renal tubular secretory defect.

 THERAPEUTICS

- Prevention is preferred.
- Asymptomatic patients with low (1.5–2.5 mg/dl), but not depleted, phosphorus concentrations may not need phosphate treatment.
- If caused by insulin administration or hyperalimentation, administer supplemental phosphorus.
- Severe hypophosphatemic (<1.5 mg/dl) patients need hospitalization and monitoring for hemolysis or hemolytic crisis. Intravenously administer isotonic electrolyte solution without calcium, supplemented with potassium phosphate.
- Fresh whole-blood transfusion for severe hemolytic crisis.

Medications

Drug(s) of Choice

- Potassium phosphate (3 mmol phosphate/ml and 4.4 mEq potassium/ml) given intravenously.
- Sodium phosphate (3 mMol phosphate/ml and 4 mEq sodium/ml) given intravenously.
- Dosage – 0.01–0.12 mMol/kg/hour CRI. Monitor serum phosphorus level every 6–8 hours.
- Discontinue therapy when serum phosphorus concentration reaches 2 mg/dl in order to avoid iatrogenic hypocalcemia and hyperphosphatemia.

Contraindications

- Hyperphosphatemia.
- Hypocalcemia.
- Hypercalcemia.
- Renal failure.
- Hyperkalemia.
- Concurrent $D_{2.5}$ and D_5 in LRS and dobutamine administration.

Precautions

- Concurrent diuretic administration, especially carbonic anhydrase inhibitors.
- Renal disease.

Possible Interactions

- ACE inhibitor (e.g., enalapril) administration.
- Cardiac glycoside (e.g., digoxin) administration,
- Potassium-sparing diuretics (e.g., spironolactone).

Alternative Drug(s)

- Oral phosphate supplement (e.g., phospho-soda) if not vomiting.
- Milk (skim or low-fat) may be supplemented.

Follow-Up

- Measure serum phosphorus levels every 6–8 hours until within normal range.
- Monitor patients for hyperphosphatemia and discontinue treatment immediately.
- Check serum potassium level daily until both stable.

Patient Monitoring
Possible Complications
- Hemolysis.
- Respiratory depression and failure.
- Cardiac arrest.

 COMMENTS

Associated Conditions

- Concurrent hypokalemia is common in patients with diabetic ketoacidosis.
- Concurrent hypercalcemia in Keeshond dogs.

Age-Related Factors

- Usually presents in older dogs.

Zoonotic Potential

- None.

Pregnancy/Fertility/Breeding

- Concurrent hypocalcemia in the periparturient animal is caused by PTH-promoted renal excretion of phosphorus, causing hypophosphatemia.

See Also

Diabetes Mellitus with Ketoacidosis
Hyperparathyroidism

Abbreviations

ACE = angiotensin-converting enzyme
ATP = adenosine triphosphate
LRS = lactated Ringer's solution
PTH = parathyroid hormone
RBC = red blood cells

Suggested Reading

DiBartola, S.P., Autran de Morais, H. (2012) Disorders of phosphorous: Hypophosphatemia and hyperphosphatemia, in *Fluid Therapy in Small Animal Practice*, 4th edition (ed. S.P. DiBartola), Saunders, Philadelphia, pp. 195–211.

Martin, L.G., Allen-Durrance, A.E. (2015) Magnesium and phosphate disorders, in *Small Animal Critical Care Medicine*, 2nd edition (eds D.C. Silverstein, K. Hopper), Elsevier-Saunders, St Louis, pp. 281–288.

Author: Michael Schaer DVM, DACVIM, DACVECC

chapter 40

Canine Hypothyroidism

DEFINITION

- Hypothyroidism is due to decreased thyroidal production of thyroid hormones thyroxine (T4) and triiodothyronine (T3).

ETIOLOGY/PATHOPHYSIOLOGY

- Greater than 90% of cases are primary, and are due to acquired immune-mediated destruction of the thyroid gland which is preceded by thyroiditis, idiopathic atrophy or, less commonly, neoplasia. Secondary forms of the disease, including thyroid-stimulating hormone (TSH) deficiency, pituitary neoplasia, and cystic Rathke's pouch, are uncommon clinical entities. Tertiary hypothyroidism with thyrotropin-releasing hormone (TRH) deficiency has not been documented in dogs. Congenital cases have been reported in both dogs and cats.

Systems Affected

- Cardiovascular – Lethargy and exercise intolerance, bradyarrhythmias, dilated cardiomyopathy in certain breeds.
- Endocrine/Metabolic – Lethargy, decreased metabolic rate.
- Gastrointestinal – Weight gain.
- Hemic/Lymphatic/Immune – Low-grade non-regenerative anemia.
- Musculoskeletal – Epiphyseal dysplasia with congenital disease.
- Nervous – Cranial nerve deficits, vestibular disease, myxedema coma.
- Neuromuscular – Peripheral neuropathies, unilateral lameness.
- Ophthalmic – Corneal lipidosis, lipemia retinalis.
- Reproductive – Possible effects on female reproductive performance (prolonged interestrus intervals, failure to cycle, silent heats). Conflicting information on male reproductive performance.

Blackwell's Five-Minute Veterinary Consult Clinical Companion: Small Animal Endocrinology and Reproduction, First Edition. Edited by Deborah S. Greco and Autumn P. Davidson. © 2017 John Wiley & Sons, Inc. Published 2017 by John Wiley & Sons, Inc.
Companion Website: www.fiveminutevet.com/endocrinology

- Dermatologic – dry scaly skin, bilaterally symmetric alopecia, seborrhea, hyperpigmentation, ceruminous otitis, myxedema, recurrent pyodermas.

 SIGNALMENT/HISTORY

- Hypothyroidism most commonly occurs in young to middle-aged dogs, with an average age of 7 years. Dogs with autoimmune disease tend to develop hypothyroidism at a younger age. While thyroid values decrease within the reference range in senior dogs, hypothyroidism is very uncommon and other factors (see below) are likely responsible for the observed decrease in thyroid concentrations in euthyroid older patients. Spayed females and neutered males are at an increased risk when compared to sexually intact animals. Breed predispositions have been reported for Golden Retrievers and Doberman Pinschers. Thyroiditis is heritable in the Beagle, Borzoi, Golden Retriever, Great Dane, Irish Setter, Doberman Pinscher, and Old English Sheepdog.

Risk Factors

- No known environmental factors have been identified. Breed predispositions as outlined above.

Historic Findings

- As thyroid hormone regulates the metabolic rate and influences the functions of many organs, clinical signs are often non-specific and insidious in onset. Many other diseases can have similar clinical signs to hypothyroidism, which may lead to an incorrect diagnosis. As such, the laboratory testing of thyroid function is often performed as part of the diagnostic work-up in animals with non-thyroidal illness.

 CLINICAL FEATURES

- Common clinical signs include lethargy, mental dullness, weight gain, exercise intolerance, alopecia, and obesity (Fig. 40.1).

 DIFFERENTIAL DIAGNOSIS

- Many metabolic, infectious, neoplastic, congenital, degenerative, and inflammatory diseases can cause similar clinical signs and biochemical abnormalities seen with hypothyroidism.

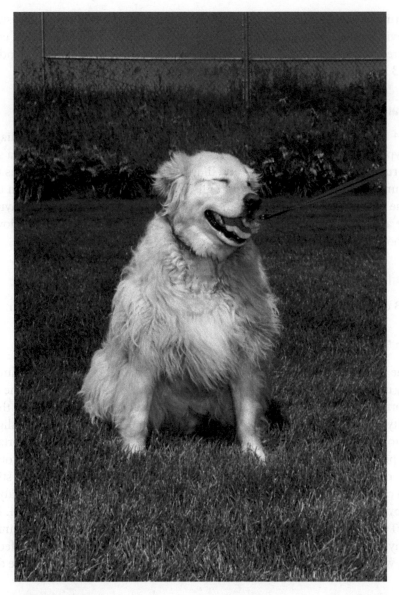

■ Fig. 40.1. Canine hypothyroidism.

DIAGNOSTICS

Laboratory Diagnosis

■ Thyroxine is the major secretory product of the thyroid, while the majority of T3 is derived from extra-thyroidal sources. Both, T4 and T3 are highly protein-bound to serum carrier proteins such as thyroid-binding globulin, transthyretin, and albumin. Only unbound (free) hormone is able to penetrate cell membranes, bind to receptors, and result in bio-logic activity. Protein-bound hormone acts as a reservoir to maintain steady concentra-tions of free hormone in the plasma, despite rapid alterations in the release and metabo-lism of T3 and T4 and changes in the plasma protein concentrations.

Serum Total T4

■ Serum T4 is a sensitive (>90–95%), but not specific (70–75%) test for the diagnosis of canine hypothyroidism. The vast majority of dogs with hypothyroidism have a serum T4 below normal, but some normal dogs and those with a variety of other problems may have a low serum T4. A diagnosis of hypothyroidism can be ruled out if the T4 is in the upper 50% of the reference range. Autoantibodies to T4 occur in about 15% of hypothyroid dogs, and these antibodies may falsely increase the serum T4 concentration from below normal into or above the normal range. In-house testing of TT4 is not recommended.

Serum Total T3

■ Serum T3 concentration is an unreliable test for evaluation of thyroid function.

Serum free T4 (fT4)

■ Thyroxine is highly (99.9%) protein-bound in the circulation. Protein binding can be altered by many non-thyroidal illnesses and by certain drugs. Measurement of the unbound or free hormone can provide a more accurate assessment of thyroid function in these cases (sensitivity >95%, specificity >97%). The sensitivity of fT4 is equivalent to or slightly bet-ter than total T4 in diagnosing hypothyroidism in routine cases. More importantly, fT4 is more specific, particularly when non-thyroidal factors that can influence total T4 are present. Free T4 is less affected by most non-thyroidal illness and drugs, but still can be altered in cases of moderate to severe illness. In addition, fT4 by equilibrium dialysis is not affected by the presence of T4 autoantibodies that will falsely elevate total T4. Measure-ment of fT4 by equilibrium dialysis should be performed when uncommon clinical signs of hypothyroidism are present, the dog is being treated with a drug that may affect thyroid function, when non-thyroidal illness is present, and if autoantibodies to T4 are detected.

Serum TSH

■ Primary hypothyroidism results in a decrease in T4 and thus decreased negative feedback on the pituitary gland. In response, the pituitary secretes more TSH such that plasma TSH levels are increased. In humans, TSH is elevated prior to any decrease of T4 or fT4 outside the normal range. In the dog, TSH concentration is elevated in only 65–75% of cases of hypothyroidism, and as such it lacks sensitivity for use as a screening test. The combina-tion of decreased total T4 or fT4 with an elevated serum TSH is diagnostic of hypothyroid-ism (specificity >95%). Therefore, whilst a normal TSH does not rule out hypothyroidism, an elevated TSH combined with a low T4 or fT4 provides a definitive diagnosis.

TSH Response Test

- The TSH response test is considered the 'gold standard' for diagnosis of hypothyroidism in the dog. The administration of TSH causes secretion of thyroid hormones, particularly T4. This test is best reserved for use when a confounding factor (non-thyroidal illness, drug administration) is present that makes diagnosis using basal hormone concentrations difficult. To perform the TSH response test, obtain a blood sample for measurement of serum T4 before and 4 hours after IV administration of 75 µg human recombinant TSH. A serum T4 concentration >30 nmol/l is considered normal. Most hypothyroid dogs have little, if any, increase in T4 following TSH administration, and typically have pre- and post-TSH T4 concentrations <20 nmol/l. Human recombinant TSH (Thyrogen®; Genzyme Corp.) can be frozen for 6 months after being reconstituted, so multiple dogs can be tested using one vial of TSH.

Diagnosis of Thyroiditis

- Antibodies against either T4 or T3 or both are sometimes present in dogs with thyroiditis, with or without hypothyroidism. The presence of these antibodies does not indicate that the dog is hypothyroid, but suggests that autoimmune thyroid disease is present. These antibodies frequently cause a false elevation of T4 or T3 concentrations that can result in marked elevation of the hormones. Autoantibodies to T4 are present in about 10–15% of hypothyroid dogs.
- Dogs with autoimmune thyroiditis may have circulating antibodies to thyroglobulin, the primary protein in the colloid of the thyroid gland. This is not a test of thyroid function, but rather a marker for the presence of autoimmune thyroiditis. In one long-term study at Michigan State University, 20% of asymptomatic, antithyroglobulin-positive dogs with normal thyroid function progressed to hypothyroidism in 1 year. The presence of these antibodies in a dog with borderline laboratory evidence of hypothyroidism and clinical signs supports a diagnosis of hypothyroidism.

Additional Considerations

Breed

- Certain breeds have normal ranges of thyroid hormones that are different from most other breeds. Few have been evaluated, but greyhounds have serum total T4 and fT4 concentrations that are considerably lower than most other breeds. Scottish deerhounds, Salukis and Whippets also have total T4 concentrations that are well below the mean concentration of dogs in general. Alaskan sled dogs have serum T4, T3, and fT4 concentrations that are below the reference range of most pet dogs, particularly during periods of intense training or racing.

Time of Day

- In one study 50% of normal dogs had a low serum T4 concentration at some time during the day.

Medications

- The drugs that are known to commonly alter thyroid function tests are glucocorticoids, phenobarbital, sulfonamides, clomipramine, aspirin, and some other NSAIDs. Glucocorticoids suppress total T4 and sometimes also fT4. Phenobarbital causes a decreased total T4 and mild increases in TSH. Sulfonamides can induce overt primary hypothyroidism, with clinical signs and thyroid function tests that support the diagnosis. The changes may be reversible when the medication is discontinued. There are dozens of drugs that affect thyroid function and thyroid function tests in humans, so many others will also likely affect dogs.

Non-Thyroidal Illness

- Illness not involving the thyroid gland can alter thyroid function tests and has been labeled 'non-thyroidal illness' or 'euthyroid sick syndrome.' Any illness can alter thyroid function tests, causing a fairly consistent decrease in total T4 and T3 concentrations in proportion to the severity of illness. Serum TSH concentration is increased in 8–10% of dogs with non-thyroidal illness. Serum fT4 measured by equilibrium dialysis is less likely to be affected, but can also be increased or decreased. However, in dogs with substantial non-thyroidal illness, the fT4 is likely to be decreased. It is recommended that testing of thyroid function be postponed until the non-thyroidal illness is resolved. If this is not possible, measurement of T4, TSH and fT4 are indicated.

Ancillary Testing: Thyroid Gland Ultrasound

- Although rarely necessary, ultrasound of the thyroid glands (performed by an experienced ultrasonographer) can be used to aid in differentiating dogs with primary hypothyroidism from those with non-thyroidal illness. Thyroid glands of hypothyroid dogs tend to be smaller, less homogeneous, and hypoechoic than those of euthyroid dogs. There is a considerable overlap with the ultrasonographic appearance and size of the thyroid glands of euthyroid and hypothyroid dogs. Thyroid ultrasound can only be used to help support a diagnosis of hypothyroidism if the thyroid glands are quite small.

Pathological Findings

- With primary hypothyroidism there is multifocal to diffuse infiltration of the thyroid parenchyma with lymphocytes, plasma cells, and macrophages. Remaining follicles are small with vacuolated colloid. The parenchyma is replaced by fibrous connective tissue with progression of thyroiditis.
- Idiopathic follicular atrophy results in loss of thyroid parenchyma and replacement by adipose and connective tissue.

 # THERAPEUTICS

Drugs

- Levothyroxine is the only hormone that appears necessary for the treatment of hypothyroidism. The frequency of levothyroxine dosing is controversial, and the only study to closely evaluate the response to treatment showed that once-daily treatment is adequate. However, in clinical practice some dogs seem to respond better to twice-daily treatment.

■ The initial starting dose is 0.02 mg/kg PO q. 24 h. In general there will never be a need to exceed 0.8 mg as an initial daily dosage, even in very large dogs. If the dog has significant cardiovascular disease, diabetes mellitus, or hypoadrenocorticism, treatment should be instituted at 25% of the standard dose, with the dosage increased by 25% every 2 weeks based on clinical response and post-pill testing. Most dogs show improvements within the first 1–2 weeks, with increased activity, improved attitude, and partial or complete resolution of neurologic signs.

■ The cutaneous manifestations of hypothyroidism may take several weeks to months to resolve. Post-treatment monitoring may be carried out, but clinical response is the most important monitoring tool. Peak T4 concentrations generally occur 4–6 hours after administration of levothyroxine and should be in the high normal to slightly above normal range (40–70 nmol/l). However, the bioavailability of thyroxine ranges from 13% to 87% in the same dog from day to day, which brings into question the utility of random post-pill monitoring of T4. It is likely more meaningful (though more expensive) to measure TSH (especially if the TSH concentration was elevated pre-treatment) or fT4 concentrations after replacement therapy has been started, especially in animals that show a poor clinical response to therapy. Serum TSH concentrations should be in the normal range or undetectable, while fT4 concentrations should be in the normal range. Serum concentrations of TSH and fT4 should not be measured until the patient has been on supplementation for at least 2 weeks. If the patient was initially started on twice-daily therapy, treatment can be reduced to once-daily treatment when a good clinical response has been obtained.

■ Hyperthyroidism is the most common complication of treatment with levothyroxine, but it is rare in dogs. Clinical signs are similar to those of hyperthyroidism in cats and the diagnosis is confirmed by documenting a substantial elevation of serum T4. Treatment consists of stopping levothyroxine treatment for 2-3 days, then instituting treatment at a lower dose.

 COMMENTS

Expected Course and Prognosis

■ Response to therapy should be observed in the first 4–8 weeks post treatment. Improvements in mentation and physical activity may be noted within the first week, though some abnormalities – especially dermatologic signs – may take several months to resolve. An absent or incomplete response to therapy may be due to an incorrect diagnosis, poor owner compliance, inadequate dosing, or poor absorption.

Suggested Reading

van Dijl, I.C., Le Traon, G., van de Meulengraaf, B.D., Burgaud, S., Horspool, L.J., Kooistra, H.S. (2014) Pharmacokinetics of total thyroxine after repeated oral administration of levothyroxine solution and its clinical efficacy in hypothyroid dogs. *J. Vet. Intern. Med.*, **28** (4), 1229–1234.

Bellumori, T.P., Famula, T.R., Bannasch, D.L., Belanger, J.M., Oberbauer, A.M. (2013) Prevalence of inherited disorders among mixed-breed and purebred dogs: 27,254 cases (1995–2010). *J. Am. Vet. Med. Assoc.*, **242** (11), 1549–1555.

Panciera, D.L., Purswell, B.J., Kolster, K.A., Werre, S.R., Trout, S.W. (2012) Reproductive effects of prolonged experimentally induced hypothyroidism in bitches. *J. Vet. Intern. Med.*, **26** (2), 326–333.

Mooney, Ct. (2011) Canine hypothyroidism: a review of aetiology and diagnosis. *N. Z. Vet. J.*, **59** (3), 105–114.

Shiel, R.E., Sist, M., Nachreiner, R.F., Ehrlich, C.P., Mooney, C.T. (2010) Assessment of criteria used by veterinary practitioners to diagnose hypothyroidism in sighthounds and investigation of serum thyroid hormone concentrations in healthy Salukis. *J. Am. Vet. Med. Assoc.*, **236** (3), 302–308.

Authors: David Bruyette DVM, DACVIM; Autumn P. Davidson DVM, MS, DACVIM (Internal Medicine)

chapter 41

Insulinoma

DEFINITION

- Functional pancreatic islet β-cell tumor that secretes an excess quantity of insulin independent of glucose concentration.

ETIOLOGY/PATHOPHYSIOLOGY

- Excessive insulin secretion leads to excessive glucose uptake and use by insulin-sensitive tissues and reduced hepatic production of glucose; this causes hypoglycemia and its associated clinical signs.

Systems Affected

- Nervous – seizures, disorientation, abnormal behavior, collapse, polyneuropathy/peripheral neuropathy, posterior paresis, and ataxia.
- Musculoskeletal – weakness and muscle fasciculations.
- Gastrointestinal – polyphagia and weight gain.

Incidence/Prevalence

- Dogs – uncommon.
- Cats – rare.

SIGNALMENT/HISTORY

Species

- Dogs and cats.

Blackwell's Five-Minute Veterinary Consult Clinical Companion: Small Animal Endocrinology and Reproduction, First Edition. Edited by Deborah S. Greco and Autumn P. Davidson. © 2017 John Wiley & Sons, Inc. Published 2017 by John Wiley & Sons, Inc.
Companion Website: www.fiveminutevet.com/endocrinology

Breed Predilections

- Dogs – Labrador Retrievers, Standard Poodles, Boxers, Fox Terriers, Irish Setters, German Shepherds, Golden Retrievers, and Collies.
- Cats – none; possibly Siamese.

Mean Age and Range

- Dogs – middle-aged to old; mean 10 years; range 3–14 years.
- Cats – mean 15 years; range 12–17 years.

 ## CLINICAL FEATURES

General Comments

- Often episodic.
- May or may not be related to fasting, excitement, exercise, and/or eating.
- Dogs generally demonstrate more than one clinical sign with progression over time.

Historic Findings

- Dogs – generalized and/or focal seizures are most common. Additional findings may include weakness, posterior paresis, collapse, muscle fasciculations, bizarre behavior, lethargy and depression, ataxia, polyphagia, weight gain, polyuria and polydipsia and exercise intolerance.
- Cats – seizures, ataxia, muscle fasciculations, weakness, lethargy and depression, anorexia, weight loss, and polydipsia.

Physical Examination Findings

- Usually within normal limits unless in a hypoglycemic crisis with the aforementioned signs.
- Obesity is common.
- Polyneuropathy can be seen rarely in dogs (paresis to paralysis, muscle atrophy, and/or hyporeflexia).

Causes

- Most dogs and cats have single insulin-producing β-islet cell carcinoma or adenocarcinoma of the pancreas. Approximately 50% or more of dogs and cats with insulinomas will develop or present with metastasis.

Risk Factors

- For hypoglycemic episodes – fasting, excitement, exercise and eating.

 # DIFFERENTIAL DIAGNOSIS

- Extrapancreatic tumor hypoglycemia – paraneoplastic hypoglycemia has been documented in dogs with numerous tumors, including hepatocellular carcinoma, metastatic mammary carcinoma, primary pulmonary carcinoma, and others; these tumors generally secrete insulin or insulin-like factors.
- Perform a complete hypoglycemic work-up and rule out causes such as iatrogenic insulin, neonatal/toy breed hypoglycemia, ingestion of oral hypoglycemic agents, hepatic failure, sepsis, hypoadrenocorticism, hunting dog hypoglycemia and glycogen storage diseases.
- Seizures and collapse – consider a variety of differentials including cardiovascular (e.g., syncope), metabolic (e.g., anemia, hepatoencephalopathy, hypocalcemia, and hypoadrenocorticism) and neurologic (e.g., epilepsy, neoplasia, toxin, and inflammatory disease).

 # DIAGNOSTICS

CBC/Biochemistry/Urinalysis

- Results often within normal limits except for hypoglycemia (<65–70 mg/dl in the majority of patients).
- Normoglycemia does not rule out the presence of an insulinoma. A small percentage of patients may be intermittently normoglycemic, which is thought to be due to counter-regulatory hormone production (e.g., epinephrine, glucocorticoids, glucagon).

Other Laboratory Tests

- Simultaneous fasting glucose and insulin determinations.
  - Upon initiating fasting (patients should always be hospitalized and monitored closely during this time due to the high risk for extreme hypoglycemia episodes), collect baseline blood samples and then hourly or bihourly for serum glucose determination and serum storage. When the serum glucose drops below 60 mg/dl, submit that serum sample for simultaneous glucose and serum insulin determination. When the insulin is elevated in the face of hypoglycemia an insulinoma is highly likely, whereas if the insulin is within normal limits in the face of hypoglycemia then insulinoma is possible. If the insulin value is below normal limits during the hypoglycemia, an insulinoma is unlikely but multiple sampling may be necessary.
  - Formulas utilizing simultaneous hypoglycemic glucose and insulin values such as the insulin:glucose ratio and the amended insulin:glucose ratio are falling out of favor due to poor specificity.

Imaging

- Thoracic and abdominal radiography – helpful for evaluation of metastatic disease and/or extrapancreatic tumor-induced causes of hypoglycemia, as well as some other differential diagnoses.
- Ultrasonography – fewer than 50% of pancreatic masses are clearly identified through ultrasonography.
- CT – superior technique for detection of primary insulinomas in dogs; however, false-positive lymph node metastases are common and problematic; should primarily be used for preoperative delineation/ confirmation of a primary pancreatic mass.
- Scintigraphy and SPECT – intermittently successful in detecting insulinomas.
- Intraoperative ultrasound – widely used for grossly occult tumor detection in human insulinomas; rarely reported in veterinary medicine.

Diagnostic Procedures

- Exploratory laparotomy – indicated when insulinoma is suspected based on the aforementioned physical, biochemical and/or imaging results.

Pathologic Findings

- Histopathologically, primary pancreatic insulinomas in dogs are generally either β-islet cell carcinomas or adenocarcinomas. Occasionally they are adenomas, but dogs with adenomas may subsequently develop metastasis, suggesting limitations with the delineation of malignancy potential with light microscopy of insulinomas. In cats, most have been malignant with metastasis commonly noted.

 # THERAPEUTICS

Appropriate Health Care

- Hospitalize for work-up and surgery since life-threatening hypoglycemia is a very real possibility.
- Outpatient if the owner declines surgery and the patient is not clinically hypoglycemic.

Nursing Care

- For emergency hypoglycemic episodes, administer 50% dextrose (1 ml/kg IV slowly over 1–3 minutes) to control seizures/severe hypoglycemic signs. Once the emergency hypoglycemia clinical signs abate, follow with fluid therapy with 2.5% dextrose (increase to 5% if needed to control clinical signs). Alternatively, if the patient can eat, frequent feedings of an appropriate diet (see below) may replace dextrose-containing fluids in many patients.

Activity

- Restricted.

Diet

- Feed four to six small meals a day.
- Food should be high in protein, fat, and complex carbohydrates, but low in simple sugars.
- Avoid semi-moist foods that dilute the aforementioned fat, protein, and carbohydrate levels.

Client education

- Owner should be educated about the signs of hypoglycemia and seek immediate attention if they occur.

Surgical Considerations

- Surgical management improves prognosis over medical therapy alone.
- Medical management to prevent severe hypoglycemia is important before an exploratory laparotomy. Most patients respond well to frequent small feedings and corticosteroids. In rare refractory cases, the use of IV fluids containing 2.5–5% dextrose and/or glucagon may be necessary.
- Objectives include confirmation of the diagnosis, elucidation of the presence/absence of any extra-pancreatic metastases and/or other disease and removal of as much cancerous tissue as possible.
- At surgery, most insulinomas can be visualized and/or palpated. If a pancreatic mass cannot be found, intraoperative ultrasound may be beneficial. In rare cases, IV 1% methylene blue (3 mg/kg added to 250 ml of 0.9% NaCl, given IV slowly over 30–45 minutes) may be used to delineate an occult pancreatic insulinoma. Hemolytic anemia, pseudocyanosis and hemoglobinuric nephrotoxicity are possible side effects of the procedure, so routine use is not recommended.
- Approximately 15% of dogs have multiple primary insulinomas, so always examine the entire pancreas.
- Biopsy the regional lymph nodes and careful evaluate the liver (and other abdominal contents) with biopsy of any abnormalities. Approximately 40–50% of dogs will have a metastasis. In one study, of 14 dogs suspected to have extra-pancreatic metastasis from a primary pancreatic insulinoma, only eight (57%) had histological evidence of metastasis. Therefore, the presence of what appears to be metastasis should be biopsied and not automatically lead to intraoperative euthanasia.

Medications

Drug(s) of Choice

- Emergency/acute therapy.
  - See 'Nursing Care' above.
- Long-term therapy
  - If dietary therapy is ineffective, glucocorticoids such as prednisone may be given at an initial dosage of 0.25 mg/kg PO q. 12 h, and increased as needed to 2–3 mg/kg PO q. 12 h.

- Diazoxide (Proglycem) stimulates hepatic gluconeogenesis/glycogenolysis and inhibits insulin secretion. Diazoxide may be given at 5–60 mg/kg PO q. 12 h (start low and increase as needed) in addition to dietary modifications and/or glucocorticoids when they are becoming less effective. Diazoxide can be difficult to locate and may be prohibitively expensive for some clients.
- Streptozotocin is a nitrosourea that semi-selectively targets pancreatic β cells. Streptozotocin may be given at 500 mg/m^2 slowly IV over 2 hours after a 3-hour 0.9% NaCl dieresis, and followed with a 2-hour diuresis. This protocol may be repeated every 3 weeks until normoglycemia is achieved. Streptozotocin is emetogenic and can be hepatotoxic and/or nephrotoxic.
- Glucagon is gluconeogenic and may be used at 5 ng/kg/minute CRI (to effect) to treat acute severe refractory hypoglycemia.
- The synthetic somatostatin analogs octreotide (10–20 μg SC q. 8–12 h) or lantreotide (no determined dose in veterinary species) may be utilized to prevent hypoglycemia in dogs refractory to conventional treatments.

Contraindications

- Insulin.

Precautions

- Dextrose boluses, when given alone, may precipitate further hypoglycemic crises.
- Glucocorticoids used at high dosages for prolonged periods can cause iatrogenic hyperadrenocorticism.
- Diazoxide may cause bone marrow suppression, gastrointestinal irritation, aplastic anemia, cataracts, thrombocytopenia and tachycardia in humans.
- Streptozotocin can cause emesis, hepatic failure, renal failure, diabetes mellitus, and pancreatitis.

Possible Interactions

- Hydrochlorothiazide can potentiate diazoxide.

Patient Monitoring

- Teach owner to monitor for return and/or progression of signs of hypoglycemia.
- In-hospital serum glucose determinations are important for monitoring for return and/or progression of insulinoma-associated hypoglycemia.

Possible Complications

- Recurrent or progressive episodes of hypoglycemia.

Expected Course And Prognosis

- Dogs that undergo exploratory laparotomy are more likely to become and remain euglycemic longer, and have longer survivals than dogs managed by medical means. Even in the presence of local metastatic disease, any reduction of tumor burden is likely to improve euglycemia control with medical therapies. The median length of euglycemic control after surgery is inversely correlated with the stage of disease, and varies from 14 months for dogs without evidence of metastasis to only 2–3 months for dogs with nodal and/or distant metastasis. The median survival time is also inversely correlated with the stage of disease, and varies from about 16–19 months (range: 2–60 months) for dogs without evidence of metastasis, to 7–9 months in dogs with evidence of nodal and/or distant metastasis. More recent studies have documented even longer median survival times of 17–18 months for all dogs with insulinoma, and 25–42 months for those dogs undergoing surgical and medical therapies.
- Limited data in cats – mean survival time about 6.5 months (range: 0–18 months). Medical management with prednisolone and diet has been reported, as well as the use of octreotide. There is no information about the use of diazoxide or streptozotocin.

 # COMMENTS

Associated Conditions

- Obesity due to hyperinsulinemia.

Age-Related Factors

- Younger dogs have shorter survival times.

Synonyms

- B-cell tumor
- Hyperinsulinism
- Insulin-producing pancreatic tumor
- Insulin-secreting tumor
- Islet cell adenocarcinoma
- Islet cell tumor

See Also

Hypoglycemia

Abbreviations

SPECT = single proton emission computed tomography

Suggested Reading

Feldman, E.C., Nelson, R.W. (2004) Beta-cell Neoplasia: Insulinoma, in *Canine and Feline Endocrinology and Reproduction*, 3rd edition (eds E.D. Feldman, R.W. Nelson), Saunders, St Louis, pp. 616–644.

Fischer, J.R., Smith, S.A., Harkin, K.R. (2000) Glucagon constant-rate infusion: a novel strategy for the management of hyperinsulinemic-hypoglycemic crisis in the dog. *J. Am. Vet. Med. Assoc.*, 36, 27–32.

Lunn, K., Page, R. (2013) Tumors of the Endocrine System, in: *Small Animal Clinical Oncology*, 5th edition (eds S.J. Withrow, D.M. Vail, R.L. Page), Elsevier, St Louis, pp. 519–521.

Madarame, H., Kayanuma, H., Shida, T., *et al.* (2009) Retrospective study of canine insulinomas: 8 cases (2005–2008). *J. Vet. Med. Sci.*, 71 (7), 905–911.

Moore, A.S., Nelson, R.W., Henry, C.J., Rassnick, K.M., Krista, O., Ogilvie, G.K., Kintzer, P. (2002) Streptozotocin for treatment of pancreatic islet cell tumors in dogs: 17 cases (1989–1999). *J. Am. Vet. Med. Assoc.*, 221 (6), 811–818.

Polton, G.A., White, R.N., Brearley, M.J., Eastwood, J.M. (2007) Improved survival in a retrospective cohort of 28 dogs with insulinoma. *J. Small Anim. Pract.*, 48 (3), 151–156.

Robben, J.H., Pollak, Y.W., Kirpensteijn, J., Boroffka, S.A., Van Den Ingh, T.S., Teske, E., Voorhout, G. (2005) Comparison of ultrasonography, computed tomography, and single-photon emission computed tomography for the detection and localization of canine insulinoma. *J. Vet. Intern. Med.*, 19 (1), 15–22.

Acknowledgment: The author and editors acknowledge the previous contribution of Phil Bergman to *Blackwell's Five-Minute Veterinary Consult: Canine and Feline*, on which this topic is based.

Author: Virginia Gill DVM, DACVIM (Oncology)

Mammary Gland Disorders: Agalactia, Galactostasis, and Mastitis

chapter **42**

DEFINITION

- Agalactia (or agalactorrhea) is an absence or failure of milk production and secretion after delivery.
- More common than agalactia is dysgalactia: the mammary glands are dysfunctional and cannot meet the demands of the litter.
- Galactostasis (also called aseptic mastitis) is the abnormal accumulation of milk in the mammary glands associated with inflammatory conditions, without infection.
- Mastitis is the septic inflammation of the mammary gland.

ETIOLOGY/PATHOPHYSIOLOGY

Agalactia

- Two forms exist. The total absence of milk production is a rare condition in dogs and cats:
  - Primary (true agalactia): there is no development of mammary gland during pregnancy; considered a defect in the pituitary ovarian mammary gland axis.
  - Secondary: occurs after concurrent systemic illness, severe stress, iatrogenic causes
- Both can be observed in the bitch and the queen in cases of:
  - Progesterone supplementation for (true or suspected) hypoluteoidism during pregnancy; this interferes with prolactin levels.
  - Stress, dystocia.
  - After premature parturition (natural or after caesarean section).
  - Very small litters that are not providing adequate suckling to stimulate milk production or excessive separation of the neonates from the dam.
  - Poor body condition caused by inadequate water and food intake, or caused by heavy parasitism.
  - Systemic diseases or hormonal imbalance.

Blackwell's Five-Minute Veterinary Consult Clinical Companion: Small Animal Endocrinology and Reproduction, First Edition. Edited by Deborah S. Greco and Autumn P. Davidson. © 2017 John Wiley & Sons, Inc. Published 2017 by John Wiley & Sons, Inc.
Companion Website: www.fiveminutevet.com/endocrinology

Galactostasis

- Lactation is a balance between the secretion of milk by the mammary tissues and the removal of accumulated milk by suckling. The emptying of the milk stock's reserve by nursing stimulates prolactin release from the pituitary gland to increase milk production. When suckling stops or is greatly reduced, resultant engorgement feeds back to the brain to decrease milk production. Galactostasis results if production exceeds removal acutely. Can predispose to mastitis.
- May be seen:
  - At weaning time.
  - When there is a loss of the litter.
  - When there is a small or feeble litter.
  - When nurslings are removed abruptly.
  - In case of maternal disease, as with concurrent mastitis, endometritis or anatomic (nipple) abnormalities.

Mastitis

- Most commonly caused by an ascending infection. Microorganisms gain entrance into the gland through the milk ducts during or after suckling.
- Other contributing factors include injury or trauma from nurslings or environmental causes.
- Can be from a hematogenous source (endometritis).
- Can occur at any time during lactation, at the end of gestation, or during false pregnancy accompanied by lactation.
- Can be acute, chronic or subclinical.
- The most common bacteria isolated are *Escherichia coli*, *Staphylococcus* spp., and *Streptococcus* spp.

Systems Affected

- Reproductive
- Skin/Exocrine
- Endocrine/Metabolic
- Hemic/Lymphatic/Immune
- Renal and liver (in case of sepsis, toxemia or shock).

 ## SIGNALMENT/HISTORY

- Agalactia: Postpartum bitch and queen:
  - Primary (true) agalactia can be suspected if the female's mammary glands do not develop in late pregnancy. Mammary underdevelopment could be an inherited defect.
  - Secondary agalactia should be evident at parturition or in the immediate postpartum period.

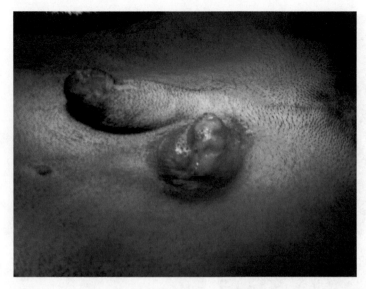

■ **Fig. 42.1.** Focal mastitis in a male dog treated with a progestational compound.

■ Galactostasis and mastitis: Post-partum and pseudopregnant bitch and queen associated with milk secretion.
■ Mastitis occurs more frequently in bitches than in queens.
■ Rare cases of mastitis have been reported in male dog with galactorrhea caused by synthetic hormone therapy for hypersexuality or prostatic hyperplasia or with a functional Sertoli cell tumor (Fig. 42.1).
■ Rare cases with profound hypothyroidism associated with galactorrhea secondary to elevated TRH levels inducing hyperprolactinemia.

Risk Factors

■ **Agalactia**
  • Underlying disease.
  • Inadequate feeding of the dam or heavily parasitized animals.
  • Congenital abnormality of the mammary endocrine system.
  • Side effects of some drugs (e.g., progestins, antiprolactins).
  • Stress.
■ **Galactostasis**
  • Congenital abnormality of the mammary duct or nipple system (Fig. 42.2A,B).
  • Nervous, painful, or stressed dam may discourage offspring from suckling, or may release stress hormones as epinephrine, blocking the oxytocin action promoting milk let-down.
  • Poor husbandry.
■ **Mastitis**
  • Unhygienic conditions or traumatic facilities causing injury of the gland.

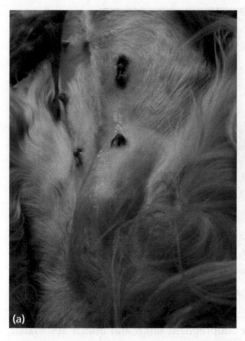
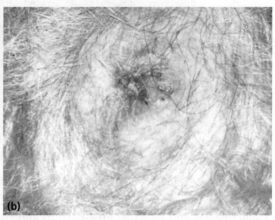

■ **Fig. 42.2.** (A) Mastitis involving a single gland in a bitch with abnormal nipple anatomy. (B) Inverted nipple found during the pre-breeding examination; this predisposes the bitch to galactostasis and mastitis.

- Poor dental care resulting in periodontitis.
- Excessive human manipulation of the mammary gland.
- May be associated with some disease conditions of the uterus (endometritis).
- Mammary glandular development and milk make an excellent growth media for bacteria.
- Systemic illness: bacteria can gain entrance from the blood; the dam's immune system is often deficient during pregnancy and lactation.
- Neonates with long nails can predispose the dam to infection due to trauma.
- Gastrointestinal inflammation is common in the post-partum period due to placental ingestion, consumption of vulvar discharge, and the neonates' eliminations. Moreover, the hormones of pregnancy stimulate intestinal parasites to come out of dormancy and enter the intestinal tract.

Historic Findings

- **Agalactia**
  - Underdevelopment of the mammary glands.
  - Neonates attempt to nurse, cry incessantly and fail to gain weight.
- **Galactostasis**
  - Should be suspected if the mammary glands are firm and swollen; milk is difficult to express due to discomfort.
  - Neonatal weight loss or failure to gain weight.

- **Mastitis**
  - Painful and enlarged mammary glands.
  - Discomfort.
  - Erythema of glands.
  - Lethargy.
  - Anorexia.
  - Poor maternal behavior.
  - Sometimes, mastitis may occur without any signs. The only sign can be fading neonates.

CLINICAL FEATURES

- **Agalactia**
  - Underdevelopment of the mammary glands without milk secretion.
  - Less milk availability than expected.
- **Galactostasis**
  - The gland will be reddened, enlarged/firm, hot, hyperemic, and sensitive.
  - There is usually no fever and the bitch/queen is not systemically ill.
- **Mastitis**
  - The disease can involve only a single or several mammary glands (Figs. 42.3 and 42.4).

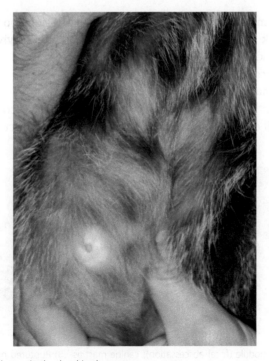

■ **Fig. 42.3.** Mastitis involving a single gland in the queen.

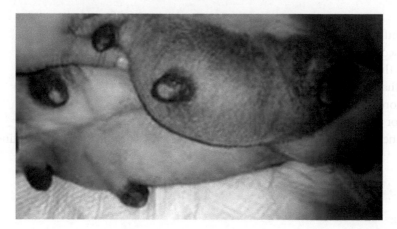

■ **Fig. 42.4.** Mastitis involving a single gland in the bitch; galactostasis in surrounding glands is evident.

- Milk can appear normal in color, or have a purulent or hemorrhagic appearance. Blood or pus can escape through the milk ducts, it can be absorbed, or it can become encapsulated by fibrous tissue and form a hematoma or abscess.
- Skin changes around the nipple can include: focal nodules, redness, cracking or ulceration (Fig. 42.5A,B).
- Gangrene and necrosis can occur.

■ **Acute mastitis**
- Signs of systemic infection (sepsis) include depression, poor maternal behavior, decreased milk production, failure of the neonates to survive, anorexia, lethargy, fever and shock.

■ **Chronic or subclinical mastitis**
- Failure of neonates to thrive.
- The glands can be firm and hard, due to the inflammatory connective tissue formation, and small cystic dilatations due to obstructed milk-ducts can be present.

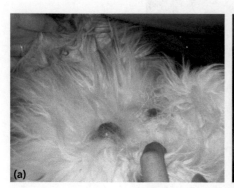
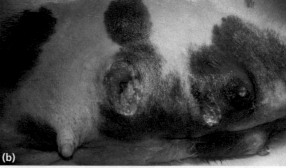

■ **Fig. 42.5.** (A) Erythemic nodule (focal abscessation); canine mastitis. (B) Ruptured mastitic abscessation; canine mastitis.

DIFFERENTIAL DIAGNOSIS

Agalactia

- Prematurity.
- Colostrum.
- Dams with inadequate lactation at term should be evaluated for metabolic or inflammatory disorders (endometritis, eclampsia, mastitis), as well as for nutritional and hydration status and parasitism.
- Lactation depression or dysgalactia.

Galactostasis

- Mastitis.
- Mammary hypertrophy.
- Mammary neoplasia or fibrocystic disease.

Mastitis

- Galactostasis.
- Insect or snake bite.
- Mammary hypertrophy, mammary neoplasia or fibrocystic disease.

DIAGNOSTICS

- A good history and complete physical examination are very important and the diagnosis is sometimes made on this basis alone.
- In case of systemic illness, additional tests may include:
    - Microscopic (cytologic) examination of milk.
    - Bacterial culture and sensitivity on milk.
    - Aspiration and cytology of masses.
    - Complete blood count (CBC).
    - Blood chemistries.
    - Urinalysis culture if (for dehydration, renal function, metabolic disorders and urinary tract infection).
    - Mammary gland ultrasound to identify abscess formation (Figs 42.6 and 42.7).
    - Blood cultures if sepsis is suspected.
    - Milk pH.

Pathological Findings

- Inflammatory exudate within the tissues.
- Polymorphonuclear leukocytes, necrotic tissues, microorganisms in milk.
- Leukocytosis (neutrophilia).

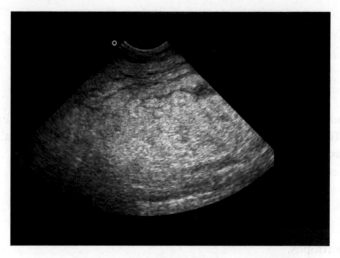

■ **Fig. 42.6.** Ultrasonographic image of mammary cellulitis; no fluid pocket is evident. Image courtesy of T.W. Baker.

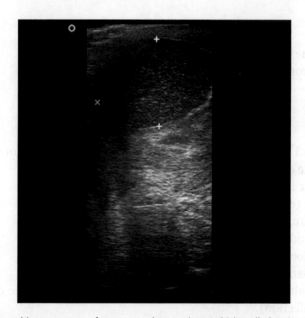

■ **Fig. 42.7.** Ultrasonographic appearance of mammary abscessation. A thick-walled cavitated site with fluid content is visible (cursors). Image courtesy of T.W. Baker.

  THERAPEUTICS

Agalactia

- Lactating dam should eat two to three times more than usual, and needs an excellent hydration; dams may need to be fed in the nest box.

- Milk let-down can be stimulated by oxytocin (0.5–1.0 U SC q. 4 h for 24 h), but this is unlikely to be effective in primary agalactia.
- Adequate supplemental feeding for neonates is required to support their nutrition, but not excessively to diminish suckling completely.
- Neonates deprived of colostrum can receive adult blood serum, ideally from own mother (22–100 ml/kg PO if within 24 hours of birth, or SC thereafter).
- Gentle hand stripping of the mammary glands should take place if suckling is not vigorous enough.
- Concurrent administration of metoclopramide (0.1–0.2 mg/kg SC or PO q. 12 h) may promote prolactin release. Symptoms such as dystonic reactions, excitation and anxiety may develop and require discontinuation of the therapy if higher doses are used.
- Side effects of domperidone (Motilium®) are similar to metoclopramide but less common; availability may be problematic.
- Acepromazine may stimulate prolactin secretion and help in cases of nervous or reluctant dams, encouraging them to permit nursing; high doses could cause hypotension, decreased respiratory rate, and bradycardia. A paradoxical reaction (hyperexcitation) may occur in some animals; at low doses (0.01 mg/kg PO or SC q. 6–12 h; sedation of the neonates is not appreciable.
- Cimetidine may induce galactorrhea.
- Local application of warm compresses.
- Introduce neonates to the dam as soon as is possible; encourage bonding.
- Restrict visitors and traffic during the first 2 weeks post-partum for limiting stress stimulus.
- Many veterinarians report success with acupuncture therapy.

Galactostasis

- Anti-inflammatory drugs can be used only with caution in nursing dams due to uncertain disposition in the nurslings; all such drugs enter the mammary glands.
- Encourage nursing and exposing all mammary glands to the nurslings.
- If there are no nurslings, or the offspring can be weaned, engorged glands should not be milked out. Administration of antiprolactin compounds such as cabergoline (2.5–5 µg/kg q. 12–24 h PO) or (Galastop ®) is indicated.
- If nursing is desired, therapies decreasing milk production without stopping it, can be used (e.g., Galastop®) in one dose (2.5–5 µg/kg PO).
- An Elizabethan collar or shirt covering the dam's thorax may decrease milk production caused by the bitch's self-stimulation inducing hormonal-negative feedback to the brain to reduce milk production.
- Mild diuretics.
- If decreasing milk production is not desired, the glands should be regularly milked out by hand or by the nurslings, and antiprolactin medications should not be used unless mastitis occurs.
- Narcotic analgesics as indicated.
- Topical cabbage leaves may be soothing; mechanism unknown.

Mastitis

- Severely systemically ill patients should be stabilized, with intravenous fluids and antibiotics, and early weaning instituted to allow the mammary glands to regress as indicated.
- Necrotic or gangrenous tissues should be debrided, often in stages; abscess management is best dictated by ultrasound findings (Fig. 42.8A,B).
- The entire gland may need to be removed (mastectomy) in rapidly progressing cases.
- Topical wound care, shaving the hair from around the teats and trimming the nails of the nurslings is helpful.
- The decision to continue to permit nursing depends on the severity of illness in the dam. Neonates avoid nursing from mastitic glands as milk is difficult to obtain. Neonates are likely already exposed to the causative bacteria. A resistant, potentially pathogenic bacterium may be an indication for weaning. Analgesia with narcotics (tramadol up to 10 mg/kg PO divided q. 24 h) is indicated, and owners should monitor for maternal aggression resulting from pain. Sometimes total separation is needed; however, galactostasis and worsening of mastitis can result. Sedation of the neonates is not recognized.
- Short-acting steroid or non-steroidal anti-inflammatory drugs are indicated in order to reduce swelling if weaning has occurred.
- Sedation with phenothiazine should be avoided as they can increase prolactin secretion if weaning has occurred.

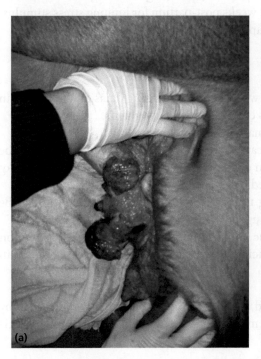 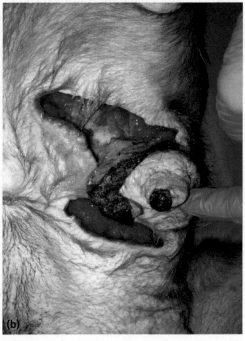

■ **Fig. 42.8.** (A) Marked necrosis/gangrene in canine mastitis; the nipple is viable. (B) Staged debridement in gangrenous canine mastitis can preserve the gland.

- If the neonates are not allowed to nurse:
  - Bitches should be prevented from self-stimulation, and the glands should not be manipulated.
  - Withholding food and rationing water to half normal intake for 24 hours might reduce milk production.
- Administration of anti-prolactin compounds is recommended (cabergoline 2.5–5 μg/kg PO q. 12–24 h); this dopamine agonist could have some side effects (vomiting and diarrhea), but these could be minimized by starting at a low dose and increasing slowly, or by dividing the dose by two and giving it BID.
- Mibolerone and progestogens should not be used.
- Antibiotics should be selected according to the antimicrobial sensitivity. A broad-spectrum antibiotic will be started until culture and sensitivity results are available.
- Factors influencing the choice of antibiotic are lipid solubility, pH, integrity of the blood–milk barrier (acute or chronic mastitis).
- Weak bases and antibiotics with high lipid solubility will better concentrate into milk. As in acute mastitis, the milk–plasma barrier is disrupted, antibiotics are able to concentrate into milk better than in cases of chronic mastitis.
- Safe for nurslings.

Mastitis with Nursing Offspring

- **Note** : avoid aminoglycosides, chloramphenicol, thiamphenicol, tetracyclines, clindamycin, lincomycin and quinolones.
- The amoxicillin/clavulanic acid combination (Clavaseptin®, Clavamox® and Synulox®) for at least 10 days is a good choice until culture and sensitivity results are available.
- Erythromycin is considered safe without apparent complication for nurslings.
- Cephalosporins are an additional good empiric choice.

Mastitis without Nursing Offspring

- The amoxicillin/clavulanic acid combination (e.g., Clavaseptin®, Amoxyclav® and Synulox®) for at least 10 days is a good choice until culture and sensitivity results are available.
- Quinolones such as ciprofloxacin (Ciproxine®), marbofloxacin (Marbocyl®), and enrofloxacin (Baytril ®).
- Chloramphenicol.
- Clindamycin (Antirobe®).
- Erythromycin.
- Cephalosporins.

Drug(s)

- Oxytocin: Administered SC at 0.25–2.0 U/dose depending on the body weight, for several days; or nasal spray (Syntocinon®). The neonates should be removed from the dam prior to each injection and returned 30 minutes later.
- Metoclopramide 0.1–0.2 mg/kg, SC or PO, BID–TID for 5 days.

- Acepromazine 0.01 mg/kg PO q. 6–24 h.
- Cimetidine 2 mg/kg PO BID–TID.

 COMMENTS

Agalactia

- Determination that lactation is adequate should be performed prior to elective cesarean section.
- Daily weight gain of neonates of at least 10% of body weight (after the first 24 hours) indicates adequate lactation.
- The best time to start nursing is a few minutes after birth or cesarean section.
- Ovariohysterectomy should not have a negative effect on bitches and queens with adequate lactogenesis.

Galactostasis

- Whelping and queening should happen in a familiar area.
- Unfamiliar surroundings may interfere with milk let-down.
- Cleaning nurslings after every meal if the maternal instincts fail.

Mastitis prevention

- In the kennel, whelping areas should be cleaned once a day and the bedding should be replaced once or twice daily; box surfaces should be impervious.

See Also

Feline Mammary Hyperplasia

Suggested Reading

Johnston, S.D., Root Kustritz, M.V., Olson, P.N.S. (2001) *Periparturient Disorders in the Bitch; Canine and Feline Theriogenology.* WB Saunders Co., Philadelphia, pp. 131–134.

Feldman, E.C., Nelson, R.W. (1996) *Canine and Feline Endocrinology and Reproduction,* 3rd edition, Saunders, Philadelphia, PA.

Freshman, J.L. (2016) *Mastitis; Blackwell's Five-Minute Veterinary Consult Canine and Feline,* 6th edition, pp. 851.

Linde-Forsberg, C., Eneroth, A. (2010) *Textbook of Veterinary Internal Medicine: Abnormalities in Canine Pregnancy, Parturition, and the Periparturient Period.* 7th edition, Vol. 2 (eds S.J. Ettinger, E.C. Feldman), WB Saunders, Philadelphia, pp. 1890–1901.

Rebuelto, M., Loza, M.E. (2010) Antibiotic treatment of dogs and cats during pregnancy. *Vet. Med. Int.,* **2010,** article ID 385640. Available at: http://dx.doi.org/10.4061/2010/385640

Wiebe, V.J., Howard, J.P. (2009) Pharmacologic Advances in Canine and Feline Reproduction, in *Topics in Companion Animal Medicine: Reproduction* (ed. A.P. Davidson), Elsevier Saunders, Philadelphia PA, vol. 24 (2), pp. 71–99.

Author: Giovana Bassu DVM, DECAR

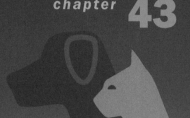

chapter 43

Feline Mammary Hyperplasia

DEFINITION

- Feline mammary hyperplasia (FMH) is a benign but clinically significant condition of the cat (and rarely dog) mammary gland.
- FMH is a rapid but non-cancerous fibroglandular proliferation of the mammae of the cat (and rarely dog). Most affected cats are either in diestrus, pregnant or being treated with exogenous progesterone at the time of presentation. Diagnosis is often straightforward, and prompt treatment is indicated to limit progression leading to local necrosis. The prognosis is favorable if appropriate medical therapy is available, making surgery rarely necessary.

ETIOLOGY/PATHOPHYSIOLOGY

- FMH results in rapid mammary fibroglandular proliferation, either diffuse or conscripted, with the development of intralobular ducts and connective tissue stroma. This is in contrast to pregnancy, in which the mammary glandular structures are growing and the stroma is regressing.
- The exact etiopathogenesis remains uncertain. Indeed, many of the hormones and growth factors involved in FMH lesions are similar to those regulating normal mammary development.
- Progesterone and its analogs are mainly implicated in the disease (Fig. 43.1). Prolonged administration of progestins orally or by injection can be sufficient to induce FMH that is refractory to treatment. Rare cases of FMH encountered in males or ovariohysterectomized females can remain unexplained, and the role of progesterone precursors should be considered.

Systems Affected

- Reproductive – mammary glands.
- Cardiovascular – tachycardia associated with pain, sepsis.
- Skin – ulceration of the mammary skin.

Blackwell's Five-Minute Veterinary Consult Clinical Companion: Small Animal Endocrinology and Reproduction, First Edition. Edited by Deborah S. Greco and Autumn P. Davidson. © 2017 John Wiley & Sons, Inc. Published 2017 by John Wiley & Sons, Inc.
Companion Website: www.fiveminutevet.com/endocrinology

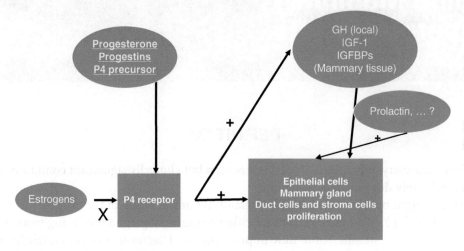

■ **Fig. 43.1.** The etiopathogenesis of FMH.

 ## SIGNALMENT/HISTORY

- Intact young queens (aged <2 years) following their first or second estrous cycle.
- Pregnant queen rarely during gestation (commonly the second month).
- Mainly diffuse fibroepithelial hyperplasia: general enlargement of the mammary gland or glands (Figs 43.2 and 43.3).
- Cats of any age, gender, and reproductive status if treated with progestagens.
- Mainly lobular hyperplasia (also called intraductal papillar hyperplasia): proliferation of the mammary gland duct (Fig. 43.4).

Risk Factors

- Progestagens.
- Cattery. The presence of a tom cat sometimes promotes spontaneous ovulation (10–20% of cases) and subsequent progesterone production (pseudo-pregnancy).

Historic Findings

- Estrus in the last 2–6 weeks. Affected female cats may or may not have a history of mating.
- Progesterone therapy in the previous weeks (males or females).
- One or more mammary glands (often all glands) undergo diffuse enlargement over 2–4 weeks.

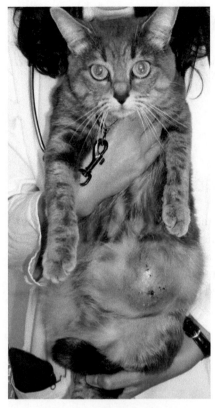

■ **Fig. 43.2.** Diffuse FMH involving a single mammary gland.

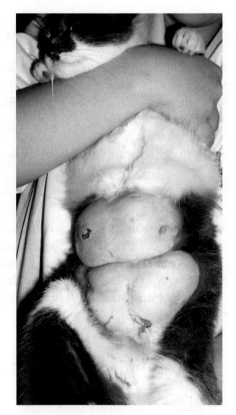

■ **Fig. 43.3.** Diffuse FMH involving multiple mammary glands.

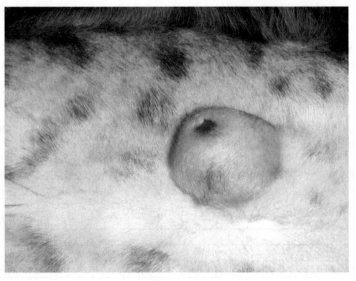

■ **Fig. 43.4.** Discrete lobular ulcerated mammary nodule.

CLINICAL FEATURES

- Single or multiple enlarged, uniform, firm, non-painful mammary masses (Figs 43.2 and 43.3).
- Simple cyst/nodule in one mammary gland (Fig. 43.4).
- Erythemic skin ulceration (Fig. 43.4).
- Anorexia.
- Hyperthermia.
- Death due to acute ischemic necrosis or thrombosis.

 # DIFFERENTIAL DIAGNOSIS

- Mammary neoplasia; can be confused with FMH, but malignant mammary tumors occur rarely in young cats, and benign mammary tumors do not grow as fast as FMH. Neither do they seem to be correlated with diestrus (or progestin administration).
- In the case of mass persisting more than 5 weeks after initialization of medical therapy, excision of the mass with histopathology should be performed to exclude the presence of a tumor.
- Mastitis.
- Pseudopregnancy.

 # DIAGNOSTICS

- Cytology of mammary mass.
- FNA and cytologic examination can help rule out malignancy (Table 43.1).
- Progesterone evaluation.
- Progesterone level remains above 5 ng/ml during the first 40 days following ovulation. A high level confirms the cycle status (diestrus), increasing the probability of FMH.
- However, basal plasma progesterone levels cannot exclude FMH. Synthetic progesterone cannot be assayed. FMH can then occur without diestrus or pseudopregnancy.

Pathological Findings

- Histopatholigically, FMH consists of well-demarcated, unencapsulated, benign fibroglandular proliferation. Necrosis can be present in advanced cases.

TABLE 43.1. Cytologic differentiation of malignant versus benign mammary masses.

Malignant tumor	Benign tumor or FMH
Anisokaryosis	Nuclei of uniform size
Nuclear pleomorphism	Regular nuclei
Heterogeneous chromatin	Homogeneous chromatin
Nucleolus: Increase in size and number	Nucleolus: single size
Increased mitotic index	Increased mitotic index
Atypical mitosis	Normal mitosis

THERAPEUTICS

- The objective of therapy is to decrease progesterone activity which is responsible for FMH.

Surgery

- Ovariectomy induces a rapid decline in the endogenous secretion of progesterone. During the second part of FMH diestrus, or in case of an unwanted pregnancy, an ovariohysterectomy is recommended. Ovariectomy during diestrus can promote pseudopregnancy due to rebound prolactin elevation.
- Mastectomy is not recommended at time of diagnosis, even in cases with skin ulceration while under the ongoing influence of progesterone. It is essential to ensure the cessation of mammary proliferation before any surgical intervention. Mastectomy may be complicated by early wound dehiscence secondary to enlargement of other mammae, and skin closure may be very complex (or impossible) in cases of severe FMH. Death at the time of surgery is also reported due to cardiovascular shock.

Medical

- Oral progestagen administration must be immediately discontinued.
- Long-acting injectable progestagens persist for several weeks.
- The progesterone antagonist aglepristone is ninefold more selective for progesterone receptors than natural progesterone, and promotes a rapid reduction of mammary development in the first week and a complete reduction in 80% of cases by 4–9 weeks (Fig. 43.5).

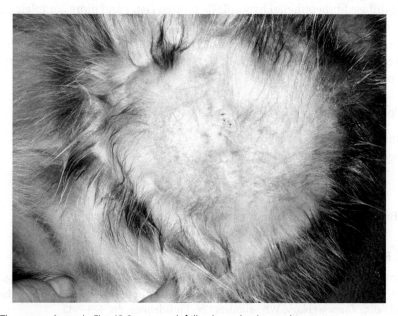

■ **Fig. 43.5.** The queen shown in Fig. 43.2, one week following aglepristone therapy.

- Aglepristone seems to be more effective than neutering, and is therefore recommended in first line in all clinical cases.
- The availability of aglepristone is not universal.
- Broad-spectrum antibiotics for secondary infection.
- Appropriate analgesics, anti-inflammatories.
- Antiprolactin therapy (cabergoline) can be helpful as prolactin is a luteotroph promoting P4 production.

Drug(s)

- Aglepristone. Alizine®, Virbac:
    - 10 mg/kg on days 1 and 2, then 10 mg/kg for 4–6 weeks.
    - 20 mg/kg/week for 4–6 weeks.
- Cabergoline (Galastop ® [Virbac, France]):
    - 5 µg/kg bodyweight, PO, q.24 h or divided BID to effect.

COMMENTS

- None.

Expected Course and Prognosis

- FMH may regress spontaneously within a few weeks when minor. However, this is not predictable, and the disease may worsen ; therefore treatment is always recommended.
- Reducing diffuse fibroepithelial hyperplasia is often faster and more complete than lobular hyerplasia.
- A partial reduction in the first week is often noted after an aglepristone injection.
- Complete remission occurs in >80% of cases after prolonged medical treatment with aglepristone.

Abbreviations

FMH = Feline mammary hyerplasia
P4   = Progesterone

See Also

Feline Pre-Breeding Examination and Breeding Husbandry

Suggested Reading

Lévy, X. (2007) La fibro-adénomatose mammaire ou mastose. *Le Point vétérinaire*, **38** (273), 54–57.
Johnston, S.D., Root Kustritz, M.V., Olson, P.N. (2001) Disorders of the mammary glands of the queen, in *Canine and Feline Theriogenology*, WB Saunders Co., Philadelphia, pp. 474–485.

Simon, D., Schoenrock, D., Nolte, I. *et al.* (2009) Cytologic examination of fine-needle aspirates from mammary gland tumors in the dog: diagnostic accuracy with comparison to histopathology and association with postoperative outcome. *Vet. Clin. Pathol.*, **38** (4), 521–528.

Görlinger, S., Kooistra, H.S.,Van den Broek, A., *et al.* (2002) Treatment of fibroadenomatous hyperplasia in cats with aglepristone. *J. Vet. Intern. Med.*, **16**, 710–713.

Jurka, P., Max, A. (2009) Treatment of fibroadenomatosis in 14 cats with aglepristone – changes in blood parameters and follow-up. *Vet. Rec.*, **165**, 657–660.

Author: Xavier Lévy DVM, DECAR

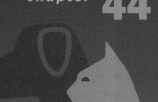
Medical Manipulation of the Estrous Cycle

DEFINITION

- Estrous cycles are primarily managed surgically by ovariectomy or ovariohysterectomy in dogs and cats.
- Especially in situations where irreversible sterilization is desirable, for example, for reasons of population control, this is still the method of choice.
- Medical manipulation of estrous cycles, however, is indicated in several situations: primarily if a reversible method is needed (e.g., in breeding animals) but also in cases when surgical methods are not available or contraindicated, such as in cases of severely increased anesthetic risk.
- Additionally, acceptance of gonadectomy is diminishing and its value as a means to effectively control pet overpopulation is being questioned; therefore, many scientists are currently involved in the development of a new, non-surgical method for sterilization (http://www.acc-d.org). The release of new methods, mainly for the indication prevention of estrus, may be expected in the future.
- In bitches, being mono-estrous, shortening of the relatively long interestrous interval (IEI) is relatively often indicated, mainly in animals intended for breeding, but it is also quite complicated.
- This is mainly due to differences in estrous cycle regulation in bitches compared to polyestrous species such as cattle, and the relative lack of knowledge on this topic in the bitch.
- In cats, however, being poly-estrous, medical estrus cycle manipulations in private practice are chiefly aimed at temporary prevention or reduction of estrus.

SHORTENING THE IEI IN BITCHES

Indications

- Management of breeding:
  - Limited availability of stud dog.
  - Seasonal activities, such as work or sports competition.

Blackwell's Five-Minute Veterinary Consult Clinical Companion: Small Animal Endocrinology and Reproduction, First Edition. Edited by Deborah S. Greco and Autumn P. Davidson. © 2017 John Wiley & Sons, Inc. Published 2017 by John Wiley & Sons, Inc.
Companion Website: www.fiveminutevet.com/endocrinology

- Compliance to rules and regulations concerning maximal allowed age for breeding.
- Efficiency of use of available staff and facilities in canine large breeding operations.
- Primary or secondary anestrous, in cases where a complete diagnostic work-up does not result in a definitive diagnosis.

Assessment

- Before onset of treatment, assess the actual stage of the estrous cycle, based on:
  - Accurate owner information regarding previous estrous cycles.
  - In cases of doubt or incomplete/lacking owner information a clinical examination should be performed to assess the actual stage of the estrous cycle.
    - □ A complete gynecological examination in order to assess presence of estrus (a follicular phase), by detecting signs indicative of increased plasma estradiol-17β concentrations.
    - □ If no signs of estrus are present, measurement of the plasma progesterone concentration helps differentiate between metestrus (the luteal phase) and anestrus:
      - ○ [progesterone]$_{plasma}$ <6 nmol/l or <1 ng/ml = anestrus.
      - ○ [progesterone]$_{plasma}$ >6 nmol/l or >1 ng/ml = metestrus/pregnancy

 # THERAPEUTICS

Drugs

- In bitches, the IEI can be shortened by continuous treatment with dopamine agonists:
  - Cabergoline (Galastop ®; Virbac, France), 5 µg/kg body weight, PO, once daily.
  - Bromocriptine (Parlodel ®; Meda Pharma, the Netherlands), 20 µg/kg body weight, PO, BID.
- Treatment should be started during the second half of metestrus or anestrus, that is, from 4 weeks after ovulation onwards, and needs to be continued until the start of estrus.
- Duration of treatment depends on the cycle stage at the start of treatment; that is, it will be shorter if the treatment is started closer to the expected onset of the next estrus.
  - For example, the mean IEI in Beagles treated with bromocriptine (20 µg/kg body weight, PO, BID) starting at 28 days after ovulation was 96 ± 6 days, significantly shorter than in untreated control cycles (216 ± 9 days).
- The induced premature estrus period has an unchanged fertility compared with a spontaneously occurring estrus as long as an adequate anestrual period occurred.

Precautions/interactions

- Dopamine agonists are not registered for the indication shortening of the IEI in bitches; no registered alternatives exist.
- Bromocriptine and cabergoline are registered for the treatment of pseudopregnancy in bitches in different countries.

- Accidental treatment of pregnant bitches with dopamine agonists should be avoided because of the high risk of induction of abortion due to inhibition of prolactin secretion.
- Dopamine agonists, especially bromocriptine, might induce nausea and vomiting; reduction of the bromocriptine dosage by 50% during the first 4 days of treatment usually prevents this side effect (i.e., 10 μg/kg body weight, PO, BID).
- Bromocriptine should be administered during or shortly after a meal.
- Reversible coat color changes have been reported after use of cabergoline.
- Dopamine agonists are contraindicated in animals with cardiovascular disease or liver dysfunction.

Alternative drugs

- Contrary to the dopamine agonists, the serotonin antagonist metergoline (Contralac®; Virbac, France) **does not** shorten the IEI.
- A follicular phase may also be induced by administration of GnRH, gonadotropins, eCG, hCG, and estrogens.
- Although many protocols exist for estrus induction in bitches, the fertility results of these methods, with the exception of administration of dopamine agonists, are variable and generally poor.
- Some methods are also too costly or labor-intensive to be suitable for veterinary practice.
  - GnRH agonists as slow-release formulations, such as the currently marketed deslorelin (Suprelorin®; Virbac, France, 4.7 mg/implant, SC), which is registered for use in male dogs and ferrets in France, reliably induces estrus, usually within 4–6 days if administered during anestrus or frequently even during the luteal phase.
  - However, with the current knowledge the use of these implants for the indication 'shortening of the IEI in bitches' is not advised, based on several disadvantages. The clinically most relevant of these are the inconsistent ovulation rate, a risk of induction of persistent (pro-)/estrus, and abortion due to luteal failure.
- Aglépristone, a progesterone-receptor antagonist, and prostaglandin $F_{2\alpha}$ have also been reported to shorten the IEI if administered during the luteal phase. However, these drugs are not recommended for the indication 'shortening of the IEI'; this results when these agents are used to terminate pregnancy or diestrus (during therapy for pyometra).

SHORTENING OF THE IEI IN QUEENS

Indications

- Management of breeding in cats with spontaneously occurring long IEI or induction of estrus in cats during anestrus.
  - Cats are poly-estrous with an IEI of 3 weeks, with some variation, so shortening of the IEI in cats that are not in anestrus is not often necessary.

Assessment

- Before onset of treatment, assess the actual stage of the estrous cycle, based on:
  - Accurate owner information regarding previous estrous cycles.
  - In cases of doubt or incomplete/lacking owner information a clinical examination should be performed.
    - □ A gynecological examination in order to assess presence of estrus (a follicular phase), by detecting signs indicative of increased plasma estradiol-17β concentrations.
    - □ In cats, mainly behavioral changes can be observed during estrus. Additionally, cytology of a vaginal smear will show a relative increase of superficial cells during estrus.
    - □ If no signs of estrus are present, measurement of the plasma progesterone level helps differentiate between postestrus/anestrus and metestrus (the luteal phase) or pregnancy:
      - ○ [progesterone]$_{plasma}$ <6 nmol/l or <1 ng/ml = anestrus/postestrus.
      - ○ [progesterone]$_{plasma}$ >6 nmol/l or >1 ng/ml = metestrus/pregnancy.

 THERAPEUTICS

Drugs

- eCG (Folligonan®; MSD, The Netherlands), 50 IE per cat, SC/IM, q. 48 hours, until onset of estrus, but with a maximum number of three administrations:
  - eCG is a gonadotropin with primarily FSH-like effects.
  - eCG administration should be initiated in postestrus or anestrus.
  - A pre-ovulatory LH surge will usually be induced by mating (several matings are necessary to ensure a sufficient LH surge and subsequent ovulation).

Precautions/Interactions

- eCG is not registered for the indication 'shortening of the IEI in queens'; no registered alternatives exist.
- eCG administration might induce superovulation followed by pregnancy of more fetuses than can be carried to term by the queen. This risk is especially present if higher doses and/or more administrations than described are utilized.

PREVENTION OF ESTROUS CYCLE IN BITCHES

Indications

- Breeding animals, temporary prevention of proestrus/estrus, such as:
  - Seasonal activities, such as work or sports competition, for which estrous bitches are excluded.
  - Social indications.

- Non-breeding animals:
  - Short-term prevention of proestrus/estrus, such as:
    - Requirements of boarding facilities, such as pensions, for temporary stays such as during holidays.
  - Long-term prevention of estrous cycles, such as:
    - Contraindications for surgical estrus prevention.
    - Increased anesthetic risk such as congenital heart disease.
    - Prevention of possible complications after gonadectomy, such as increased aggression in already dominant animals.

 ## THERAPEUTICS

Drugs

- Proestrus/estrus prevention can be accomplished with several types of drugs, of which progestogens and androgens are most important, depending on availability and desired duration of action.
- Short-term estrus prevention
  - Medroxyprogesterone acetate (MPA):
    - Oral administration of MPA is the most common progestogen for short- term estrus prevention in the bitch.
    - Administered orally, the MPA dosage is 5 mg per bitch, once daily with a maximum of 21 days (10 mg during the first 5 days for large bitches). Estrus suppression will last for 2–9 months.
  - Mibolerone or compounded androgens:
    - Oral administration of the androgen mibolerone is an alternative to progestogens in areas where it is registered for this indication in bitches.
    - Mibolerone is **not** recommended for use in bitches before the first estrus and in bitches intended for breeding.
    - Dosage: for bitches weighing 0.5–11.5 kg, 30 μg once daily PO; 11.5–23 kg, 60 μg once daily PO; 23–45 kg, 120 μg once daily PO; >45 kg and German Shepherds (and their crossbreds) 180 μg once daily PO. Mibolerone can also be given with a small amount of food.
    - Mibolerone should be administered during anestrus, at least 30 days before onset of the expected follicular phase.
    - After discontinuation of treatment, estrus will occur anywhere between 1 week and 8 months, with an average of 2.5–3 months.
    - Controlled studies are lacking; availability complicated by potential for human abuse in some countries.
- Long-term estrus prevention:
  - Proligestone (PROL)
    - Because of the relatively low potency with matching low incidence of side effects, PROL (Delvosteron®; MSD Animal Health, The Netherlands) is the progestogen most suitable for longer-term estrus prevention in the bitch.

   □ The single SC dose of PROL, as recommended by the manufacturer, ranges from 30 mg/kg for a 3-kg bitch to 10 mg/kg for a bitch of 60 kg.
   □ After the administration of PROL estrus is usually suppressed for 9–12 months. If a continuation of estrus suppression is desired the treatment can be repeated using the following scheme:
      ○ 1st interval, 3 months;
      ○ 2nd interval, 4 months;
      ○ subsequent intervals of 5 months.
- Progestogens should be administered during anestrus, approximately 1 month before onset of the expected follicular phase.
- Mibolerone
   □ Continuous daily oral administration of the androgen mibolerone is an alternative to progestogens for longer-term estrus prevention. However, bitches should not be treated for longer than 24 months.
   □ Details on dosage: see 'Short-term estrus prevention.'

Precautions/interactions

- Use of progestogens for estrus prevention may lead to the following side effects:
  - Development of cystic endometrial hyperplasia (CEH) – endometritis.
  - Increased risk of neoplastic transformation of mammary tissue, ranging from hyperplasia, adenomatous hyperplasia, and adenomas to malignant tumors. The progestogen-induced transformation begins with proliferation of undifferentiated terminal ductal structures, so-called terminal end buds, which increases susceptibility of the mammary tissue to malignant transformation.
  - Hypersecretion of growth hormone, which may lead to diabetes.
  - Prolonged gestation if conception occurs after a progestogen is administered subcutaneously at the onset of the follicular phase or during pregnancy; Cesarean section may be needed
- With the exception of prolonged pregnancy, these side effects are largely dependent on the total progestogen exposure. Using the recommended doses the exposure may be greater with MPA and MA than with proligestone, the latter being a rather weak progestogen. Therefore, bitches treated with PROL might still show estrus in a situation where a treated bitch is housed together with estrous bitches.
- It is not recommended to administer progestogens during the follicular phase.
- Side effects of mibolerone that have been reported are clitoral hypertrophy, vaginitis, and behavioral changes.
- Furthermore, it causes birth defects in when administered to pregnant bitches (teratogenic effect).
- Mibolerone should not be used in patients with liver or kidney disease, or in patients with androgen-dependent tumors, such as perianal adenomas.
- Mibolerone should not be used in cats due to a narrow therapeutic range.

Alternative drugs

- For long-term estrus suppression in dogs, MPA, administered parenterally, can be used. The single SC dose is 2 mg/kg (maximum 60 mg per animal).
  - After the parenteral administration of MPA, estrus may be suppressed for as long as 2–3 years. For that reason MPA is not recommended for use in animals intended for breeding at a later date.
- GnRH agonists in a slow-release formulation might seem to be a good alternative to progestagens for the prevention of estrus, especially for long-term treatment (if administered repeatedly); However, several considerations should be taken into account before this drug is used for this indication in bitches:
  - GnRH agonists administered in high doses over a long period of time prevent estrus by pituitary downregulation.
  - The early stimulatory effect of GnRH analogs may cause signs of estrus, if administered during anestrus, and sometimes even if administered during the luteal phase: this is the 'flare-up effect.'
  - The GnRH agonist deslorelin (Suprelorin®; Virbac, France) is registered in some countries for contraceptive use in male dogs and ferrets, and may also induce suppression of estrus. Available implants contain 4.7 mg or 9.4 mg per implant, given SC, but the implants are not registered for the indication. This compound's availability varies by country and has limited availability for companion animal contraceptive use in many countries.
  - The initial induction of estrus (flare-up effect) is a serious limitation for the use of deslorelin for reasons of estrus prevention. The following preventive measures have been studied:
    - □ Administering a GnRH agonist to pre-pubertal bitches at 4 months of age, but not at 7 months, prevents flare-up. However, reproductive function might be prevented for 1 year or even longer, without certainty of spontaneous occurrence of puberty.
    - □ The prior administration of progestogens does not consistently prevent the flare-up effect. Rather, it appears to depend on the interval between the beginning of progestogen treatment and the implantation, the stage of anestrus, the dose of progestogen, and the type of GnRH analog. Furthermore, adding progestogens to prevent the initial stimulation of GnRH agonists cancels the advantage of not administering progestogens for estrus prevention.
- Potential side effects that should also be considered before use of GnRH agonists for estrus prevention in the bitch are:
  - risk for induction of persistent estrus;
  - risk for induction of endometritis, especially in older animals.
- At present information on fertility of subsequent estrus periods after treatment with GnRH agonist implants is scarce, so extra prudence is in order when bitches are treated that are intended for breeding.

PREVENTION OF ESTRUS IN QUEENS

Indications

- Breeding animals, temporary prevention of estrus, such as:
  - group housing with intact tom cats;
  - social indications.
- Non-breeding animals.
  - Long-term prevention of estrus, such as:
    - □ contraindications for surgical estrus prevention.
    - □ increased anesthetic risk, e.g., congenital heart disease.

 # THERAPEUTICS

Drugs

- In cats, estrus prevention is mainly accomplished with progestogens administered orally, and increasingly with slow-release GnRH agonists.
- The GnRH agonist implants are not registered for this indication but, depending on availability, cost and desired duration of effect, they might be an alternative in selected cases.
- Progestogens
  - For short-term and longer-term delay of estrus, MPA (5 mg per animal per week, PO) and MA (2 mg per animal per week PO) can be used.
  - Treatment should be started during postestrus or (the end of) seasonal anestrus, not during estrus.
  - The dose needed for an individual cat can be lower, so if longer-term treatment is anticipated, the lowest dose that still prevents estrus should be found in order to decrease the cumulative exposure to progestogens, for example by diminishing the weekly dose given or increasing the dosing interval.
- GnRH agonist in a slow-release formulation.
  - Longer-term suppression of estrus can be achieved by treatment with the GnRH agonist deslorelin (Suprelorin®; Virbac, France). Available implants contain 4.7 mg or 9.4 mg, administered SC.
  - GnRH-agonist implants are not registered for the prevention of estrus in queens; availability is variable in many countries.
  - Duration of effect is highly variable in queens, and may last from 16 months to >37 months, with an average of 23 months (deslorelin, 4.7-mg implant).
  - In order to facilitate future removal of implants, such as in cases of prolonged duration of effect, it is advised to place the implant subcutaneously at a site where it can easily be retrieved, such as in the umbilical area.

Precautions/interactions

- Progestogens
  - Cats should not be treated with progestogens before the first estrus because of an increased risk for endometritis and fibroadenomatous hyperplasia of the mammary glands.
  - Use of progestogens formulated for parenteral use is not advised in cats.
    - ☐ The duration of estrus suppression is highly variable.
    - ☐ There is a risk of prolonged gestation if the cat was pregnant at the moment of treatment.
      - ○ Prolonged pregnancy is a realistic risk, mainly in cats that are (partly) allowed outdoors as pregnancy cannot yet be determined at the moment of treatment (during postestrus).
- GnRH agonist in a slow-release formulation
  - Information on return to fertility after treatment in cats is scarce, but as yet the effect of GnRH implants seems to be reversible, without negative remnant effects on subsequent fertility.
  - Contrary to bitches, queens less often show a 'flare-up' effect after implantation. If measured, the plasma estradiol concentration initially increases with a concomitant increase of superficial cells in vaginal smears, but behavioral estrus is often not shown.
  - Fertile mating after deslorelin-induced estrus might occur.

Alternatives

- Increasing the IEI:
  - SHAM-mating. Stimulating the vagina several times within 1 hour during estrus, using a glass rod or cotton swab, induces a pre-ovulatory LH surge of sufficient amplitude to induce ovulation. Subsequently, a luteal phase (pseudopregnancy) of approximately 6–7 weeks may be expected.
  - GnRH agonist: A single administration of a short-acting GnRH agonist (e.g., gonadorelin; Fertagyl®; Merck Animal Health, USA, 10 µg/kg body weight, SC/IM), or buserelin; Receptal®; Merck Animal Health, USA, 0.4 µg/kg body weight, SC/IM) induces an LH surge and ovulation followed by pseudopregnancy, if administered to estrous queens.
  - Pseudopregnancy is characterized by an increased IEI.
- Photoperiod:
  - In temperate areas cats show least estrous periods in the months with a short photoperiod.
  - In cats kept under artificial light, changing the photoperiod abruptly from long to short day length might induce anestrus (e.g., from 16 hours to 8 hours of continuous light per day).

Abbreviations

eCG   = equine chorionic gonadotropin
GnRH = gonadotropin-releasing hormone

hCG = human chorionic gonadotropin
IEI = interestrous interval
IM = intramuscular
MPA = medroxyprogesterone acetate
MA = megestrol acetate
PO = oral administration
PROL = proligestone
SC = subcutaneous

See Also

Diabetes Mellitus without Complications – Cats
Diabetes Mellitus without Complications – Dogs
Estrous Cycle Abnormalities
CEH, Hydrometra, Mucometra and Pyometra
Canine Breeding Management
Feline Pre-Breeding Examination and Breeding Husbandry

Suggested Reading

Beijerink, N.J., Dieleman, S.J., Kooistra, H.S., Okkens, A.C. (2003) Low doses of bromocriptine shorten the interestrous interval in the bitch without lowering plasma prolactin concentration. *Theriogenology*, **60**, 1379–1386.

Galac, S., Kooistra, H.S., Dieleman, S.J., Cestnik, V., Okkens, A.C. (2004) Effects of aglepristone, a progesterone receptor antagonist, administered during the early luteal phase in non-pregnant bitches. *Theriogenology*, **62**, 494–500.

Goericke-Pesch, S., Wehrend, A., Georgiev, P. (2014) Suppression of fertility in adult cats. *Reprod. Domest. Anim.*, **49** (Suppl. 2), 33–40.

Gobello, C., Castex, G., Broglia, G., Corrada, Y. (2003) Coat colour changes associated with cabergoline administration in bitches. *J. Small Anim. Pract.*, **44**, 352–354.

Kutzler, M.A. (2007) Estrus induction and synchronization in canids and felids. *Theriogenology*, **68**, 865–870.

Leyva, H., Madley, T., Stabenfeldt, G.H. (1989) Effect of light manipulation on ovarian activity and melatonin and prolactin secretion in the domestic cat. *J. Reprod. Fertil.*, **39** (Suppl.), 125–133.

Maenhoudt, C., Santos, N.R., Fontaine, E., Mir, F., Reynaud, K., Navarro, C., Fontbonne, A. (2012) Results of GnRH agonist implants in oestrous induction and oestrous suppression in bitches and queens. *Reprod. Domest. Anim.*, **47** (Suppl. 6), 393–397.

Maenhoudt, C., Santos, N.R., Fontbonne, A. (2014) Suppression of fertility in adult dogs. *Reprod. Domest. Anim.*, **49** (Suppl. 2), 58–63.

Okkens, A.C., Kooistra, H.S. (2006) Anoestrus in the dog: a fascinating story. *Reprod. Domest. Anim.*, **41**, 291–296.

Romagnoli, S.E., Camillo, F., Cela, M., Johnston, S.D., Grassi, F., Ferdeghini, M., Aria, G. (1993) Clinical use of prostaglandin F2 alpha to induce early abortion in bitches: serum progesterone, treatment outcome and interval to subsequent oestrus. *J. Reprod. Fertil.*, **47** (Suppl.), 425–431.

Selman, P.J., Mol, J.A., Rutteman, G.R., van Garderen, E., van den Ingh, T.S., Rijnberk. A. (1997) Effects of progestin administration on the hypothalamic-pituitary-adrenal axis and glucose homeostasis in dogs. *J. Reprod. Fertil.*, **51** (Suppl.), 345–354.

Sokolowski, J.H., Zimbelman, R.G. (1974) Canine reproduction: effects of multiple treatments of medroxy-progesterone acetate on reproductive organs of the bitch. *Am. J. Vet. Res.*, **35**, 1285–1287.

Rubion, S., Desmoulins, P.O., Riviere-Godet, E., Kinziger, M., Salavert, F., Rutten, F., Flochlay-Sigognault, A., Driancourt, M.A. (2006) Treatment with a subcutaneous GnRH agonist containing controlled release device reversibly prevents puberty in bitches. *Theriogenology*, **66**, 1651–1654.

Russo, I.H., Russo, J. (1991) Progestagens and mammary gland development: differentiation versus carcinogenesis. *Acta Endocrinol. (Copenh.)*, **125** (Suppl. 1), 7–12.

Sung, M., Armour, A.F., Wright, P.J. (2006) The influence of exogenous progestin on the occurrence of proestrous or estrous signs, plasma concentrations of luteinizing hormone and estradiol in deslorelin (GnRH agonist) treated anestrous bitches. *Theriogenology*, **66**, 1513–1517.

Trigg, T.E., Doyle, A.G., Walsh, J.D., Swangchan-uthai, T. (2006) A review of advances in the use of the GnRH agonist deslorelin in control of reproduction. *Theriogenology*, **66**, 1507–1512.

van Os, J.L., van Laar, P.H., Oldenkamp, E.P., Verschoor, J.S. (1981) Oestrus control and the incidence of mammary nodules in bitches, a clinical study with two progestogens. *Vet. Q.*, **3**, 46–56.

Wright, P.J., Verstegen, J.P., Onclin, K., Jöchle, J., Armour, A.F., Martin, G.B., Trigg, T.E. (2001) Suppression of the oestrus responses of bitches to the GnRH analogue deslorelin by progestin. *J. Reprod. Fertil.*, **57** (Suppl.), 263–268.

Author: J De Gier DVM, DECAR

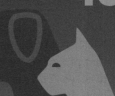

chapter 45

Medical Abortion, Canine and Feline

DEFINITION

- Medical abortion, or mismating, in the bitch is commonly requested by clients when a mating to an undesired male (a stray, another breed, an undesirable male or a too closely related male) is actually observed; when a bitch deemed too young to breed is actually observed to be mated; or when a bitch is actually observed to be bred by a potentially desirable male but the potential puppies are unwanted or the timing of the litter is undesirable.
- It is also common for clients to request a medical abortion when their bitch, presumed to be in estrus, has been missing for period of time and mating is presumed, but has not actually been observed.
- The request for medical abortion in the queen is not as common as in the bitch.
- Medical pregnancy termination can be indicated in certain metabolic disorders of pregnancy, such as pregnancy ketosis or pregnancy diabetes.

ETIOLOGY/PATHOPHYSIOLOGY

- Unwanted pregnancies in bitches and queens are a universal problem where intact, estrual females are allowed to freely roam and become exposed to intact males. However, unwanted matings may also occur in well-managed kennels and catteries.
- For a pregnancy to occur, an estrual female must be mated to a fertile male. Bitches normally attain puberty between 5 and 24 months and queens between 4 and 24 months. Signs of estrus in the bitch include a swollen vulva, a red or straw-colored vaginal discharge, and attracting males. The average duration of proestrus is about 9 days, during which time the vulva may be enlarging, there is a red vaginal discharge, and males may be attracted. Bitches will not normally mate or be fertile at this time. Estrus, the time of sexual receptivity and maximum fertility, lasts approximately 9 days and is associated with an enlarged vulva, possibly a straw-colored discharge and receptivity to the male.

Blackwell's Five-Minute Veterinary Consult Clinical Companion: Small Animal Endocrinology and Reproduction,
First Edition. Edited by Deborah S. Greco and Autumn P. Davidson. © 2017 John Wiley & Sons, Inc.
Published 2017 by John Wiley & Sons, Inc.
Companion Website: www.fiveminutevet.com/endocrinology

Diestrus occurs immediately after estrus, and may begin with a dark bloody discharge that progresses to no discharge. The bitch will not normally accept mating by the male in diestrus. The duration of estrus in the queen is generally 8–10 days with signs of estrus including vocalization and lordosis when stroked on the back. The interestrus interval (IEI) in the bitch is normally ≥6 months, with a 3-month mandatory endometrial repair period occurring after each diestrus or pregnancy. Seasonally, queens will return to a fertile estrus approximately 2–6 weeks after parturition, 1–10 days after an anovulatory estrus, and 2–6 weeks after an induced 40-day luteal period.

Systems Affected

- Reproductive

 ## SIGNALMENT/HISTORY

- The animal must be sexually intact and attained puberty (old enough to begin having estrous cycles). The age of first estrus varies but ranges from 5 to 24 month in bitches, to 4 to 24 months in queens. The bitch or queen must be in estrus in order to become pregnant or have been in estrus to be pregnant at the time of examination.
- Since the IEI in the bitch is normally ≥6 months, with a 3-month mandatory endometrial repair period occurring after each diestrus or pregnancy, owners concerned about a mismate within 4 months of the previous estrus should be advised that pregnancy is an unlikely outcome. With queens returning to a fertile estrus approximately 2–6 weeks after parturition, 1–10 days after an anovulatory estrus, and 2–6 weeks after an induced 40-day luteal period, the chances of a fertile mating are greatly increased.

Risk Factors

- Intact, estrual females allowed to freely roam and become exposed and mated with intact males. Unwanted matings may occur in well-managed kennels and catteries, with mistakes made by caretakers when estrual females are incorrectly intermingled with intact males or isolation from males not being fail-proof.

Historic Findings

- The owner may report that the bitch was seen interacting with or actually 'tied' with a male for a period of 10–20 minutes. This is a case of a bitch obviously in estrus; however, the owner may report that a bitch is presumed to be in estrus and has been missing for minutes to hours to days. The signs the owner may interpret as estrus include vaginal discharge and attracting males. These signs are not definitive signs of estrus, however. The owner may be able to give accurate dates of the last estrus, the last litter, or the dates that the bitch was observed being mated or was missing and presumed to have been mated. The owner also may also observe that the bitch is becoming larger or 'fatter' or having mammary gland development for some unknown reasons, or possibly after a known or presumed estrus.

- With the above possibilities in mind, clients will present animals in estrus and known to have been mated, in estrus and suspected to have been mated, or at some later date after a suspected estrus with an unwanted pregnancy being a concern. Since many cases presented for mismate may not have been in estrus, may not have been bred, or may not have become pregnant, a pregnancy examination by ultrasound should be made at least 30 days after the suspected estrus before mismating therapy is considered.

 ## CLINICAL FEATURES

- An enlarged vulva and straw-colored vaginal discharge may be seen if the bitch is in estrus. Also when in estrus, the bitch may 'flag' its tail when the area lateral to the tail-head is stroked. If the bitch is in proestrus the vulva may be enlarged and the vaginal discharge may be bloody. If the bitch has entered diestrus, the vulvar enlargement may still be evident and the vaginal discharge may be a dark-red color. Vaginal cytology can confirm estrus versus diestrus.
- The estrual queen will display lordosis when the back is stroked and the neck is grasped firmly.
- If pregnancy is suspected by the owner, the abdomen may appear enlarged and there may be mammary development in both the bitch and queen.

 ## DIFFERENTIAL DIAGNOSIS

Observed Mating

- If a true 'tie' has been observed, it is reasonable to assume that the bitch is truly is in estrus. The veterinarian should confirm that the bitch is in estrus by performing a vaginal cytology examination within 1–2 days of the suspected mating. If the bitch was bred in late estrus, examination 1–2 days later may show an abundance of non-cornified cells and many PMNs typical of diestrus. If a queen is observed to be mated by a tom (biting the neck and treading over the queen) and the queen performing the typical post-mating 'aftercry' and rolling, the queen can be considered in estrus. Vaginal cytology is not as useful at confirming estrus in the queen as it is in the bitch.

Suspected Mating

- If a bitch is suspected to be mated the owner needs to be questioned as why mating was suspected. If the bitch is gone for 10 minutes or less the chances of the bitch actually being mated is slim, as a true 'tie' can take 10–20 minutes. A short time away does not preclude that the bitch has been mated, however. If an unknown mating is suspected, estrus should be confirmed by performing a vaginal cytology examination. The presence of sperm cells in the vaginal cytology examination confirms that a mating has taken place, but their absence does not preclude it. If a queen is suspected of being mated, the signs of estrus can be checked by grasping the neck and stroking the back. The estrual queen will normally display lordosis when this is done. Although vaginal cytology is not a straightforward way to check for estrus in the queen, the presence of sperm cells in the vaginal cytology exam confirms that mating has taken place, but their absence does not preclude it.

Vaginal Discharge

- Vaginal discharge, which the client may assume to be a sign of estrus, may originate from several distinct sources, depending in part on the age and reproductive status of the patient. It may arise from the urinary tract, uterus, vagina, vestibule, clitoris, or perivulvar skin. A vaginal cytology examination will determine if the bitch is in estrus or has vaginitis. Endoscopic examination of the vestibule and vagina may differentiate urinary tract discharge from vaginal discharge. An ultrasound examination of the uterus may help rule out a pyometra. Careful examination of the vulva will rule out perivulvar vaginitis.

Pregnancy

- Establishing that the bitch is actually pregnant should be done before any mismate protocol is initiated. Several methods for pregnancy diagnosis are available, but ultrasound usually yields the most information for the veterinarian and the earliest detection of pregnancy.

Pseudopregnancy (Overt Pseudopregnancy or Psuedogenetra)

- After the luteal phase approximately 60 days after estrus, it is not uncommon to see a bitch with mammary gland enlargement, build a 'nest,' start to lactate, and 'adopt' inanimate objects as puppies, even though they are not pregnant and did not whelp. These clinical signs are associated with the normal decline in progesterone after the luteal period with a concomitant rise in prolactin. These hormonal events occur in all bitches at the conclusion of diestrus, though most do not present with any clinical signs. Bitches that present with clinical signs may have an increased concentration of prolactin or may be more sensitive to the normal concentration of prolactin.

 ## DIAGNOSTICS

Vaginal Cytology

- A vaginal cytology swab can be made by moistening a 15-cm cotton tip swab, inserting the swab into the dorsal commissure of the vulva to avoid the urethra, and then inserting the swab into the cranial vagina. The swab can then be removed, the cotton tip rolled onto a slide, and the slide stained with a commercial fast-staining technique. Estrogen, from the growing follicles during proestrus, causes the vaginal epithelium to become hyperplastic and individual cells to become cornified. The vaginal cells seen when doing a vaginal cytology consist of parabasal, intermediated, superficial and anuclear cells. Cornification is determined by the percentage of superficial and anuclear cells. Anuclear cells have a large angular cytoplasm with no apparent nucleus; and superficial cells have the same large angular cytoplasm, however a dark-staining pyknotic nucleus is present. Non-cornified cells are the parabasal and intermediate cells and have a rounded or a slightly angular cytoplasm; however, the nucleus will be stippled and not pyknotic. If the vaginal cytology slide is 90–100% cornified the bitch is in estrus. If the vaginal cytology slide does not contain cornified cells, the bitch is not in estrus (the bitch may have progressed into diestrus). Mating can be confirmed by the presence of sperm cells in the vaginal cytology; however, the absence of sperm cells in the vaginal cytology does not preclude that the bitch has been mated. Sperm cells normally are not evident more than 24 hours after mating, and bitches mated within 24 hours of obtaining the vaginal smear will likely have sperm heads in the sample. If sperm cells are not seen, a moistened cotton swab can be left in the vagina for 1 minute, the tip of the swab placed into a small tube containing 0.5 ml saline for 10 minutes, the swab tip squeezed dry into the tube, and the fluid in the tube centrifuged at $2000 \times g$ for 10 minutes. The sediment can then be stained using the same technique as a vaginal cytology. Using this technique, approximately 75% of bitches mated within the previous 48 hours will have sperm heads visible.

- Vaginal cytology in the queen is not performed as commonly as it is in the bitch. Because ovulation induction is a risk using a cotton swab, it is advisable to instill a small amount of saline into the vagina, then aspirate the saline, place it on a slide and stain. During estrus the background clears and the cytology changes from mostly intermediate and superficial cells to anuclear and superficial cells.

Progesterone

- Serum progesterone values may have some use in determining if a bitch is in early estrus, at the LH peak, ovulating or at the end of estrus, or in diestrus. Different laboratories and different progesterone assay techniques will give slightly varying results. In our laboratory the LH peak is around 2–3 ng/ml, at ovulation around 4–8 ng/ml, and diestrus begins around 25 ng/ml. Vaginal cytology and serum progesterone testing permit evaluation of the risk of pregnancy, but do not make the diagnosis. Both, pregnant and non-pregnant bitches in diestrus have elevated progesterone levels. In bitches with a history of mismating, progesterone levels <1.0 ng/ml suggest anestrus, ruling out pregnancy.

Pregnancy Tests

- A commercially marketed relaxin test is available to diagnose pregnancy. Relaxin is first observed at 22–28 days after ovulation (24–30 days after the LH peak). Care must be taken that the duration of gestation is long enough to preclude running the test too early, resulting in a false-negative diagnosis. Because fertile matings can occur earlier than the LH peak, it is advisable to perform the test approximately 7 days later than the earliest date recommended by the manufacturer. Small litters may give a false negative and call a pregnant bitch non-pregnant.

Palpation

- Transabdominal palpation can be used to tentatively diagnose pregnancy from around 21 to 31 days after the first day of diestrus (29–39 days after the LH peak). During this window the distinct gestational vesicles can be palpated; however, segmental pyometras and fetal resorption cannot be differentiated from viable pregnancies. After this stage the gestational sacs become more confluent and lose their distinction to palpation. After day 50 the puppies may be palpated directly. Some bitches are too large to palpate, some tense their abdomen and make palpation difficult, and some carry the pregnancy more cranial, making palpation very difficult. Mammary gland enlargement at the end of gestation may also make palpation difficult.

Ultrasound

- Ultrasound has become the standard of care for pregnancy diagnosis. Gestational sacs are visible as black, hypoechoic structures as early as 18–20 days (bitch) or 16 days (queen) after the LH peak (Fig. 45.1a). Fetuses with visible heartbeats are normally seen around 23–25 days after the LH peak, and fetal movement can be seen 34–36 days past the LH peak to term (Fig. 45.1b). The presence of fetal heartbeats and movement can accurately establish fetal viability. The normal heart rate in the fetus is approximately 200 beats per minute, and an increase or decrease in the fetal heart rate may indicate fetal stress. The absence of a heartbeat indicates fetal death (Fig. 45.2). Because fertile matings can occur earlier than the LH peak, it is advisable to perform the first ultrasound examination approximately 7 days after earliest date recommended by the literature (>30 days after the breeding). This will help avoid a false-negative diagnosis. If the pregnancy diagnosis is performed too late, however, a true abortion (fetal expulsion) rather than a fetal resorption may occur with mismate therapy.

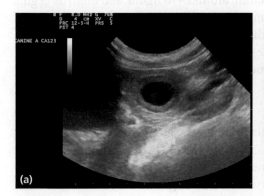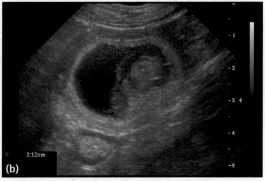

■ **Fig. 45.1.** (a) Transverse ultrasound image of a canine gestational sac 26 days post LH peak. The fetus is not visible in this image. (b) Transverse ultrasound image of a canine pregnancy 35 days post LH peak. Cursors mark the gestational sac. Image courtesy of T.W. Baker.

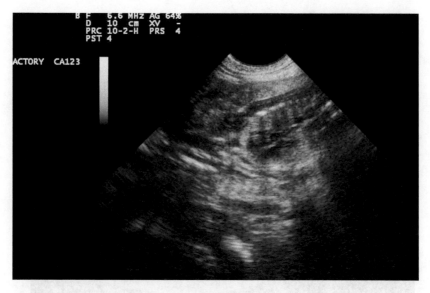

■ **Fig. 45.2.** Sagittal ultrasound image of a non-viable canine pregnancy (fetal thorax with cardiac structure) 53 days post LH peak. Lack of cardiac motion would indicate fetal death.

Radiographs

- Radiographs can be taken to determine pregnancy, though the fetal skeleton only becomes visible 43–46 days after the LH peak. Earlier than this, a non-pregnant uterus cannot be distinguished from a pregnant uterus. Fetal death is also difficult to diagnose radiographically until several days after demise.

 THERAPEUTICS

- The objective of a medical abortion is to provide a 100% efficacy in pregnancy termination after one treatment when given at any stage of estrus or pregnancy, cause no vaginal discharge, have no adverse side effects, not impair future fertility, and be readily available and inexpensive. Most treatments are compromises of these goals. Since the canine pregnancy is totally reliant on luteal progesterone, most medical abortion protocols are designed to lyse, or destroy, the corpora lutea or to block effects of progesterone on the uterus. With any protocol, it is imperative that complete abortion is confirmed (usually by ultrasound), and that the protocol not be stopped until confirmation of pregnancy loss is made. Fetal loss can be expected when a mild brownish vaginal discharge is observed (starting 2–3 days after treatment starts, using PGF) and becoming abundant on days 4–5 (after the start of PGF treatment). Ultrasound can be used to confirm fetal loss. About 3 days after treatment with PGF fetuses still have heartbeats, but by 5 days after starting PGF no fetuses or fluid are generally seen (Figs 45.3–45.5).

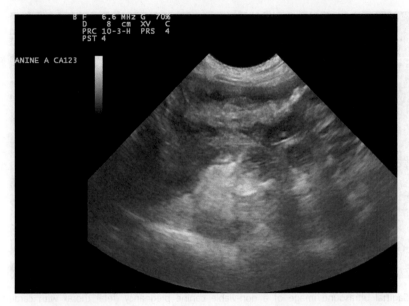

■ **Fig. 45.3.** Sagittal ultrasound image of a terminated canine pregnancy 57 days post LH peak showing a placental site.

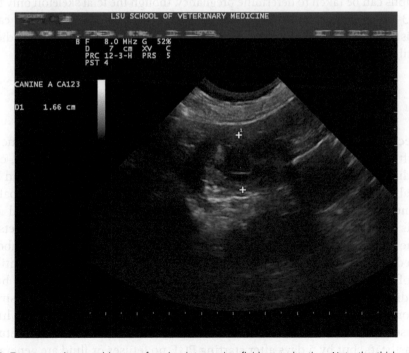

■ **Fig. 45.4.** Transverse ultrasound image of canine intrauterine fluid post abortion. Note the thickened, irregular uterine wall (cursors) as compared to the image in Fig. 45.1a.

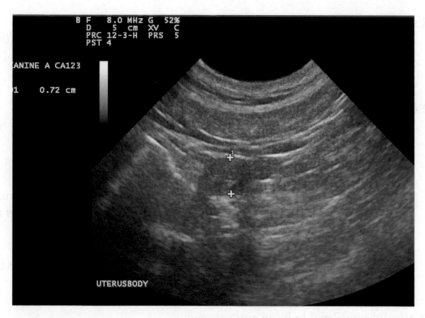

■ **Fig. 45.5.** Transverse ultrasound image of a normal, homogenous canine uterine body.

Drug(s)

Bitch

■ Mismate during estrus
  • Not actually a medical abortion.
  • Approximately 38–60% of bitches presented for elective pregnancy termination may not actually be pregnant, so treating all bitches presented for possible mismate during estrus may result in treating potentially non-pregnant bitches.
  • It is recommended that the animal have an ultrasound pregnancy examination performed approximately 30 days after mating to determine if pregnancy was the outcome. If pregnant, very safe, effective alternatives exist to terminate the pregnancy.
  • Estrogens
    □ Estrogen use for mismate is not endorsed by the author as the safest, most efficacious method to terminate pregnancy. Many animals that are not actually pregnant will be unnecessarily treated and exposed to potential drug toxicities.
    □ The estrogens commonly used for mismate include estradiol cypionate (ECP®), estradiol benzoate, and diethylstilbestrol (DES). Using DES is not effective as a mismate therapy.
    □ Side effects are purported to be prolonging estrual signs, pyometra, and aplastic anemia.
    □ Must only be used during cytologic estrus (before pregnancy can be confirmed). Administration during diestrus increases the potential for inducing a pyometra.
    □ Not approved for mismating. Not recommended by the author as safer and more effective alternatives are available.

- Estradiol cypionate
  - □ A single dose of 44 µg/kg ECP® during estrus resulted in no bitches (0/4) bred to a fertile male becoming pregnant, no pyometras, and no evidence of aplastic anemia at 25 days after treatment in one report.
  - □ No longer marketed for veterinary use.
- Estradiol benzoate
  - □ A single dose of estradiol benzoate at 0.2 mg/kg IM 2 days after breeding (5 days after known ovulation) to 10 bitches prevented pregnancy.
    - ○ Treatment delayed embryonic descent through the uterine tubes.
    - ○ No uterine or hematologic side effects were noted.
  - □ A lower dose of estradiol benzoate administered at 0.01 mg/kg intramuscularly at 3 and 5 days (and occasionally 7 days) after mating in 358 bitches resulted in only 16/358 (4.5%) of the bitches actually whelping.
    - ○ None of the bitches had bone marrow aplasia reported.
    - ○ There was a 7.3% incidence of pyometra, which was the same as the 'normal' incidence in the population.
- Tamoxifen
  - Normally considered to be an anti-estrogen.
  - Has estrogenic activity in the dog.
  - Tamoxifen citrate (Taxol, Bristol-Meyers, Squibb, New York, NY) administered at 1 mg/kg orally twice-daily for 10 days, starting either in proestrus, estrus, or the second, 15th, and 30th days of diestrus, had a 100% (12/12) efficacy for preventing pregnancy when administration began before the 15th day of diestrus.
    - □ When administered on the fifteenth day of diestrus or later it was not effective at preventing pregnancy.
      - ○ Side effects include pyometra, endometritis, and cystic ovaries when administered during all estrous cycle stages, except early diestrus.
      - ○ Half (2/4) of the bitches treated during proestrus developed pyometra.
      - ○ Poor efficacy and side effects make it an uncommon choice for medical abortion.

Medical Abortion

- Luteolytics
  - Prostaglandins
    - □ Prostaglandins are luteolytic, causing destruction of the copra lutea and a resulting decline in serum progesterone.
    - □ Serum progesterone must drop to <2 ng/ml for 24 hours for abortion to occur.
    - □ Prostaglandins are not approved for inducing medical abortion in the bitch so client consent must be obtained, forewarning them of potential complications, prolonged treatments, and the need for multiple abdominal ultrasound examinations. However, treatment is accepted as a standard therapy and is supported by multiple publications.

◻ The interestrus interval may be about 1 month shorter than anticipated if diestrual luteolysis occurs, so the client needs to be forewarned in order to prevent another mismate.

◻ PGF2α

  ○ The natural prostaglandin is the most common drug (Lutalyse, Zoetis, New York, NY).

  ○ A single dose of natural prostaglandin will not result in luteolysis.

  ○ Side effects include vomiting and diarrhea, but these usually only last about 30 minutes and tend to wane as the treatment continues.

  ○ Some recommend hospitalization for the treatment duration or at least 30 minutes after each treatment.

  ○ To minimize caloric loss from emesis it is best to feed the bitches at least 1 hour after treatment.

  ○ Bitches have had normal litters after abortion with PGF2α.

  ○ A dose of 0.1–0.25 mg/kg is administered subcutaneously two to three times a day until complete abortion is confirmed.

  ○ A dose of 0.1 mg/kg subcutaneously every 8 hours for 2 days, and then 0.2 mg/kg SC every 8 hours until abortion is complete (usually by 9 days after treatment starts) has been found to have few side effects.

  ○ A dose of 0.012 mg/kg SC every 6 hours has been found to be efficacious and have no noticeable side effects, with fetal heartbeats stopping after 3 days and no fetuses remaining after 5 days.

• Synthetic prostaglandins include cloprostenol, fluprostenol, and alfaprostol.

  ◻ These have a greater affinity for the prostaglandin receptors and a longer half-life than natural prostaglandins. A much smaller dose is therefore needed.

  ◻ These cause fewer smooth muscle contractions than natural prostaglandins, therefore reducing side effects.

  ◻ Cloprostenol at a dose of 1.0 to 2.5 µg/kg SC once daily for 4–5 days was 100% effective at inducing abortion after a 4- to 7-day treatment regimen. At the low dose of 1 µg/kg the side effects of cloprostenol were noted to be minimal to none.

  ◻ A 2.5 µg/kg dose of cloprostenol given every 48 hours for three doses resulted in 53 of 67 bitches aborting after 1 day. After a second treatment 2 days later, 62 of 67 bitches had aborted.

  ◻ A single dose of 50–150 µg/kg fenprostolene administered subcutaneously 25 days after ovulation caused 100% abortion (16/16) at 3 to 13 days after treatment. Interestingly, only half the treated bitches became pregnant on the subsequent estrus, whereas all the control bitches became pregnant.

  ◻ An alternative drug delivery method is to inject 15 µg of cloprostenol into a single embryonic vesicle. This resulted in fetal death in 100% (10/10) of bitches in 3.1 ± 1.2 days.

• Side-effect amelioration

  ◻ A combination of atropine sulfate at a dose of 0.025 mg/kg, prifinium bromide at a dose of 0.1 ml/kg, and metopimazine at a subcutaneous dose of 0.5 mg/kg.

- □ 15 minutes before a 2.5 µ/kg dose of cloprostenol given every 48 hours.
- □ Prevented side effects in 58% of bitches (39/67).
- Dopaminergics
  - Prolactin inhibitors
    - □ Prolactin is luteotrophic during the second half of gestation.
    - □ Lowering the prolactin concentration will cause luteal demise and result in medical abortion.
  - Bromocriptine
    - □ A dose of 62.5 µg/kg orally twice daily at 43–45 days post ovulation resulted in only two of four aborting (tablets can be crushed and dissolved in oil to ease dosing, but the drug is inactivated by water).
    - □ Side effects
      - ○ Two episodes of emesis in three of the four approximately 3 hours after treatment.
      - ○ Loose stools.
    - □ As a sole medical abortifacient it does not appear to be a good choice. It is more commonly used in combination with a prostaglandin product. Side effects are problematic for clients.
  - Cabergoline
    - □ Given after 40 days of gestation daily for 7 days at 60 µg orally to a 32-kg German shepherd dog, resulted in abortion with no side effects.
    - □ Available in Europe as a veterinary product.
    - □ Only an oral 0.5 mg tablet is available in the United States, making administration difficult because the dose for a 10 kg dog is only 0.05 mg. An oral solution, much like that with bromocriptine (see above) could be formulated. Expense of the initial purchase may be a factor with this drug.
    - □ Compounded drug readily available in United States. Suggested dosage is 2.5–5.0 µg/kg/day for 7 days.
  - Metergoline
    - □ A dose of 0.6 mg/kg orally twice daily, starting on day 28 after the onset of cytological diestrus resulted in abortion in 88% of bitches (8/9).
    - □ Abortions occurred at an average of 12.5 ± 6.4 days after treatment started, and were completed in 2.2 ± 2.7days.
    - □ No side effects were seen.
    - □ Available in Europe, but not the US.
- Progesterone blockers
  - Competitively bind to progesterone receptors, but have no progesterone actions themselves, thereby preventing progesterone action.
  - Aglepristone (Alizine) is available in Europe, but not the US, for medical abortion in the bitch.
    - □ Two doses of 10 mg/kg given subcutaneously 24 hours apart at 45 days after mating caused uncomplicated abortions within 7 days in 100% (35/35) and 95.7% (66/69) of bitches, respectively.

- If in mid-pregnancy a brown mucoid vaginal discharge was seen 24 hours before fetal expulsion.
- Other side effects included slight depression, transitory anorexia, and mammary gland congestion.
- Bitches have become pregnant after treatment.
□ Two doses of 0.10 mg/kg subcutaneously 24 hours apart in seven bitches in early pregnancy and seven bitches in mid-pregnancy.
- All bitches (14/14) terminated their pregnancies.
- Embryonic death occurred in the early-gestation group.
- Fetal expulsion in the mid-gestation group.
- Treatment did not reduce plasma concentrations of progesterone.
□ A single dose of 110 μg/kg SC or a 330 μ/kg single dose SC.
- Mid-pregnancy administration.
- 14/14 aborted.
  - 6/6 at 7 ± 1.9 days for the 110 μ/kg group.
  - 8/8 at 6.4 ± 1.3 days for the 330 μ/kg group.
- Progesterone decreased in treated animals at a varying rate.
- Progesterone was baseline at the time of abortion.
- Concluded that decreased progesterone caused abortion.
- No side effects seen.
□ A 20 mg/kg total dose, given at 10 mg/kg SC on two consecutive days.
- Mid-pregnancy.
- 21/22 (95%) terminated pregnancy 1 to 8 days after treatment.
- Side effects
  - Vaginal discharge was evident in 17/22 (77%).
  - Parturition was seen in nine (41%).
  - 8/22 (36%) developed anorexia.
  - 2/22 (9%) had an injection site reaction.
- Unknown action methods
  - Dexamethasone
    □ The exact mechanism of action is not known, but progesterone concentration fell to less than 1 ng/ml by the fourth day after treatment was initiated.
    □ Administered after 30–50 days of gestation, an oral 10-day dose regimen was as follows: 0.2 mg/kg twice daily for 7 days, 0.16 mg/kg in the morning of the 8th day, 0.12 mg/kg in the evening of the 8th day, 0.08 mg/kg in the morning of the 9th day, 0.04 mg/kg in the evening of the 9th day, and 0.02 mg/kg the morning of the 10th day. (At the author's and editor's institutions a dose of 0.2 mg/kg twice daily for 10 days is used, with no tapering of the dose and no more than the anticipated side effects are seen.)
    □ Fetal death
      - 5–9 days after start of treatment.
      - Live fetuses seen as long as 8–12 days after start of treatment.
      - Abortion or resorption was generally complete 10–23 days after the treatment was initiated.

- ○ Pregnancies less than 40 days of gestation generally had no fetuses expelled.
- ○ The majority had no external signs of pregnancy loss
- ○ Mild vaginal discharge seen in about 20% (26/75) of the bitches that resorbed.
- □ Treatment failure of a blindly followed protocol may occur if the animal is not re-examined for fetal loss.
- □ If the initial treatment fails, a second treatment regimen or continued therapy may cause abortion, but some bitches treated a second time carried puppies to term, so prostaglandin treatment may be advisable.
- □ Side effects – polydipsia and polyuria that generally subsided 3–4 days after the termination of treatment.
- □ Potentially immunosuppressive.
- □ Metritis is a possible complication.
- □ Successful pregnancies were obtained in 18 of 20 bitches bred during the first estrus after treatment and in 2 of 2 on the second estrus.

Drug combinations

- ▪ May reduce side effects of individual drugs.
- ▪ Cloprostenol and cabergoline.
  - • Cloprostenol at 1.0 or 2.5 µg/kg/day SC and cabergoline at 1.65 µg/kg/day SC daily for 5 days from mid-gestation.
    - □ 100% effective (5/5).
    - □ Side effects
      - ○ Less severe than with cloprostenol alone.
      - ○ In the group treated with the low dose, no adverse side effects were noted.
  - • Cloprostenol at 1 µg/kg SC and cabergoline at 5 µg/kg daily for 7 days in the food and during mid-gestation.
    - □ Abortion in 12/13 bitches after 4.6 ± 0.7 days.
    - □ Abortion or fetuses were not observed, but a mucoid sanguinous vulvar discharge was observed for 5–8 days in aborting bitches.
  - • Cloprostenol at 1 µg/kg every other day until fetal death (mean of three injections) and oral cabergoline at 5 µg/kg/day given (at 1 hour after cloprostenol) until 2 days after fetal death, starting at 25 days after the LH peak.
    - □ Mean fetal death was after 9 days and resulted in 100% (5/5) of bitches resorbing fetuses.
    - □ No side effects of treatment.
    - □ A serosanguinous discharge lasted an average of 16 days.
  - • Cloprostenol – a single SC injection of 2.5 µg/kg and cabergoline at 5 µg/kg orally for 10 days.
    - □ Started 28 days after the LH surge.
    - □ 5/5 resorbed without overt abortion.
    - □ Some had red cells, neutrophils, and cellular debris in the vaginal cytology smears for 4 to 21 days after treatment.
    - □ All became pregnant on the subsequent estrous cycle.

- □ Subsequent estrous cycle occurred sooner than normally anticipated.
- □ Side effects of treatment included those commonly seen with prostaglandin (vomiting and diarrhea).
- Cloprostenol – two SC injections of 1.0 μg/kg and cabergoline at 5 μg/kg orally for 10 days.
  - □ Cloprostenol on 28 and 32 days after the LH surge.
  - □ 5/5 resorbed, but one had an overt abortion.
  - □ Some had red cells, neutrophils, and cellular debris in the vaginal cytology smears for 4 to 21 days after treatment.
  - □ All became pregnant on the subsequent estrous cycle.
  - □ Subsequent estrous cycle occurred sooner than normally anticipated.
  - □ No prostaglandin side effects were seen.
- Cloprostenol – two SC injections of 1.0 μg/kg and bromocriptine at 30 μg/kg three times a day for 10 days, plus two doses of 1 μg/kg cloprostenol.
  - □ Cloprostenol on 28 and 32 days after the LH surge.
  - □ 5/5 resorbed without overt abortion.
  - □ Some had red cells, neutrophils, and cellular debris in the vaginal cytology smears for 4 to 21 days after treatment.
  - □ All became pregnant on the subsequent estrous cycle.
  - □ Subsequent estrous cycle occurred sooner than normally anticipated.
  - □ Side effects of treatment included those commonly seen with prostaglandin (vomiting and diarrhea).
- Dinoprost tromethamine at 0.1–0.2 mg/kg SC every 24 hours, and bromocriptine mesylate at 15–30 μg/kg orally every 12 hours.
  - □ 25/25 aborted.
  - □ Side effects:
    - ○ Vomiting and diarrhea.
    - ○ Mucoid sanguineous vulvar discharge for 3–10 days.
    - ○ Pseudopregnancy.
- Cloprostenol sodium at 1 μg/kg SC every 48 hours, and bromocriptine mesylate at 15–30 μg/kg orally every 12 hours.
  - □ 25/25 aborted.
  - □ Side effects.
    - ○ Mucoid sanguineous vulvar discharge for 3–10 days.
    - ○ Pseudopregnancy.
- Prostaglandin at 0.1 mg/kg SC three times a day for 2 days, and then at a dose of 0.2 mg/kg SC three times a day to effect, plus misoprostol (Cytotec, Pharmacia, Peapack, New Jersey) at 1–3 μg/kg, deposited into the cranial vaginal vault once daily using a cat pilling device.
  - □ 9/9 aborted.
  - □ Mean time to complete abortion was 5 days.
- Aglepristone at 10 g/kg SC for 2 days, cabergoline at 5 μg/kg orally every day until completion of abortion, and misoprostol at 200 μg for ≤20 kg bitches or 400 μg for >20 kg bitches, daily intravaginally, until completion of abortion.

        ◻ 25–35 days gestation.

        ◻ 6/7 (85.7%) aborted by 8–10 days.

        ◻ No side effects.

- Aglepristone at 10 mg/kg SC for 2 days, and misoprostol at 200 μg for ≤20 kg bitches or 400 μg for >20 kg bitches, daily intravaginally, until completion of abortion).
  - ◻ 25–35 days gestation.
  - ◻ 7/7 (100%) aborted by 6 days.
  - ◻ No side effects.
- Aglepristone at 10 mg/kg SC for 2 days and cloprostenol at 1 μg/kg SC for 2 days, combined with the aglepristone injections.
  - ◻ 25–35 days gestation.
  - ◻ 3/7 (42.8%) aborted by 8–10 days.
  - ◻ Severe vomiting after each treatment and until the end of abortion.
- Alfaprostol at 10 μg/kg SC at day 3 of treatment, and cabergoline at 10 μg/kg daily orally until abortion was complete ($n = 6$).
  - ◻ 22–40 days post mismate.
  - ◻ 5/6 (83.3%) aborted.
  - ◻ Cervical dilatation time 5.4 ± 2.8 days.
  - ◻ Side effects – transient anorexia, weakness, mild vomiting and diarrhea or low-grade hair loss seen in 30.3%.
- Alfaprostol at 10 μg/kg SC at days 0 and 3 of treatment, and cabergoline at 10 μg/kg daily orally until abortion was complete ($n = 9$).
  - ◻ 22–40 days post mismate.
  - ◻ 7/9 (77.7%) aborted.
  - ◻ Cervical dilatation time 5.5 ± 2.5 days.
  - ◻ Side effects – transient anorexia, weakness, mild vomiting and diarrhea or low-grade hair loss seen in 54.3%.
- Alfaprostol at 10 μg/kg SC at days 0 and 3 of treatment, cabergoline at 10 μg/kg daily orally until abortion was complete, and misoprostol at 400 μg for bitches ≤20 kg or 600 μg for bitches >20 kg every other day, intravaginally ($n = 7$).
  - ◻ 22–40 days post mismate.
  - ◻ 7/7 (100%) aborted.
  - ◻ Cervical dilatation time 3.1 ± 0.9 days.
  - ◻ Side effects – transient anorexia, weakness, mild vomiting and diarrhea or low-grade hair loss seen in 54.0%.

Queen

- Lyteolytics
  - Prostaglandins
    - ◻ Not considered effective until 40 days of gestation, although estimating gestation duration may be more difficult than in the dog.
    - ◻ PGF2α at 2 mg/cat subcutaneously for 5 days.

- ○ 3/3 aborted fetuses within 6 days.
      - ○ Side effects – nausea, vomiting, diarrhea, and prostration starting 10 minutes after treatment and continuing for an hour.
    - ☐ PGF2α at 0.2 mg/kg SC given twice the first day, followed by 0.5 mg/kg twice daily for up to 5 days.
      - ○ Four at 30 days of gestation; 1/4 aborted.
      - ○ Four at 45 days of gestation; 3/4 aborted.
      - ○ Aborting queens had had progesterone values less than 1.0 ng/ml.
- ■ Prolactin Inhibitors
  - • Cabergoline at 5 to 15 μg/kg to feral cats for 4 to 9 days.
    - ☐ 36–40 days of pregnancy.
    - ☐ 41/41 aborted.
- ■ Progesterone inhibitors
  - • Aglepristone at 10 mg/kg on two consecutive days.
    - ☐ Mid-gestation.
    - ☐ 6/6 aborted in 5 ± 2 days.
    - ☐ Progesterone plasma concentration did not decrease, but increased after aglepristone injection.
    - ☐ A hemorrhagic vaginal discharge was observed in all queens during the abortion and for a week thereafter.
    - ☐ The next estrus after abortion averaged 24.6 ± 6.6 days.

Drug combinations

- ■ Cloprostenol at 5 μg/kg SC every 2 days, and cabergoline at 5 μg/kg orally every day.
  - • Started on 30th day after coitus.
  - • 5/5 aborted after an average of 9 days of treatments.
  - • No side effects were seen.
  - • Queens that were bred subsequently became pregnant.

Procedures

- ■ The client should be carefully counseled to ensure that future pregnancies are indeed desired for viable reasons. If not, the best option to terminate a pregnancy and prevent future pregnancies is surgical sterilization (ovariohysterectomy or ovariectomy if not pregnant) if the animal is not a valuable breeder.

 ## COMMENTS

- ■ Dosage, treatment duration, relative costs for initial purchase, and actual drug cost for the most commonly available abortifacients available in the United States are shown in the following table.

Drug name	Trade name	Manufacturer	Drug unit	Number/ pack	Initial cost/pack	Dose/kg	Days Rx	Rx/day	Efficacy	Hospitalize for treatment?	Drug cost alone
Cabergoline	Dostinex	Teva	0.5 mg tablet	8	$$$	0.005	7	1	100% (1/1)	No	$$
Cloprostenol	Estrumate	Intervet	250 µg/ml	20	$$	0.025	5	1	100% (?)	Yes	$$
Dexamethasone		Various	4 mg tablet	100	$	0.22	10	2	100% (18/18)	No	$
Prostaglandin F$_{2\alpha}$	Lutalyse	Pfizer	5 mg/ml	30	$$	0.25	9	3	100% (30/30)	Yes	$$$
Cloprostenol/ Cabergoline	Estrumate	Intervet	250 µg/ml	20	$$	0.025	10	1	100% (5/5)		
Combination	Dostinex	Teva	0.5 mg tablet	8	$$$	0.005	10	1		Yes	$$$

- If the bitch has been mated to an unknown stray male, the possibility of exposure to *Brucella canis* or Transmissible Venereal Tumor may exist.

Expected Course and Prognosis

- With appropriate medical management, most cases will resolve with resorption of the litter and minimal vaginal discharge. If the procedure is done very late in pregnancy, overt abortion can occur, necessitating euthanasia of the neonates. The chance of metritis occurring is rare, but if there is underlying uterine pathology, uterine rupture could occur. With most treatments, prognosis for pregnancy during the next estrus has shown to be good.

Abbreviations

LH   = Luteinizing hormone
PGF = Prostaglandin $F_{2\alpha}$

See Also

Pregnancy Diabetes
Pregnancy Ketosis

Suggested Reading

Eilts, B.E. (2010) Contraception and Pregnancy Termination in the Dog and Cat, in *Textbook of Veterinary Internal Medicine*, 7th edition (eds S.J. Ettinger, E.C. Feldman), Saunders Elsevier, St Louis, pp. 1906–1913.

Feldman, E.C., Davidson, A.P., Nelson, R.W., Nyland, T.G., Munro, C. (1993) Prostaglandin induction of abortion in pregnant bitches after misalliance. *J. Am. Vet. Med. Assoc.*, **202**, 1855–1858.

Sutton, D.J., Geary, M.R., Bergman, J.G.H.E. (1997) Prevention of pregnancy in bitches following unwanted mating – a clinical trial using low-dose estradiol benzoate. *J. Reprod. Fertil., Suppl.*, **51**, 239–243.

Tsutsui, T., Mizutani, W., Hori, T., Oishi, K., Sugi, Y., Kawakami, E. (2006) Estradiol benzoate for preventing pregnancy in mismated dogs. *Theriogenology*, **66**, 1568–1572.

Wanke, M., Loza, M.E., Monachesi, N., Concannon, P. (1997) Clinical use of dexamethasone for termination of unwanted pregnancy in dogs. *J. Reprod. Fertil. Suppl.*, **51**, 233–238.

Whitacre, M.D., Yates, D.J., Vancamp, S.D., Meuten, D.J. (1992) Detection of intravaginal spermatozoa after natural mating in the bitch. *Vet. Clin. Pathol.*, **21**, 85–87.

Author: Bruce Eilts DVM, DACT

chapter 46

Neonatal Resuscitation and Early Neonatal Care

DEFINITION

- Neonatal resuscitation (NR): restoration to life of a puppy or kitten apparently dead and returning them to consciousness by applying cardiopulmonary resuscitation (CPR), emergency procedure used to treat puppies or kittens of cardiac and respiratory arrest. No attention from dam within 60 seconds of a natural delivery warrants attention. Also indicated post Caesarean section due to maternal anesthesia, sometimes complicated by previous dystocia.
- Neonate: a newborn puppy or kitten from parturition through the first 2 weeks of life.
- Neonatal care: procedures employed to maintain life and growth of a puppy or kitten neonate the first 2 weeks of life.

ETIOLOGY/PATHOPHYSIOLOGY

- Neonate: fatal abnormalities in heart or lungs, intestinal abnormalities, airway obstruction, navel cord twist or breakage, anesthetic agents.
- Dam: placental abnormalities (pre-partum hemorrhage), premature detachment of placenta from the endometrium leading to the appearance of greenish-black-stained discharge. These conditions result in anoxia leading to asphyxia. Intrauterine infection or intoxication may lead to weak or dead puppies.

SIGNALMENT/HISTORY

Risk factors

- Previous manual birth assistance or cesarean section. Dead puppy or kitten in uterus or other dystocia, leading to prolonged time between start of stage 2 (expulsion phase) to delivery. Neonatal loss is strongly correlated to the duration of stage 2 labor.

Blackwell's Five-Minute Veterinary Consult Clinical Companion: Small Animal Endocrinology and Reproduction, First Edition. Edited by Deborah S. Greco and Autumn P. Davidson. © 2017 John Wiley & Sons, Inc. Published 2017 by John Wiley & Sons, Inc. Companion Website: www.fiveminutevet.com/endocrinology

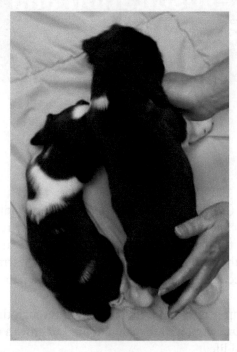

■ **Fig. 46.1.** Sibling neonates illustrating low birth weight (left).

- Opioid (or other sedatives/tranquilizers) administration to dam prior to surgery predisposes to respiratory depression in puppies.
- Primary inertia in the bitch (overweight, older dams, large litters, very small litters), excess use of oxytocin to stimulate contractions, resulting in overdosing of oxytocin that may negatively affect puppies.
- Low-weight puppies or kittens weighing less than 50% of mean litter weight (average weight of kittens 100 g, average puppy weights vary by breed from 150 to 650 g. Last kitten or puppy in large litter (Fig. 46.1).
- Meconium-stained neonates indicative of intrauterine stress.
- Incompatibility between blood types (B queens to A sires) in cats causing neonatal isoerythrolysis (NI) if predisposed kittens are allowed to nurse.

Incidence/Prevalence

- Need for NR: exact data is not available, probably dependent on kennel management and breeding stock. Frequently in cases with dystocia, from one to two neonates to whole litter, depending on litter size and duration of parturition.
- Feline NI: Rare in the general population, but the most common cause in newborn kittens that have suckled their mothers. A survey on kitten mortality (from birth to 16 weeks of age), revealed that the majority of deaths in the perinatal period (<1 day) was due to NI.

DIAGNOSTICS

Clinical Signs

- Normal newborn puppies vocalize and often struggle vigorously when picked up. Vocalization is less frequent in kitten neonates. Both are firm to the touch, unstained by meconium, and have a soft pink color around the nose, of the oral mucosa, on the abdomen, and on the extremities. Newborns should react to pinching between toes and display a suction reflex (Fig. 46.2). Heart rate should be >200 beats per minute (bpm).
- Compromised puppies and kittens appear dead or flaccid, feel cold to the touch, mouth open or shut, do not breathe, may be meconium-stained (brown color), hardly vocalize or not at all, and are pale blue (cyanotic) to white in color of the nose area, mucosa and paws. No pinching reflex or suction reflex. Heart rate <150 bpm.
- In NI, once kittens drink colostrum they start to show clinical signs within hours to days: stop nursing, fail to thrive, develop hemolytic anemia within 1–2 days after birth, and some or all of the litter will die. Early clinical signs are pigmenturia (dark red-brown urine). Affected kittens will be anemic, jaundiced, and depressed. Immune-mediated hemolysis, disseminated intravascular coagulation, acute renal failure, and anemia cause death.

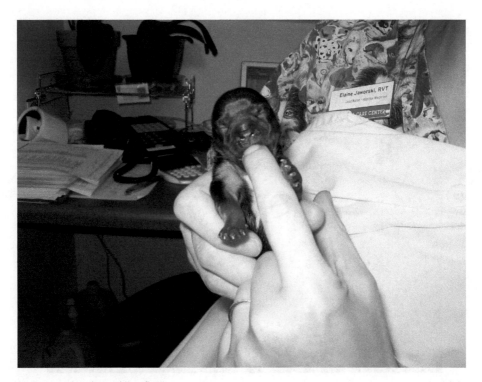

■ Fig. 46.2. Assessing the suckle reflex in a neonate.

Equipment (Fig. 46.3)

- Oxygen delivery system.
- Heating pad, heating lamp, warm air bags or incubator T = 28–30 °C (80–90 °F) if not with dam.
- Fluid administration sets, syringes (tb), acupuncture needles, small-gauge needles (25–27).
- Navel disinfectant (tincture of iodine), ligature for sealing umbilical cord cut in 5-inch (12-cm) lengths.
- Towels.
- Thermometer (digital).
- Stethoscope with pediatric-size bell (2 cm) and diaphragm (3 cm).
- Epinephrine freshly diluted 1:9, 50% dextrose freshly diluted to 5%.
- Small face masks, piglet resuscitators, 'first puff' ventilator system.
- Suction (pediatric bulb syringes, DeLee aspirators).
- Puppy box (Styrofoam) with heat support.
- Multiple clean mosquito forceps and small scissors.
- Bowls for warm water baths.
- Doppler for pulse or heartbeat detection.
- Neonatal scale.

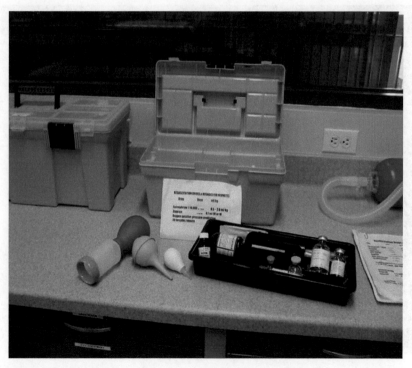

■ **Fig. 46.3.** Neonatal resuscitation kit.

THERAPEUTICS

- Immediate action is required due to respiratory depression causing anoxia or hypoxia as the neonate may not have drawn its first breath.
  - First, remove the amniotic membrane and fluid from the mouth and airways, while keeping puppy or kitten head slightly lower than hindquarters, before clamping or tearing/cutting navel cord or the attached placenta (Fig. 46.4a,b). Removal of thicker or residual secretions from the mouth can be done by using airway suction, allowing controlled suction and inspection of pharynx (Fig. 46.5a–e). After removal of oral contents, stimulate spontaneous breathing with gentle, brisk rubbing of the thorax and muzzle with a warm towel. If spontaneous breathing does not occur within 30–60 seconds, apply a small face mask and supply positive-pressure ventilation (~30–60 breaths per minute) for 3–4 minutes, take a 1-minute break and repeat (Fig. 46.6a). Mouth-to-mouth can be attempted but is less hygienic. If unsuccessful, intubation with a 2-mm endotracheal tube may be attempted. Jen chung acupressure can also be attempted to stimulate ventilation (Fig. 46.6b). Assure that the airways are free of fluids by repeating suction with the head lower than the thorax.
  - Cardiac stimulation should follow ventilation if bradycardia persists; however bradycardia is likely due to myocardial hypoxemia and improved ventilation is indicated first. Rub the neonate gently but rapidly with clean towel and try applying a direct pressure to the chest. Administration of 20–40 µg/kg epinephrine IV in umbilical vein or via an interosseous (IO) route can be attempted for cardiac standstill (Fig. 46.7).

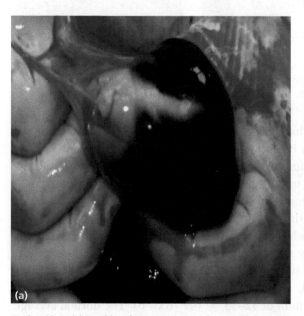
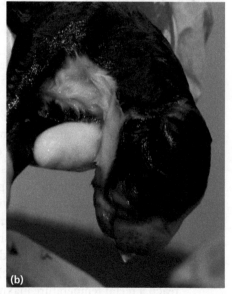

■ **Fig. 46.4.** (a) Breaking the amniotic membrane. (b) Draining amniotic fluid from the airways.

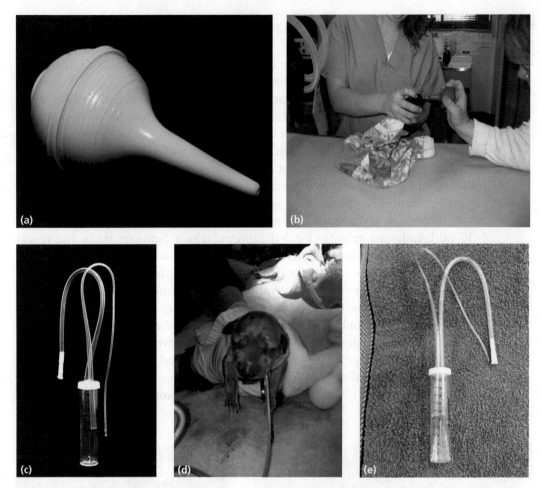

■ **Fig. 46.5.** (a) Preemie neonatal bulb syringe. (b) Aspirating pharyngeal fluid using a bulb syringe. (c) Dee aspirator, unused. (d) Aspirating airway fluid using the Dee aspirator. (e) Amniotic fluid recovered from a neonate's airway with a Dee aspirator.

- After ventilation and heart rate have become acceptable, clamp the navel cord and remove it with attached placenta by cutting with blunt scissors approximately 2 cm (0.8 in) from the base. Tear or cut navel cord from the pup's side opposite its placenta to avoid damage to pup's umbilical area. Use disinfectant and ligate cord to control bleeding and prevent a portal for bacterial ascension (Fig. 46.8a,b).
- All handling should be done within a warm environment, using water-heated bottle, warm-air blanket, warm hands, bare skin to neonate body contact (inside your shirt). The latter simultaneously enables rubbing and keeping the neonate warm. A warm-water bath can be used if neonatal chilling is significant, and also permits ongoing rubbing (Fig. 46.9a–c). Hypothermic pups should be warmed gently to reach a rectal temperature maximum of 32–33 °C (99–100 °F). The normal average body temperature the first 7 days is 35.6 ± 0.7 °C (96 ± 1.5 °F).

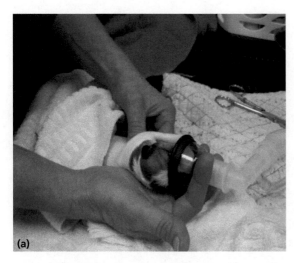
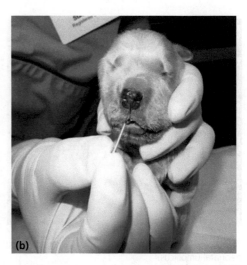

■ **Fig. 46.6.** (a) Positive-pressure ventilation using a snug face mask and oxygen source. (b) Jen chung acupressure point for stimulating breathing.

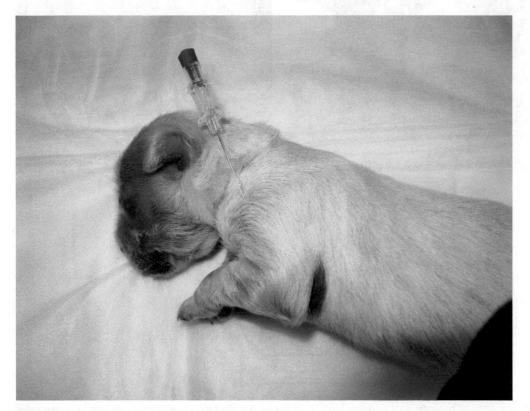

■ **Fig. 46.7.** Interosseous catheter placement, proximal humerus.

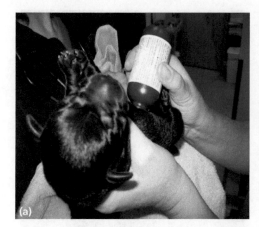

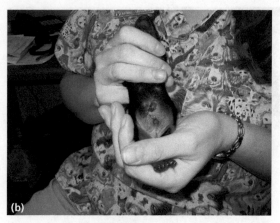

■ **Fig. 46.8.** (a) Dunking the umbilicus with 2% tincture of iodine. (b) Appearance of properly ligated and disinfected neonatal umbilicus.

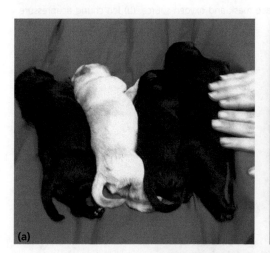

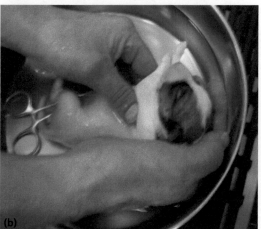

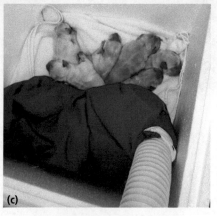

■ **Fig. 46.9.** (a) Neonates on a warm-air blanket. (b) Neonatal resuscitation in a warm-water bath. (c) Resuscitated neonates in an insulated box with a warm-air blanket.

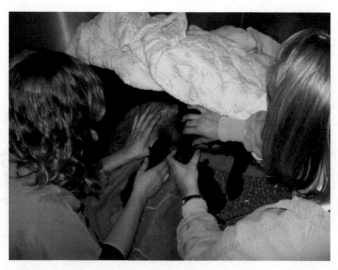

■ **Fig. 46.10.** Supervised nursing of colostrum.

- If breathing commences, measure heart rate and temperature, and evaluate need for supportive fluid therapy. Once neonates are pink and are breathing well on their own, place in warm environment and allow neonates to nurse as soon as possible. This requires supervision if the dam is groggy from anesthesia and normal maternal behavior not yet established reliably (Fig. 46.10).
- Revival of puppies and kittens with depressed respiration after C-section may require medical therapy, such as naloxone 0.1 mg/kg IM if narcotics were used in the dam's anesthesia. Do not use in other cases of apneic hypoxic patients. Doxapram is unlikely to be beneficial in neonates with a hypoxic brain due to its diminished effect on central stimulation in hypoxic neonates. Atropine is contraindicated as it exacerbates myocardial hypoxemia.
- NI: Do not allow kittens to nurse. Even if the kittens are removed from dam as soon as the first clinical signs develop, the mortality rate will be high. Prevention is the preferred 'treatment' for NI. Affected kittens need supportive care, blood transfusions. However, prognosis is guarded.

Fluid therapy

■ Use balanced multiple electrolyte solution with 2.5% dextrose (isotonic).
■ *Warmed fluid* can be administered orally, intraperitoneally (IP), intravenously (IV), or by interosseous cannulation (IO) in the femur/humeral head or wing of the ileum (Fig. 46.11). IV fluids can be given at an initial rate of 1 ml per 30 g over 5–10 minutes.
■ Maintenance requirements IV are 60–200 ml/kg/day. Glucose replacement therapy in hypoglycemic neonates: 0.5–1.0 g/kg body weight (2–4 ml/kg) of a 5–10% dextrose solution.

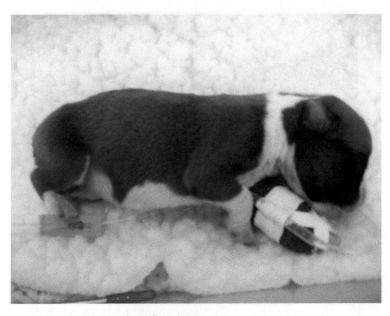

■ **Fig. 46.11.** Intravenous catheterization for IV fluid therapy.

 COMMENTS

- Puppies and kittens should be examined for gross abnormalities and trauma and weighed soon after birth. They subsequently should be weighed twice daily on a digital scale to accurately measure weight gain. Caloric requirement from days 1 to 7 is 30–140 calories/kg/day. Neonates should gain 10–15% of birth weight per day and double their body weight in 10 days. If healthy and satiated, neonates should feel warm and firm; skin turgor is not always reliable due to increased water content and decreased fat content of the skin. They should appear pink, have rounded soft abdomen, be quiet unless disturbed, and show activated sleep (sleep with small twitches in limbs and head). The umbilical area is slightly pink and dry, and the desiccated cord should be lost in 2–3 days (Fig. 46.12). If awake, they should rapidly seek the udder and nurse frequently. Righting and suckling reflexes are normal. Normal respiratory rate is 15–30 breaths per minute. Sick puppies often vocalize (less common in kittens), and they may feel hot (hyperthermia) or cold (hypothermia) to the touch, be flaccid, have a flat or distended abdomen, have a lower than 150-bpm heart rate, and may show less activated sleep, sleeping away from littermates.

Client Education

- Inform clients on the benefits of accurate ovulation timing for mating and term of delivery. Discourage breeding in first estrus females, females older than 8 years, or females with more than two previous cesarean sections. Cat breeders should be aware of NI.

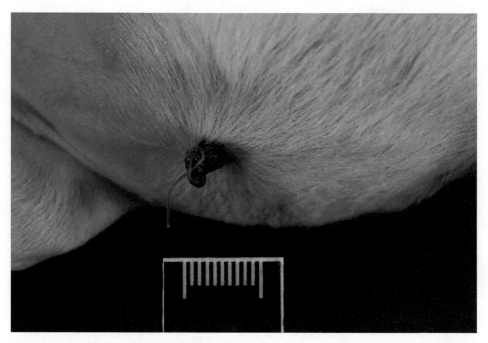

■ **Fig. 46.12.** Normal umbilicus 24 hours post-partum.

See Also

Caesarean Section Elective and Emergency
Breeding Management: Canine
Feline Prebreeding Examination and Breeding Husbandry
Nutrition of the Breeding Dog and Cat

Suggested Reading

Johnson, C.A., Casal, M.L. (2012) Neonatal resuscitation: Canine and Feline, in *Management of Pregnant and Neonatal Dogs, Cats and Exotic Pets* (ed. C. Lopate), Wiley-Blackwell, Ames, Iowa, pp. 677–692.
Ricard, V. (2011) Birth and the first 24h, in *Small Animal Pediatrics. The First 12 Months of Life* (eds M.E. Peterson, M.A. Kutzler), Elsevier-Saunders, St Louis, Missouri, pp. 11–19.
Silvestre-Ferreira, A.C., Pastor, J. (2010) Feline neonatal isoerythrolysis and the importance of feline blood types. *Vet. Med. Int.*, **2010**, 75376, pp. 1–8. Doi: 0.4061/2010/753726

Author: Wenche Farstad DVM, PhD, DECAR

Nutrition in Pregnancy and Lactation in the Bitch and Queen

chapter 47

DEFINITION

- Reproduction includes the most nutritionally demanding life stages.
- The goals of feeding for optimum reproduction include:
  - Optimize conception rate and litter size.
  - Optimize milk production.
  - Minimize dam/queen impact by providing adequate energy with a balanced diet.
  - Optimize puppy/kitten development and growth.
  - These goals are best achieved when the bitch/queen is provided:
    - □ adequate amounts of energy and water.
    - □ optimal concentrations of essential nutrients.

ETIOLOGY/PATHOPHYSIOLOGY

- Energy needs increase by 30–60% in the second half of gestation:
  - Depending on the breed and litter size.
  - Queens increase food intake soon after conception.
  - Gain weight in linear fashion throughout gestation.
  - Lose less than half of gestational gain at parturition.
- Bitches gain most gestational weight during last 3–4 weeks, and energy requirements do not increase until this time:
  - Energy requirements increase to about 3.0-fold resting energy requirements (RER).
  - Prevent excessive gain early in gestation and prior to confirming pregnancy.
  - At whelping, bitches should return to approximately pre-breeding weight.
- Ensure good body condition prior to breeding (Fig. 47.1):
  - Obesity increases the risk of dystocia and smaller litters.
  - Conversely, poor condition may limit performance during lactation and decrease neonatal survival.

Blackwell's Five-Minute Veterinary Consult Clinical Companion: Small Animal Endocrinology and Reproduction, First Edition. Edited by Deborah S. Greco and Autumn P. Davidson. © 2017 John Wiley & Sons, Inc. Published 2017 by John Wiley & Sons, Inc. Companion Website: www.fiveminutevet.com/endocrinology

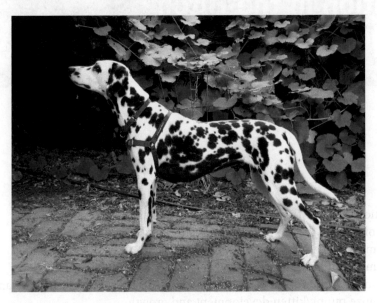

■ **Fig. 47.1.** Ideal body condition in a Dalmatian bitch.

- ■ Lactation is the most energetically demanding life stage:
  - Energy needs may double during the period of peak milk production around 3–4 weeks.
  - Often higher with larger litters.
  - Queens often lose weight during lactation, so an adequate but not excessive amount of weight gain during gestation is desirable.
  - Bitches should not fall below ideal body condition during lactation.

SIGNALMENT/HISTORY

- ■ Transient decreased appetite may be noted at peak estrus, at 3–4 weeks after mating, and at whelping in bitches, and at 2 weeks after mating and during the last week of gestation in queens.
- ■ During late gestation and throughout lactation, both bitches and queens are at risk for hypocalcemia (eclampsia):
  - It appears to be the result of an increased calcium sink into rapidly developing fetuses or into milk production.
  - It may be concurrent with hypoglycemia.
  - Larger litters may increase risk due to the increased fetal and mammary demands.
  - Highest risk at peak milk production around 3–4 weeks.
  - Uterine inertia may result if occurs at parturition.
  - Preventive supplementation with calcium is not advised and should be reserved for documented hypocalcemia.
  - Avoid suboptimal calcium intakes, either too high or too low.

CLINICAL FEATURES

- Water is critical nutrient for adequate milk production
  - Queens and bitches may be reluctant to leave litter in immediate post-natal period.
  - Ensure ample water is available very close to nursing area, but not where puppies or kittens can get into it.
- Diet should be of adequate energy density to avoid volume limitations
  - Food intake at the end of gestation may be limited by uterine encroachment.
  - Small, frequent meals recommended throughout gestation and lactation.
- Commercially available diets that have been through feeding tests for reproduction or all life stages should be offered from breeding; this information is on the pet food label.
- Provision of oral colostrum is strongly advised within the first 24–48 hours.
  - Parenteral administration of adult canine or feline serum/plasma can be substituted if necessary.
  - Commercially available milk replacers should be used with caution.
    - □ Associated with overfeeding.
    - □ Potential issues with nutritional adequacy.
    - □ Bottle use may increase risk of aspiration versus intermittent gastric tube feeding.
    - □ Do not enlarge bottle nipple holes.
    - □ Home-prepared formulas are not adequate and should only be used short term in emergency situations.
    - □ Use of foster bitch or queen is ideal (Fig. 47.2).
    - □ At 3–4 weeks of age offer soft, soaked kibble or canned growth diets in several small meals per day.

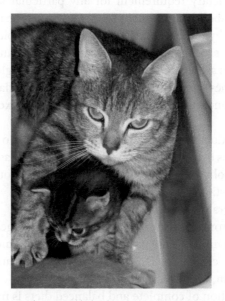

■ **Fig. 47.2.** Foster queen showing good maternal behavior.

DIAGNOSTICS

- Body condition scoring should be performed at every clinic visit.
- Diet history should be collected at every clinic visit.
- Puppies and kittens should be regularly weighed (daily) during lactation to ensure adequate growth.

THERAPEUTICS

- In addition to energy and water, nutrients important for reproduction and growth include:
  - Protein
    - ☐ Supplies nitrogen and amino acids.
    - ☐ Synthesis of dispensable amino acids, protein (muscle, enzymes, etc.), and a wide variety of metabolic compounds.
  - Fat
    - ☐ Supplies essential fatty acids, cell membrane components, other metabolic components.
    - ☐ Requirement for long-chain omega-3 fatty acids is suspected for growth and reproduction.
    - ☐ Docosahexaenoic acid (DHA) important for early neurological development:
      - ○ Impacts diet palatability.
      - ○ Major factor in energy density of diet.
  - Carbohydrate
    - ☐ No specific dietary requirement for any particular starch or sugar; however, absolute metabolic requirement for glucose must be met.
    - ☐ Dietary carbohydrate is conditionally essential for bitches.
    - ☐ Protein requirements are higher during gestation and lactation when low/no carbohydrates are fed to bitches in order to supply gluconeogenic precursors.
    - ☐ Feeding bitches some carbohydrate may be beneficial for optimum reproductive performance unless protein content of diet exceeds around 45% on an energy basis.
    - ☐ Tests of reproductive performance using diets with no carbohydrate and protein concentrations between 27% and 45% on an energy basis have not been reported.
    - ☐ Effect of carbohydrate on reproduction in queens not tested but unlikely to be required if dietary protein is adequate.
  - Vitamins and minerals
    - ☐ Multiple micronutrients essential during all life stages.
    - ☐ Vitamins and minerals are used for wide variety of metabolic functions: essential cofactors, critical for DNA synthesis and structure, necessary for metabolism of protein, fat, carbohydrate.
    - ☐ Supplementation of complete and balanced diets is not recommended.
    - ☐ Excesses and nutrient interactions may have adverse effects.

See Also

Canine Breeding Management
Feline Pre-Breeding Examination and Breeding Husbandry

Suggested Reading

Corbee, R.J., Tryfonidou, M.A., Beckers, I.P., *et al.* (2012) Composition and use of puppy milk formulas in German shepherd puppies in the Netherlands. *J. Anim. Physiol. Anim. Nutr. (Berlin)*, **96** (3), 395–402.

Fascetti, A.J., Delaney, S.J. (2012) Feeding the healthy dog and cat, in *Applied Veterinary Clinical Nutrition* (eds A.J. Fascetti, S.J. Delaney), Wiley-Blackwell, West Sussex, UK, pp. 75–94.

Kienzle, E., Meyer, H. (1989) The effects of carbohydrate-free diets containing different levels of protein on reproduction in the bitch, in *Nutrition of the Dog and Cat* (eds I.H. Burger, J.P.W. Rivers), Cambridge University Press, Cambridge, UK, pp. 243–257.

Ad hoc Committee on Dog and Cat Nutrition (2006) Nutrient Requirements of Dogs and Cats. National Academies Press, Washington, DC.

Author: Jennifer Bones Larsen DVM, MS, PhD, DACVN

chapter 48

Ovarian Remnant Syndrome/ Hyperestrogenism

DEFINITION

- Ovarian remnant syndrome (ORS) refers to the presence of functional ovarian tissue in a previously ovariectomized animal.
- Hyperestrogenism/estrogen toxicity refers to a syndrome characterized by physiologically inappropriate elevations in serum concentrations of estrogens (estradiol, estriol, or estrone).

ETIOLOGY/PATHOPHYSIOLOGY

- Elevated serum estrogen may occur secondary to exogenous or endogenous estrogens.
- Exposure to exogenous sources of estrogen may occur via known administration (diethylstilbestrol, estradiol cypionate), or by unintentional exposure during handling to transdermal hormone replacement products used by a human.
- Sites of endogenous estrogen production include ovarian follicles, follicular ovarian cysts, Leydig cells, and the adrenal cortex (zona glomerulosa and reticularis). Can also occur as a result of peripheral conversion of excessive androgens, or in association with an ovarian or testicular tumor – more commonly granulosa cell tumors and Sertoli cell tumors but also noted with other ovarian and testicular tumors.
- The physiologic roles of estrogen are numerous, and in the female include normal sexual behavior and development and function of the female reproductive tract. In the male, estrogens are responsible for Leydig cell function.
- Estrogen receptors are found in a wide variety of non-reproductive tract tissues including brain, lung, bone, kidney, and intestine.
- In the female reproductive tract, estrogens potentiate the stimulatory effect of progesterone in the endometrium and permit cervical relaxation; these two effects increase the risk of cystic endometrial hyperplasia and (stump) pyometra. In the male reproductive tract, estrogen potentiates the action of androgens in the prostate.
- Estrogens increase osteoblastic activity, retention of calcium and phosphorus, and total body proteins and metabolic rate.

Blackwell's Five-Minute Veterinary Consult Clinical Companion: Small Animal Endocrinology and Reproduction,
First Edition. Edited by Deborah S. Greco and Autumn P. Davidson. © 2017 John Wiley & Sons, Inc.
Published 2017 by John Wiley & Sons, Inc.
Companion Website: www.fiveminutevet.com/endocrinology

- High serum estrogen levels can interfere with stem cell differentiation in the bone marrow and erythrocyte iron metabolism.
- Serum estrogen provides a source of negative feedback at the level of the pituitary due to decreased sensitivity to gonadotropin-releasing hormone (GnRH), and is thus associated with low levels of serum luteinizing hormone (LH).
- At the time of follicular development, elevations in serum estrogen, *in conjunction with progesterone*, provide positive feedback to both GnRH and LH, resulting in the peri-ovulatory spike in LH,

Systems Affected

- Hemic/Lymphatic/Immune: bone marrow suppression.
- Nervous: behavioral alteration with respect to expression/suppression of sexual behavior.
- Reproductive: vulvar and clitoral enlargement, ovarian or testicular mass, signs of estrus, uterine stump pyometra.
- Renal/Urologic: stranguria, pollakiura, hematuria.
- Skin/Endocrine: alopecia, hyperpigmentation.

 # SIGNALMENT/HISTORY

Ovarian Remnant Syndrome

- Presentation typically due to signs of estrus in a previously ovariohysterectomized female.
- More commonly noted in dogs due to vulvar edema and vaginal discharge, especially if concurrent uterine stump/pyometra; feline estrual behavior prompts presentation.
- More frequently associated with the right ovary.
- Presentation typically one year after ovariohysterectomy but may present immediately or several years (>8) after surgery.

Hyperestrogenism/Estrogen Toxicity

- Presentation typically due to prolonged signs of estrous (female), hair loss and hyperpigmentation (male).

Endogenous

- Older male dogs (secondary to testicular tumors).
- Older female dogs (secondary to granulose cell tumors or other ovarian tumor types, follicular ovarian cysts).
- Young female dogs (follicular ovarian cysts).

Exogenous

- All species and ages in association with estrogen administration or exposure.
- Toy breed dogs (lap dogs) exposed to owner's transdermal hormone replacement therapy.

Risk Factors

- Dogs are more likely to experience ovarian remnant syndrome; in part this is thought to be due to the increased adipose tissue around the canine ovary as compared to the feline ovary, increasing surgical error.
- Feline ovarian remnant not related to surgical experience.
- Follicular ovarian cysts.
- Functional ovarian tumor (granulosa cell tumor and other ovarian tumors).
- Testicular tumor (specifically Sertoli cell tumor but also may occur secondary to Leydig and interstitial cell tumors).
- Exogenous estrogen administration more commonly occurs due to unintentional exposure to owner transdermal hormone replacement treatments.

Historic Findings

Ovarian Remnant Syndrome
- Onset of signs of estrous in the dog.
- Increased vocalization, affection, grooming, agitation in the cat.
- Lordosis (this may be reported by the owner as lumbar pain).
- Occasionally owners with present cat due to signs of 'seizures' or extreme pain which are actually misinterpreted normal components of sexual behavior (yowling, flicking tail, rolling, twitching, biting).

Hyperestrogenism/Estrogen Toxicity

- Attractive to male/other dogs.
- Vulvar bleeding or enlargement.
- Prolonged proestrus and estrus (female).
- Hair loss.
- Hyperpigmentation.
- Decreased libido (male).
- Nymphomania.
- Hematuria (in association with benign prostatic hyperplasia or thrombocytopenia).

 CLINICAL FEATURES

Ovarian Remnant Syndrome

Canine
- Vulvar swelling/edema.
- Vaginal discharge – variable depending on presence of endometrial tissue.
- Behavioral changes associated with sexual receptivity.

Feline

- Vulvar swelling and discharge are not a feature of ovarian remnant syndrome in the cat.
- Lordosis in response to genital stimulation or petting.
- Increased vocalization.
- Behavioral change – aggression and/or increased affection may be noted.

Hyperestrogenism/Estrogen Toxicity

- Non-pruritic, symmetric alopecia (endocrine alopecia); stud dog tail.
- Hyperpigmentation.
- Testicular mass or testicular asymmetry (in association with a tumor mass or testicular atrophy).
- Testicular atrophy – may be unilateral in contralateral non-tumor-containing testicle, or bilateral, as seen in association with exogenous hyperestrogenism.
- Cryptorchidism.
- Prostatomegaly (due to squamous metaplasia).
- Vulvar edema/discharge.
- Gynecomastia.
- Pale mucous membranes (anemia), petechiation or hemorrhage (thrombocytopenia), fever (secondary to neutropenia).

 DIFFERENTIAL DIAGNOSIS

Non-Pruritic, Symmetric Alopecia (Endocrine Alopecia)

- Hypothyroidism – diagnosis based on appropriate clinical sings in conjunction with typical hematologic and biochemical abnormalities (normocytic normochromic nonregenerative anemia, hypercholesterolemia, and thyroid function testing (total T4, free T4, cTSH).
- Hyperadrenocorticism – clinical signs usually included polyuria, polydipsia; CBC may reveal leukocytosis and erythrocytosis and thrombocytosis; serum biochemistry abnormalities include elevated ALP, ALT and cholesterol, and decreased BUN; additional testing includes urine cortisol creatinine ratio, LDDS test, ACTH stimulation test, endogenous ACTH, abdominal ultrasonography.
- Adrenal sex hormone dermatosis – clinical signs typically are similar to hyperadrenocorticism but polyuria and polydipsia are variable; LDDS and ACTH stimulation cortisol testing are normal, but extended ACTH stimulation testing including sex hormones is abnormal.

Attractive to Male Dogs/Other Dogs

- Vaginitis – may be differentiated from hyperestrogenism via examination of vaginal cytology, which will reveal a lack of epithelial cell cornification.
- Behavioral abnormality – diagnosis of exclusion.

- Genitourinary tract infection, inflammation (foreign body), or neoplasia – diagnosis based on ruling out estrogen influence by examination of vaginal cytology, urine culture and sensitivity, and vaginal examination including vaginoscopy.

Infertility

- Testicular degeneration/atrophy/immune-mediated orchitis – diagnosis based on physical examination, lack of testicular or intra-abdominal masses, semen evaluation (azoospermia), and testicular FNA cytology or biopsy.
- Intersex abnormalities – uncommon; diagnosis is supported by physical examination findings (abnormal external genitalia), karyotype examination and histologic examination of the reproductive tract.

 ## DIAGNOSTICS

Ovarian Remnant Syndrome

- A key component to a diagnosis of ovarian remnant syndrome is documentation of the presence of estrogen, *and* ovarian tissue in a previously ovariohysterectomized female.

CBC/Biochemistry/Urinalysis

- Typically normal; increased RBC may be noted in voided urine samples if a sanguineous vaginal discharge is present.

Vaginal Cytology/Serum Hormone Evaluation/Stimulation Testing

- Vaginal cytology
  - Vaginal cytology is the initial diagnostic of choice if estrogen effect is present (signs of heat), and represents an easy, cost-effective, point of service, endogenous bioassay for estrogen; in the cat, vaginal cytology is best achieved using a vaginal flush technique rather than swab.
  - Epithelial cell cornification with anuclear or pyknotic nuclei is consistent with estrogen influence (Fig. 48.1).
  - With ORS, signs of heat are usually periodic (unless functional ovarian follicular cysts or neoplasia are present).
  - With exogenous estrogen exposure, signs of heat are usually continuous.
- Progesterone levels
  - If the female is not clinically showing signs of heat/estrogen influence, serum progesterone can be of use in the bitch to evaluate the diestrual hormone profile (post-ovulation); however, it is only of significance if >2 ng/ml, as both the ovariectomized and anestrous females will have low serum progesterone (<1.0 ng/ml).
  - In the queen, ovulation may, or may not, occur spontaneously or after coital contact. Progesterone levels are unreliable indicators of ovarian tissue unless elevated (>2 ng/ml).

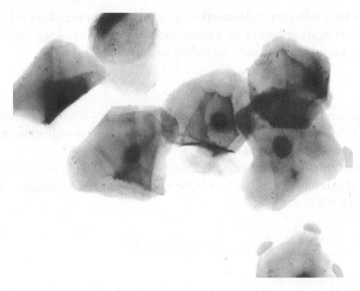

■ **Fig. 48.1.** Superficial vaginal epithelial cells with anuclear or pyknotic nuclei is consistent with estrogen influence.

- Luteinizing hormone
  - Luteinizing hormone (LH) is negative (<1 ng/ml) in intact bitches/queens or those with ORS at any point in the estrous cycle, except the time of the LH surge (lasting 12–24 hours; spontaneous in the bitch, usually induced by coitus in the queen).
  - LH is also negative in bitches/queens exposed to exogenous estrogen (LH testing does not differentiate endogenous versus exogenous estrogen exposure); it cannot be used to differentiate ORS and hyperestrogenism/estrogen toxicity.
  - The current recommendation is not to perform LH testing if the patient is currently showing signs of estrogen stimulation to avoid measuring a positive LH during the LH surge in an intact female or female with ORS; however, two positive tests performed several days apart (to ensure that the sample was not taken during the LH surge) provide conclusive evidence that ovarian tissue is not present.
  - A negative result in a non-estrogenized bitch/queen is consistent with the presence of ovarian tissue.
  - Major veterinary laboratories perform LH tests, and an LH test kit is also available (Witness LH; Zoetis.com) for in-house use.
- Anti-Mullerian hormone
  - An assay for anti-Mullerian hormone (AMH) expressed by granulosa cells of the ovary is now commercially available, and is reliable in post-pubertal bitches and queens; AMH is produced solely by the ovaries in females, so its measurement can be used to distinguish between intact and completely ovariectomized individuals.
  - AMH is not suppressed by estrogen and can be used at any time in post-pubertal bitches/queens to evaluate for the presence of ovaries/ovarian remnant (positive result).
  - AMH is negative in ovariectomized bitches/queens under exogenous estrogen exposure; it can be used to differentiate ORS and hyperestrogenism/estrogen toxicity.

- The AMH ELISA is currently performed at the Animal Health Diagnostic Center at Cornell University; the Clinical Endocrinology Laboratory at University of California, Davis; and AViD Laboratories.
- The in-house lateral flow test is not recommended for ORS screening as it is not sensitive enough to detect some ORS cases.

■ GnRH hCG

- Both, GnRH and hCG stimulation testing have been described to evaluate cases of ORS; results are variable.
- Recent studies suggest that GnRH (10 µg/kg) IV (or 200 IU for dogs <15 kg, 300 IU for dogs >15 kg) may be used in the dog to confirm ovarian remnant tissue; samples should be collected at time zero and 90 minutes and evaluated for estrogen. This is only of value if vaginal cytology is unrewarding.
- The use of hCG is described for feline patients (250 IU IM once during presumed estrous) with serum progesterone evaluation 2–3 weeks later. Functional ovarian tissue is present if the serum progesterone concentration is >2 ng/ml.

■ Endoscopy

- Visualization of the canine cervix may be achieved with the use of an extended-length cystourethroscope.
- Can be of benefit to document the presence of a cervix, localize the source of hemorrhagic discharge and/or drainage of mucopurulent discharge for those cases associated with a stump pyometra or granuloma.
- Can be of benefit to evaluate for vaginal mucosal edema in association with estrogen effect (Fig. 48.2).

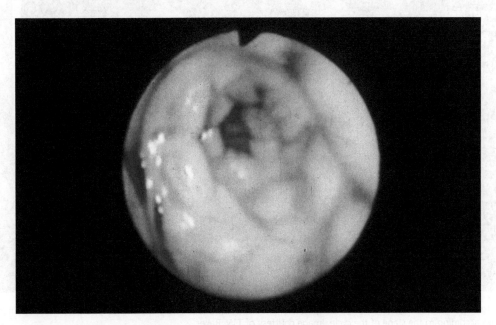

■ **Fig. 48.2.** Vaginoscopic view of estrogen influence (mucosal edema) in the bitch.

- Imaging
  - Abdominal ultrasound should be performed while the animal is showing signs of heat; ovarian remnants will appear as a small round cystic/hypoechoic nodules (Fig. 48.3), and are typically located in the vicinity of the ovaries – it is prudent not to assume only one remnant source.

Hyperestrogenism/Estrogen Toxicity

CBC/Biochemistry/Urinalysis

- Changes are variable and dependent upon exposure duration and dose, and the time delay between insult and testing.
- Generally, in the initial 2–3 weeks both thrombocytopenia and thrombocytosis may be noted with progressive anemia, and leukocytosis. (The WBC count may exceed 100 000/µl).
- After 3 weeks, pancytopenia and aplastic anemia may be noted.
- Hematuria may occur secondary to thrombocytopenia.

Serum Hormone Evaluation/Stimulation Testing

- Serum estrogen (estradiol) concentrations may be evaluated via RIA; however, vaginal and preputial cytology are considered more accurate and reliable as an endogenous biomarker.

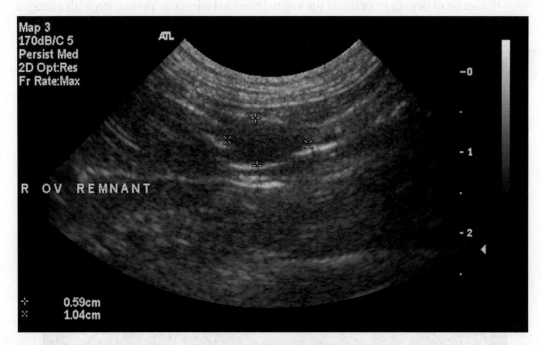

Fig. 48.3. Ultrasonographic image of hypoechoic follicles in an ovarian remnant. The appearance of a remnant varies according to the stage of the cycle. Image courtesy of T.W. Baker.

- Estrogen will result in the predominance of cornified epithelial cells either anuclear, or with a pyknotic nuclei.
- A single serum concentration above 20 pmol/ml is consistent with elevated physiologic levels; serum values may be affected by lipid, and assay sensitivity varies.
- Pathologic follicular cysts typically do not respond to GnRH or hCG reliably.
- Fluid aspirated from a follicular cyst may be submitted for hormone analysis to aid diagnosis.
- LH and AMH testing (see above).
- ACTM stimulation testing with sex hormone analysis may be used to detect altered adrenal sex hormone function.

Endoscopy

- Typically of limited use; however, under the influence of estrogen, vaginoscopy should reveal an edematous and pink vaginal mucosa (Fig. 48.2).

Imaging

- Ultrasonography of the ovaries or testes is advised to detect mass and cystic lesions, in addition to changes in echogenicity or architecture.
- CT offers another modality for evaluation.
- Follicular cysts may be aspirated and the fluid submitted for hormone analysis; however, as the cyst structure itself remains, clinical resolution is not expected.
- It is prudent to evaluate the size and echotexture of regional lymph nodes and other intra-abdominal organs.
- Three-view chest films are advised for evaluation of metastatic disease.

Clinical/Anatomic Pathology Evaluation

- Fine-needle aspirate cytology of testicular masses may provide a cytologic diagnosis prior to pursuing surgery.
- Bone marrow aspirate cytology and bone biopsy if needed, are helpful to evaluate erythroid and myeloid precursor populations.
- Fine-needle aspirate cytology of enlarged lymph nodes should be evaluated for metastatic disease, as indicated by imaging.
- Skin biopsy may be used to confirm endocrine alopecia (telogen arrest, orthokeratotic hyperkeratosis, epidermal atrophy and melanosis, sebaceous gland atrophy).

Surgery

- Neoplastic masses, and affected lymph nodes may be excised completely by exploratory celiotomy or laparoscopy where available.

THERAPEUTICS

Ovarian Remnant Syndrome

- The treatment of choice is surgical exploration, and removal of all gonadal tissue.
- Histopathology of all tissue removed is advised to confirm that it is indeed gonadal tissue and to evaluate for neoplasia.
- Many ovarian remnants are small, and difficult to locate (Fig. 48.4); thus, surgeon experience is invaluable for the successful identification and removal of ovarian remnant tissue.

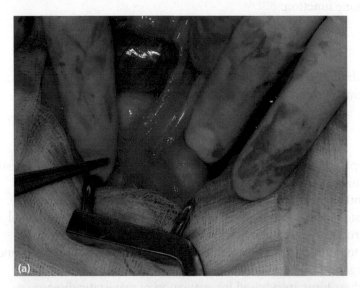

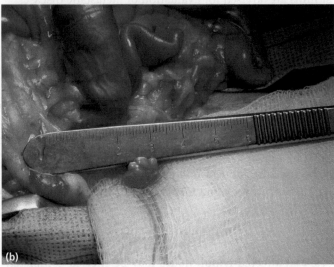

■ **Fig. 48.4.** Intraoperative images of an ovarian remnant. (a) Small remnant at ovarian pedicle. (b) Excised ovarian remnant measures ~ 1.0 cm.

Hyperestrogenism/Estrogen Toxicity

- The treatment of choice for endogenous hyperestrogenism in the intact female and male is surgical neutering.
- Unilateral orchiectomy or ovariectomy of the affected neoplastic testicle or ovary, or cystic ovary, may be considered in valuable breeding animals; the use of prosthetic devices is not advised and is not ethical.
- Endometrial changes secondary to prolonged estrogen exposure can occur and contribute to subfertility, even if the abnormal ovary had been removed making the prognosis for fertility guarded.
- Histopathology should always be performed to evaluate neoplastic changes and to confirm or negate local metastases.
- For those cases of exogenous estrogen exposure, stopping estrogen administration and preventing access, should result in clinical cure. It should be noted that in cases of exogenous estrogen exposure, clinical signs might take several weeks to resolve.

Drug(s) of Choice

- Supportive care for those cases with bone marrow involvement may include blood produces and antimicrobials.
- Synthetic erythropoietin, G-CSF, GM-CSF may be considered to stimulate erythroid and granulocytic production at the level of the bone marrow.
- GnRH is unlikely to induce ovulation in cases of follicular cysts.
- Iron dextran should be administered 10 mg/kg IM once a month to facilitate erythropoiesis as needed.

Precautions/Interactions

- Administration of chemotherapeutic agents for treatment of metastatic testicular or ovarian neoplasia should be pursued with caution due to increased risk of bone marrow suppression secondary to hyperestrogenism.

 COMMENTS

Patient Monitoring

- Repeat serial CBC analysis – to evaluate response to therapy and progression of disease for those cases with bone marrow change.
- Repeat serial bone marrow aspiration cytology – to evaluate erythroid and myeloid lineage response to removal of estrogen compounds and treatment.

Prevention/Avoidance

- ORS has been documented to occur due to revascularization of ovarian tissue that is surgically removed, but left in the abdomen at time of spay.

Possible Complications

▪ Lack of resolving pancytopenia and continued bone marrow hypoplasia 3 weeks after removal of estrogen source is associated with a grave prognosis.

Expected Course and Prognosis

▪ Clinical signs associated with exogenous estrogen should resolved within 2–6 weeks of source removal.
▪ Clinical signs of male feminization syndrome should resolve within 2–6 weeks.
▪ Surgical removal of ovarian remnant tissue is curative, and clinical signs should resolve promptly post surgery.

Abbreviations

ACTH = adrenocorticotropic hormone
ALP = alkaline phosphatase
ALT = alanine aminotransferase
AMH = anti-Mullerian hormone
fT4 = free total thyroxine
GCSF = granulocyte colony-stimulating factor
GH = growth hormone
GMCSF = granulocyte-macrophage colony-stimulating factor
GnRH = gonadotropin-releasing hormone
hCG = human chorionic gonadotropin
LDDS = low-dose dexamethasone suppression test
LH = luteinizing hormone
ORS = ovarian remnant syndrome
RBC = red blood cell
T4 = total serum thyroxine
TSH = thyroid-stimulating hormone
WBC = white blood cell

See Also

TVT
Sertoli Cell Tumors
Prostatic Adenocarcinoma
Prostatic Transitional Cell Neoplasia

Suggested Reading

Ball, R., Birchard S., May, L., *et al.* (2010) Ovarian remnant syndrome in dogs and cats: 21 cases (2000–2007). *J. Am. Vet. Med. Assoc.*, **236** (5), 548–553.
Buijels, J., de Gier, J., Kooistra, H., *et al.* (2011) The pituitary-ovarian axis in dogs with remnant ovarian tissue. *Theriogenology*, **75** (4), 742–751.

Rohlertz, M., Strom Holst, B., Axner, E. (2012) Comparison of the GnRH-stimulation test and a semiquantitative quicktest for LH to diagnose presence of ovaries in the female domestic cat. *Theriogenology*, **78** (9), 1901–1906.

Löfstedt, R., VanLeeuwen, J. (2002) Evaluation of a commercially available luteinizing hormone test for its ability to distinguish between ovariectomized and sexually intact bitches. *J. Am. Vet. Med. Assoc.*, **220** (9), 1331–1335.

Ongoing safety review of Evamist (estradiol transdermal spray) and unintended exposure of children and pets to topical estrogen. FDA Drug Safety Communication. Available at: http://www.fda.gov/Drugs/DrugSafety/PostmarketDrugSafetyInformationforPatientsandProviders/ucm220185.htm; accessed January 2015.

Place, N.J., Hansen, B.S., Cheraskin, J.L., *et al.* (2011) Measurement of serum anti-Müllerian hormone concentration in female dogs and cats before and after ovariohysterectomy. *J. Vet. Diagn. Invest.*, **23**, 524–527.

Nett, T.M., Turzillo, A.M., Baratta, M., *et al.* (2002) Pituitary effects of steroid hormones on secretion of follicle-stimulating hormone and luteinizing hormone. *Domest. Anim. Endocrinol.*, **23**, 33–42.

Author: Sophie A. Grundy BVSc, MACVSc, DACVIM (Internal Medicine)

chapter 49

Pheochromocytoma

DEFINITION

- APUDomas are tumors of the cells known as amine precursor uptake and decarboxylation (APUD) cells.
- APUDomas are peptide-secreting cells that synthesize and metabolize biogenic amines; they are located throughout the body (thyroid, adrenal medulla) and the gastrointestinal tract.
- Pheochromocytomas consist of chromaffin cells that originate from neural crest cells within the adrenal medulla or sympathetic ganglia (paragangliomas).

ETIOLOGY/PATHOPHYSIOLOGY

- Clinical signs develop as a result of the space-occupying nature of the tumor and its metastases, or from excessive secretion of catecholamines (e.g., hypertension, tachycardia).
- Signs of hypertension and tachycardia may be constant or paroxysmal.

Incidence/Prevalence

- Uncommon disease in dogs; rare in cats.

SIGNALMENT/HISTORY

Species

- Dogs and rarely cats.

Breed Predilections

- Boxers, miniature poodles, and German Shepherd dogs.

Blackwell's Five-Minute Veterinary Consult Clinical Companion: Small Animal Endocrinology and Reproduction, First Edition. Edited by Deborah S. Greco and Autumn P. Davidson. © 2017 John Wiley & Sons, Inc.
Published 2017 by John Wiley & Sons, Inc.
Companion Website: www.fiveminutevet.com/endocrinology

Mean Age and Range

- Median age in dogs is 11 years; range is 1–16 years.
- Older cats.

 CLINICAL FEATURES

General Comments

- The predominant signs result from alpha-mediated vasoconstriction and beta-mediated cardiac effects that cause systemic hypertension or tachyarrhythmias.
- Signs of hypertension may be constant or paroxysmal. Signs may be present for more than a year, or develop suddenly resulting in death.
- Some 30% of cases are asymptomatic and only identified at necropsy.

Historic Findings

- Clinical signs are often episodic or acute.
- Generalized weakness and lethargy are common.
- Anorexia.
- Vomiting.
- Weight loss.
- Panting, dyspnea.
- Diarrhea.
- Whining, pacing.
- Ascites, edema.
- PU/PD.
- Shakes/shivers.
- Epistaxis.
- Adypsia.

Physical Examination Findings

- May be normal.
- Lethargy, depression.
- Tachypnea, dyspnea.
- Thin, emaciated.
- Weakness.
- Peripheral edema.
- Ascites.
- Cardiac arrhythmias.
- Systolic murmur.
- Rales.

- Pale or hyperemic mucous membranes.
- Abdominal mass.
- Dehydration.
- Blindness.
- Abdominal pain.

 # DIFFERENTIAL DIAGNOSIS

- Hyperadrenocorticism.
- Hyperaldosteronism.
- Essential hypertension (cats).
- Renal disease with secondary hypertension.

 # DIAGNOSTICS

CBC/Biochemistry/Urinalysis

- Non-regenerative anemia.
- Hemoconcentration.
- Leukocytosis.
- Mild hyperglycemia.
- Mild uremia.
- Increased liver enzymes.
- Hypoalbuminemia.
- Hypocalcemia.
- Proteinuria.

Other Laboratory Tests

- Arterial blood pressure – systolic >180 mmHg or diastolic >95 mmHg is diagnostic for hypertension. Only 50% of animals with pheochromocytoma are hypertensive when blood pressure is measured because of the episodic nature of secretion of some tumors.
- Electrocardiography – sinus tachycardia is the most common arrhythmia; ventricular premature contractions less common.

Imaging

Abdominal Radiography

- Abdominal mass (30%).
- Calcification of the adrenal mass (10%).
- Hepatomegaly.
- Renal displacement.
- Abnormal renal contour.

- Ascites.
- Enlargement of the caudal venal cava.

Thoracic Radiography
- Generalized cardiomegaly.
- Pulmonary congestion or edema.

Abdominal Ultrasonography
- Unilateral adrenal mass.
- Tumor invasion of the caudal vena cava and other adjacent structures.
- Intra-abdominal and liver metastasis.

Other Imaging Modalities

- CT scan and MRI.
- Scintigraphy using iodine-123 – metaiodobenzylguanidine scan.

Diagnostic Procedures

- Plasma catecholamines
  - >2000 pg/ml supports diagnosis or pheochromocytoma.
- Urinary catecholamine and catecholamine metabolites:
  - Total excretion over 24 hours is required.
  - No vanilla ingestion, drugs, or radiographic contrast agents prior to obtaining the urine sample.
  - 10–15% false positives.
  - Urine must be acidified (pH <3).
  - Low sensitivity as a test for pheochromocytoma (0.42) compared with plasma catecholamines (0.97).
  - VMA – normal <7.0 µg/day.
  - Metanephrine/nor-metenephrine – normal <1.3 µg/day.
  - Total urinary catecholamines – normal <250 µg/day.
- Inhibin – Not recommended as yet. Levels similar to those in neutered dogs, normals not established in dogs.
- Phentolamine test:
  - Used in hypertensive patients to evaluate the dependence of catecholamines on maintaining hypertension.
  - After a stable arterial blood pressure is obtained, an IV bolus of phentolamine (0.5–1.5 mg) is given.
  - Blood pressure is recorded every 30 seconds for the first 3 minutes, and every minute thereafter for an additional 7 minutes.

- Test is positive if the fall in blood pressure is greater than 35 mmHg systolic or 25 mmHg diastolic, and the decline lasts at least 5 minutes.
- High incidence of false-positives and hypotension.
■ Provocative tests:
  - Histamine, tyramine, glucagon may cause hypertensive crisis.

Pathologic Findings

■ Immunohistochemical staining of tumor tissues with chromogranin A or synaptophysin allows differentiation of pheochromocytomas from other tumor types.

 # THERAPEUTICS

Appropriate Health Care

■ Surgical removal of the tumor is the treatment of choice.
■ Medical therapy is most commonly used to stabilize patients prior to surgery.

Client Education

■ Survival times may be as long as 3 years following successful resection of tumor. In cats, removal of tumor is often curative; these are often benign as opposed to the malignant tumors seen in dogs.

Surgical Considerations

Preoperative Care
■ Phenoxybenzamine (0.2–1.5 mg/kg PO, q. 12 h) 1–2 weeks prior to surgery.
■ Atenolol, a β_1-selective antagonist (0.2–1.0 mg/kg PO, q. 12–24 h), can be used to control clinically significant supraventricular tachycardia.

Complications and Patient Monitoring
■ Common complications – hypertension, severe tachycardia, other cardiac arrhythmias, and hypovolemia/hypotension.

Anesthesia
■ Induce anesthesia with a narcotic agent or propofol.
■ Maintain anesthesia with isoflurane.

Surgery
■ Unilateral adrenalectomy and often thrombectomy. Manipulation of the tumor may cause severe hypertension if patient is not properly premedicated.

Medications

Drug(s) of Choice

- Preoperative and intraoperative hypertension can be treated with phentolamine (0.02–0.1 mg/kg IV to effect).
- Cardiac arrhythmias and severe tachycardia – common problems; usually respond to β-blocking agents such as esmolol (0.5 mg/kg slow IV bolus, followed by 0.05–0.2 mg/kg/minute IV infusion).

Contraindications

- Anesthetic agents – morphine, meperidine, xylazine, and ketamine.
- Severe hypertension can develop if a non-selective β-blocker (e.g., propranolol) is used without prior alpha-adrenergic blockade (e.g., phentolamine, phenoxybenzamine).

Precautions

- Non-selective beta-blockade can lead to fatal hypertension.

Alternative drug(s)

- Not available.

Patient Monitoring

- Blood pressure, central venous pressure, and ECG are closely monitored in the immediate postoperative period (24–72 hours).

Possible Complications

- Postoperative – intra-abdominal hemorrhage, hypotension, peritonitis, sepsis.

Expected Course and Prognosis

- Prognosis is guarded to fair.

 COMMENTS

Associated Conditions

- Multiple endocrine neoplasia Types II and III.

See Also

Hypertension, Systemic

Abbreviations

APUD = amine precursor uptake and decarboxylation
CT   = computed tomography
ECG   = electrocardiogram
MRI   = magnetic resonance imaging
PU/PD = polyuria/polydipsia
VMA   = vanillylmandelic acid

Suggested Reading

Greco, D.S. (2001) APUDomas and other emerging feline endocrinopathies, in *Consultations in Feline Internal Medicine IV* (ed. J.R. August), Saunders, Philadelphia, pp. 181–185.

Kyles, A.E., Feldman, E.C., De, Cock, H.E.V., *et al.* (2003) Surgical management of adrenal gland tumors with and without associated tumor thrombi in dogs: 40 cases (1994–2001). *J. Am. Vet. Med. Assoc.*, **223**, 654–662.

Author: Deborah S. Greco DVM, PhD, DACVIM

Post-Partum Metritis/ Subinvolution of Placental Sites (SIPS)

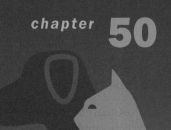

chapter 50

DEFINITION

- Both conditions present in the post-partum period with a complaint of vulvar discharge. In the case of post-partum metritis this discharge can be bloody or sanguino-purulent, and is often malodorous. In SIPS the discharge is sanguinous or serosanguinous.
- Post-partum metritis is a bacterial uterine infection that develops in the immediate (3–7 days) post-partum period in the bitch or queen.
- SIPS is the delay or failure of normal post-partum uterine involution that normally requires 12–15 weeks to complete, and occurs only in bitches.

ETIOLOGY/PATHOPHYSIOLOGY

- Post-partum metritis is inflammation of the endometrium and myometrium, usually due to an ascending bacterial invasion through the open cervix; the large, flaccid post-partum uterus is particularly susceptible to bacterial growth. Hematogenous spread from mastitis is another route of infection. Most commonly, a Gram-negative organism (*Escherichia coli*) is found. Conditions that increase the risk of post-partum metritis include dystocia, prolonged labor, obstetric manipulation, and retained placentas or fetuses.
- Post-partum metritis often presents as systemic illness and can lead to sepsis.
- SIPS is due to the failure of fetal trophoblastic or maternal decidual cells to regress (usually occurs by 2 weeks post-partum), rather invading the maternal endometrium and myometrium, causing vascular damage.
- SIPS, in most cases, is a self-limiting illness, but in rare cases can result in blood loss that is significant enough to cause serious anemia necessitating ovariohysterectomy.

Systems Affected

Cardiovascular

- Post-partum metritis, when severe, can cause dehydration and hypovolemic shock, as well as endotoxic shock from septicemia.

Blackwell's Five-Minute Veterinary Consult Clinical Companion: Small Animal Endocrinology and Reproduction, First Edition. Edited by Deborah S. Greco and Autumn P. Davidson. © 2017 John Wiley & Sons, Inc. Published 2017 by John Wiley & Sons, Inc. Companion Website: www.fiveminutevet.com/endocrinology

Gastrointestinal

- Post-partum metritis often causes anorexia and may, if infection is severe, result in diarrhea secondary to endotoxemia.

Hemic/Lymphatic/immune

- Post-partum metritis usually results in a CBC with a leukocytosis with left shift, although leukopenia occurs in severely ill bitches and queens.
- In rare cases of SIPS blood loss may be significant enough to require transfusion or ovariohysterectomy.

Reproductive

- Post-partum metritis, if severe, may cause enough uterine damage that future reproductive success is compromised. Milk production and mothering of offspring may be compromised enough to require foster dam or supplementation/hand-raising of pups or kittens.
- In a few cases of SIPS metritis may occur as a secondary problem.

 ## SIGNALMENT/HISTORY

- SIPS has been reported variously to occur most commonly in bitches aged <3 years, and in bitches with an average age of 4.5 years. SIPS is not reported in queens.
- Post-partum metritis is not reported to have a breed or age predilection. However, as it is associated with dystocia, obstetrical manipulation and large litters, breeds more commonly afflicted with these conditions are at increased risk.

Risk Factors

- Post-partum metritis in the bitch and queen is associated with parturient conditions, including large litter, poor environmental hygiene, prolonged labor, dystocia, obstetrical manipulation, uterine trauma, devitalization of uterus, and retained fetuses or placentas.
- SIPS is more frequent in primiparous bitches, although it can also occur in later litters.

Historic Findings

- In post-partum metritis, owners often report anorexia, lethargy, poor mothering, and a malodorous red-brown vulvar discharge.
- With SIPS, owners typically report dam and pups doing well, but that a variable amount of bloody, non-odorous vulvar discharge persists beyond 6–12 weeks post-partum.

CLINICAL FEATURES

- With post-partum metritis, the bitch or queen is often systemically ill, febrile, and dehydrated. Vulvar discharge is present in variable amounts, usually fetid and often reddish-brown. Self-grooming by the patient may make discharge difficult to see externally. Palpation of the abdomen may reveal an enlarged uterus.
- Bitches with SIPS present as normal apart from the bloody vulvar discharge. Abdominal palpation may reveal discrete uterine swellings of different sizes.

 DIFFERENTIAL DIAGNOSIS

- Post-partum metritis and SIPS are differentiated from each other by way of clinical presentation, presence or absence of systemic signs, and cytology of the vulvovaginal discharge.
- Other causes of anorexia and poor mothering in the post-parturient period include hypocalcemia and mastitis, and can be differentiated from post-partum metritis by physical examination, vaginal cytology, and serum calcium concentration. Any or all of these peri-parturient disorders may exist in combination.
- Additional differential diagnoses for the hemorrhagic vaginal discharge of SIPS include vaginitis, vaginal foreign body, vaginal mass, cystitis, trauma, and coagulopathy. Urinalysis, vaginal cytology, coagulogram, and in some cases vaginoscopy, can be used to differentiate these conditions if the patient is in the post-parturient risk period for SIPS.
- A final differential diagnosis for SIPS is vulvar discharge associated with estrogen stimulation, either endogenous from a shortened interestrous interval, exposure to topical hormone-containing products on human skin, or less commonly to adrenal production of excessive estrogen. Vaginal cytology taken from the horizontal vaginal vault will diagnose estrogen presence.

 DIAGNOSTICS

- Cytology of discharge ideally obtained from the horizontal vaginal vault is key to diagnosing both post-partum metritis and SIPS. In post-partum metritis, cytology reveals increased PMNs, usually with intracellular and extracellular bacteria. PMNs may be severely degenerated and erythrocytes may be seen. Muscle fibers from retained fetuses can be present. In SIPS, the cytology may reveal trophoblastic-like foamy cells (heavily vacuolated, polynucleated) that are diagnostic. No inflammation is seen on SIPS cytology.
- Anterior guarded vaginal culture or transcervical uterine culture for identification of organism and antibiotic choice for post-partum metritis.
- Radiography may show an enlarged uterus with post-partum metritis, but is not sufficient for evaluating fluid in the uterine lumen.

■ Ultrasound examination of the uterus for a diagnosis of both conditions. In post-partum metritis increased fluid is seen in the uterine lumen, the uterine walls may be thickened and hyperechoic with a corrugated appearance, and a retained fetus or placenta may be seen (Fig. 50.1). With SIPS, focal uterine wall thickening can be seen (Fig. 50.2).

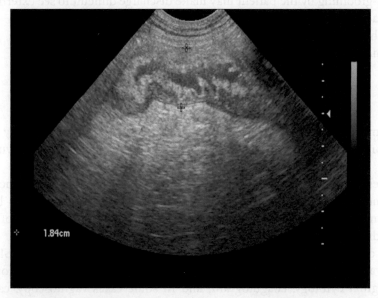

■ **Fig. 50.1.** Ultrasonographic image of post-partum metritis. Sagittal uterine horn (cursors) with corrugated endometrium and increased fluid in the lumen. Image courtesy of T.W. Baker.

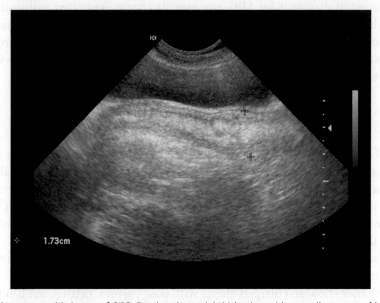

■ **Fig. 50.2.** Ultrasonographic image of SIPS. Focal endometrial thickening with a small amount of hypoechoic fluid at a placental site (cursors). Image courtesy of T.W. Baker.

Pathologic Findings

- Grossly, post-partum metritis shows a thickened uterus with bloody purulent fluid in the lumen. Histopathology reveals invasion of the endometrium and myometrium by poly-morphonuclear white blood cells and bacteria.
- Grossly, SIPS shows some blood in the uterine lumen and raw, bleeding, localized spheroid enlargement focally in the uterine wall. Histologically, these are syncytial masses of cells with foamy, eosinophilic cytoplasm invading the endometrium and myometrium.

 # THERAPEUTICS

- Treatment objectives for post-partum metritis are to treat and resolve dehydration, shock and sepsis, resolve the uterine infection, remove any retained fetal and placental tissue, and in cases where important, preserve reproductive function. Treatment objectives for SIPS are to rule out more serious problems and monitor for the rare instance of serious hemorrhage.

Drug Treatment of Post-Partum Metritis

- Intravenous balanced electrolyte solution as indicated by degree of shock or dehydration.
- Broad-spectrum antibiotics such as cephalosporins, amoxicillin-clavulanic acid (dogs, 12.5–25 mg/kg PO, q. 12 h; cats, 62.5 mg/kg PO, q. 12 h). Can administer q. 8 h with Gram-negative infections, or oxacllin (22–40 mg/kg PO, q. 8 h) to start pending culture and sensitivity results. Injectable antibiotics can be given if patient is in a critical condition. Antibiotic choices are limited if neonates are nursing, as all are secreted into the milk.
- For evacuation of uterus if <48 hours since parturition, oxytocin 0.5–1.0 IU IM, to be repeated q. 1–2 h as needed. If >48 hours or inadequate response to oxytocin for uterine evacuation, $PGF_{2\alpha}$ 100 μg/kg SC, q. 12 h or cloprostenol 1–3 μg/kg, SQ q. 12–24 h for 3 to 7 days until ultrasound reveals an absence of fluid in the uterine lumen. Evaluation of the uterus for healthy uterine wall prior to $PGF_{2\alpha}$ administration is recommended to prevent uterine rupture in cases of thin or damaged wall.

Drug Treatment of SIPS

- For SIPS, no treatment is required (or is effective) except in the rare instance of hemorrhage requiring transfusion or ovariohysterectomy.

Procedures

- If post-partum metritis is secondary to retained fetus or placenta, surgery is necessary to remove those materials.
- In patients where further breeding is not desired and the condition of the patient allows it, ovariohysterectomy can be performed.
- Flushing of uterus through the vaginal vault is not recommended. Surgical flushing of the uterus has been successful in some cases, but caution is recommended as damage to the uterus affecting future fertility is possible, as is uterine rupture and peritonitis if devitalized tissue is present.

▪ In rare cases of SIPS that have excessive hemorrhage requiring transfusion, ovariohysterectomy can be performed after stabilization of the patient.

 COMMENTS

▪ In cases of post-partum metritis where future reproductive success is desired, the earlier the treatment is initiated the better the long-term outcome will be.

Expected Course and Prognosis

▪ Post-partum metritis, when recognized and treated in a timely manner, typically has a good outcome. If fetal or placental retention is present, surgical management of those issues early on results in better outcome. Delayed recognition and treatment may affect future reproductive success. Delayed treatment may also result in chronic foci of infection in the uterus that may reactivate with the following diestrus.
  • Medical treatment can usually be managed on an outpatient basis permitting nursing of neonates at home.
▪ SIPS usually results in spontaneous resolution by the following estrus cycle. In rare cases, excessive hemorrhage necessitates ovariohysterectomy resulting in complete resolution. Recurrence is not typical.

Abbreviations

SIPS   = subinvolution of placental sites
$PGF_{2\alpha}$ = prostaglandin $F_{2\alpha}$

See Also

Eclampsia
Mammary Gland Disorders: Agalactia, Galactostasis, Mastitis
Caesarean Section Elective and Emergency

Suggested Reading

Feldman, E.C., Nelson, R.W. (2004) Periparturient diseases, in *Canine and Feline Endocrinology and Reproduction*, 3rd edition. WB Saunders, Philadelphia, pp. 808–834.
Grundy, S.A., Davidson, A.P. (2004) Theriogenology question of the month. Acute metritis secondary to retained fetal membranes and a retained nonviable fetus. *J. Am. Vet. Med. Assoc.*, **224** (6), 844–847.
Johnston, S.D., Root Kustritz. M.V., Olson, P.N.S. (2001) Periparturient Disorders in the Bitch, in *Canine and Feline Theriogenology*. WB Saunders, Philadelphia, pp. 129–145.
McEntee, K. (1990) Postpartum lesions. The Uterus: Degenerative and Inflammatory Lesions, in *Reproductive Pathology of Domestic Mammals*. Academic Press, Inc., San Diego, pp. 157–158.
Sontas, H.B., Stelletta, C., Milani, C., et al. (2011) Full recovery of subinvolution of placental sites in an American Staffordshire terrier bitch. *J. Small Anim. Pract.*, **52** (1), 42–45.

Author: Joni L. Freshman DVM, DACVIM (Internal Medicine)

Pregnancy Diabetes

DEFINITION

- Pregnancy diabetes (or gestational diabetes) is type II diabetes that develops during pregnancy (usually the second half), and is induced by elevated levels of progesterone associated with diestrus.
- The condition is more common in the bitch than the queen.
- Treatment with insulin or termination of the pregnancy is usually indicated.
- Diabetes is often temporary and will usually resolve in the days to weeks following the end of the pregnancy, however it may be permanent.
- Intrauterine fetal death and puppy/kitten mortality are increased.

ETIOLOGY/PATHOPHYSIOLOGY

- Increased levels of progesterone that occur during pregnancy or non-pregnant diestrus stimulate growth hormone secretion, and in some individuals, may lead to downregulation of insulin receptors and insulin resistance.
- Pregnant bitches/queens have a decreased ability to produce glucose, and therefore blood glucose levels are not always elevated.

SIGNALMENT/HISTORY

- Most commonly seen in middle-aged to older bitches/queens that are pregnant or have recently been in estrus (and bred if queens).
- The Nordic Spitz breed maybe over-represented.
- Obesity can predispose.

CLINICAL FEATURES

- Classic signs of diabetes mellitus including polyuria and polydipsia are often seen. Polyphagia and weight loss may also be seen.

Blackwell's Five-Minute Veterinary Consult Clinical Companion: Small Animal Endocrinology and Reproduction, First Edition. Edited by Deborah S. Greco and Autumn P. Davidson. © 2017 John Wiley & Sons, Inc. Published 2017 by John Wiley & Sons, Inc.
Companion Website: www.fiveminutevet.com/endocrinology

- Rarely, transient acromegaly (due to excessive growth hormone secretion) may develop in the bitch leading to edema of the head, throat, and legs. Voice change may also be observed due to edema of the larynx.

DIFFERENTIAL DIAGNOSIS

- Myxedema (hypothyroid).
- Pyometra (PU PD).

DIAGNOSTICS

- Diagnosis is generally made based on an elevated blood glucose concentration in the bitch, along with concurrent glucosuria.
- Diagnosis can also be based on an elevated blood insulin level in the presence of a normal blood glucose concentration.
- IGF-1 usually normal.

THERAPEUTICS

- Treatment with insulin therapy should be initiated as soon as possible in the hyperglycemic patient.
- Non-ketotic bitches can be started on neutral protamine Hagedorn (NPH) insulin at a starting dosage of 0.25–0.5 U/kg administered SC twice daily. Non-ketotic queens can be started on Glargine insulin at a starting dose of 1 U/dog, once or twice daily.
- Patients suffering from diabetic ketoacidosis should be started on regular insulin either administered as CRI or as intermittent IM or SC injection at a starting dosage of 0.1–0.2 U/kg.
- Patients should be maintained on a high-quality, high-protein diet.
- Precise blood glucose control is often not possible during pregnancy due to progesterone elevation in diestrus/pregnancy (anti-insulin effect).
- The development of acromegaly in the bitch is often life-threatening and requires termination of the pregnancy.

Surgical Considerations

- Ovariohysterectomy is recommended to avoid recurrence during diestrus of the next estrous cycle.
- Medical abortion can be performed if the bitch/queen is not stable enough for anesthesia and surgery.
- Ovariectomy or ovariohysterectomy should be performed before the next estrous cycle as the condition will likely recur even in non-pregnant diestrus.

COMMENTS

Possible Complications

■ The pregnant diabetic bitch/queen is prone to aborting her litter as a result of the effects of chronic hyperglycemia.

■ Fetal oversize resulting in dystocia can occur secondary to chronic hyperglycemia.

Expected Course and Prognosis

■ A guarded to poor prognosis is expected for the fetuses.

■ The fetuses may be undernourished, but they may also become excessively large (due to the effects of hyperglycemia), with a poor survival rate.

■ Transient neonatal hypoglycemia secondary to chronic hyperinsulinemia can be a complication in the immediate post-partum period.

■ Insulin resistance can persist during lactation due to growth hormone elevation.

See Also

Cesarean Section: Elective and Emergency
Medical Pregnancy Termination in the Bitch and Queen

Suggested Reading

Fall, T., *et al.* (2008) Gestational diabetes mellitus in 13 dogs. *J. Vet. Intern. Med.*, **22**, 296–300.

Feldman, E., Nelson, R. (2004) *Canine and Feline Endocrinology and Reproduction*. Saunders, St Louis.

Forseberg, C. (2010) Abnormalities in canine pregnancy, parturition, and periparturent period, in *Small Animal Internal Medicine*, 7th edition, Vol. 2 (eds. S.J. Ettinger, E.C. Feldman), Elsevier, St Louis, pp. 1890–1901.

Johnston, S., *et al.* (2001) *Canine and Feline Theriogenology*. Saunders, Philadelphia.

Root Kustritz, M. (2005) Pregnancy diagnosis and abnormalities of pregnancy in the dog. *Theriogenology*, **64**, 755–765.

Author: E. Freya Kruger DVM, DACVIM (Internal Medicine)

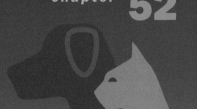

chapter 52

Pregnancy Edema in the Bitch

DEFINITION

- Edema associated with pregnancy ranges from pitting edema of the distal pelvic limbs, the ventral abdomen, mammary glands and perineal subcutaneous tissues to an increase in intrauterine amniotic/allantoic fluid accumulation.
- Abnormal fluid accumulation in the fetus/neonate, hydrops fetalis, is a separate disorder, and not a comorbidity.
- Edema in canine pregnancy has been referred to as *hydrops* by breeders; there is no evidence that the condition is comparable to hydrops in humans. The pathophysiology of the pregnancy edema syndrome in the dog has not yet been established. Hydrops allantois and hydrops amnii have been reported in mares and cows.

ETIOLOGY/PATHOPHYSIOLOGY

- Possible causes of edema include venous/lymphatic compression from an enlarged, gravid uterus; cardiogenic disease; hypoalbuminemia; vasculitis; protein-losing nephropathy; hepatopathy; or electrolyte abnormalities.
- In humans, pregnancy edema can be normal (80%), or can be associated with pre-eclampsia, pregnancy toxemia, and eclampsia (proteinuric hypertension); a placental trigger is suspected (immunologic).
- During normal pregnancy, total body water increases both extracellularly and interstitially. There is also a cumulative retention of sodium distributed between the maternal extracellular compartments and the fetus. Changes in factors governing renal sodium and water handling accompany alterations in local Starling forces, whereby there is a moderate fall in interstitial fluid colloid osmotic pressure and a rise in capillary hydrostatic pressure, as well as changes in hydration of connective tissue ground substance.

Systems Affected

- Cardiovascular.
- Endocrine/Metabolic.

Blackwell's Five-Minute Veterinary Consult Clinical Companion: Small Animal Endocrinology and Reproduction, First Edition. Edited by Deborah S. Greco and Autumn P. Davidson. © 2017 John Wiley & Sons, Inc. Published 2017 by John Wiley & Sons, Inc. Companion Website: www.fiveminutevet.com/endocrinology

- Hemic/Lymphatic/Immune.
- Hepatobiliary.
- Musculoskeletal.
- Renal/Urologic.
- Reproductive.

 SIGNALMENT/HISTORY

- Pregnancy edema occurs most commonly in bitches with very large litters, mid to late gestation. Many breeds have been affected, most commonly reported are Golden Retrievers, Labrador Retrievers, Pugs, French bulldogs, Dobermans, Bulldogs, and Bullmastiffs.

Risk Factors

- Large litter (10–12+).

Historic Findings

- Swelling/pitting edema of paws, mammary glands, perineum, vulva noted by owner.
- Abdominomegaly.
- Marked and sudden weight gain.
  - Variable anorexia, nausea and lethargy.
  - Occurs variably with previous/subsequent pregnancies.

 CLINICAL FEATURES

- Pitting edema of pelvic limbs, perineum, vulva, ventrum.
- Marked abdominomegaly.
- ± Systemic hypertension.
- ± Increased allantoic/amniotic fluid.
- ± Ascites.
- Thin/stretched uterine wall.
- Poor labor/dystocia.
- Elective cesarean section common.
- Hemorrhagic gastroenterocolitis.
- Fetal/dam morbidity and mortality.

 DIFFERENTIAL DIAGNOSIS

- Uteromegaly: closed pyometra.
- Abdominomegaly: hepatomegaly, ascites, uroabdomen, hemoabdomen, ruptured uterus.
- Hypertension: primary, secondary.

DIAGNOSTICS

- Complete blood count and serum chemistries/electrolytes including magnesium, urinalysis, urine protein creatinine ratio if proteinuric.
- Consider urine electrolyte evaluation if electrolyte abnormalities exist.
- Abdominal ultrasound with particular attention to fetal viability, and intra-abdominal intrauterine, placental, allantoic and amniotic fluid volumes.
- Echocardiography with Doppler for evaluation of cardiac disorders.
- Blood pressure measurement, serial if hypertensive.
- DNA sampling in confirmed cases for future genetic evaluation.
- Tocodynamometry to assess myometrial activity/irritability.
- Fetal HR determination with Doppler to determine fetal well-being.

Pathological Findings

- Poorly characterized; collection of deceased fetuses, placentae encouraged for histopathologic evaluation.
- Consider uterine/placental biopsy during cesarean section.
- Complete necropsy with histopathology desirable in the event of maternal death to elucidate the cause.

THERAPEUTICS

- Address life-threatening conditions (malignant hypertension, seizure/thrombosis, hypomagnesemia) first.

Drug(s) of Choice

- Hypertension
    - Hydralazine 0.5–2 mg/kg PO q. 12 h, titrate up to effect; or 0.2 mg/kg IV or IM, repeat q. 2 h as needed. Monitor for hypotension, hospitalize until normotensive. Hydralazine is the drug of choice for treatment of acute hypertension of pregnancy in humans. Pregnancy category C drug (benefit should justify potential risk, studies N/A).
- Seizure/stroke/hypomagnesemia
    - Magnesium sulfate 0.5–1 mEq/day CRI in 5% dextrose, reduce 50% in azotemia.
- Secondary conditions (edema, nausea).
    - Drug(s) considerations
        □ Edema: Treatment of edematous conditions in pregnancy in the bitch is controversial and without evidence-based data. In human medicine, diuretics are *not* advised to treat physiologic edema of pregnancy and do not prevent pre-eclampsia.
        □ Anecdotal use of the aldosterone antagonist spironolactone 1–2 mg/kg PO, q. 12 h ± loop diuretic furosemide 2–4 mg/kg PO, q. 12 h has occurred in veterinary practice.

    ☐ Spironolactone is a pregnancy category D drug (positive evidence of fetal risk, benefits must outweigh risk). There are no adequate reports or well-controlled studies in human fetuses. Spironolactone is an antiandrogen and can feminize male rats.

    ☐ Furosemide can cause a significant decrease in placental intervillous blood flow. Diuretics are contraindicated with contracted intravascular volume. Caution must be exercised if diuretic therapy is implemented.

- Nausea/anorexia
  - Metoclopramide 0.1–0.2 mg/kg SC or PO, q. 12 h.

Precautions/Interactions

- The use of diuretics can exacerbate hypertension by promoting dehydration, and at this time, use of diuretics cannot be routinely recommended unless studies demonstrate benefit to the dam/fetuses (beyond anecdotal reports).
- In humans, the role of diuretics in obstetric practice is restricted to the management of pulmonary edema in pre-eclampsia. Volume expansion therapy in pregnancy runs the risk of pulmonary or cerebral edema, particularly in the immediate puerperium. Vulval edema and erythematous edema associated with deep-venous thrombosis are rare but dangerous complications of pregnancy.
- Any drug used is likely to cross the placenta, fetal effects should be considered, and informed consent acquired.

Appropriate Health Care

- Pregnancy termination can be indicated if life-threatening hypertension, thrombosis, or coagulopathy exists unresponsive to medical therapy.

Nursing Care

- Mild distal limb edema can benefit from mild walking, hydrotherapy or massage. Elevating the limbs and avoiding further compression of the caudal abdominal veins/lymphatics can help disseminate edema.

Diet

- Mild sodium restriction if signs of congestive heart failure are present.
- Appropriate dietary protein if hypoalbuminemia or significant proteinuria present.

Surgical Considerations

- Elective cesarean section at term, or pregnancy termination via ovariohysterectomy.
- Use caution when prepping for cesarean section: do not place dam in complete dorsal recumbency until time of laparotomy incision, but rotate approximately 30°, tilting to one

side during surgical preparation. The goal is to decrease direct pressure on the abdominal vena cava and promote cardiac pre-load. Monitor and manage hypertension, hypotension, and hypovolemia.

- Medical pregnancy termination not advised due to the fragile condition of these bitches.

 ## COMMENTS

Client Education

- Consider genetic evaluation of affected dogs and their mates/parents.

Patient Monitoring

- Blood pressure evaluation until normotension maintained.
- Continued evaluation of fetal viability.

Prevention/Avoidance

- Consider pedigree evaluation. If an increased incidence occurs in related bitches, removal from a breeding program should be strongly considered.

Possible Complications

- Fetal and maternal mortality.

Expected Course and Prognosis

- Fair to guarded prognosis.

Synonyms

- None, as the syndrome is not well defined. Hydrops (allantois, amnion) has been suggested but not documented to be the equivalent disease in humans and dogs.

See Also

Pregnancy Toxemia
Pregnancy Ketosis
Cesarean Section: Elective and Emergency
Dystocia

Suggested Reading

Weiner, C.P., Buhimschi, C. (2004) *Drugs for Pregnant and Lactating Women*. Churchill Livingston, Philadelphia, PA.

Root Kustritz, M. (2005) Pregnancy diagnosis and abnormalities in the pregnant dog. *Theriogenology*, **64**, 755–765.

Davison, J.M. (1997) Edema in pregnancy. *Kidney Int. Suppl.*, **59**, 90–96.

Zamorski, M.A., Green, L.A. (2001) NHBPEP report on high blood pressure in pregnancy: a summary for family physicians. *Am. Fam. Phys.*, **64** (2), 263–270.

Davidson, A.P. (2001) Uterine and fetal monitoring in the bitch. *Vet. Clin. North Am. Small Anim. Pract.*, **31** (2), 305–313.

Davidson, A.P. (2013) Clinical Conditions in the Bitch and Queen, in *Small Animal Internal Medicine*, 5th edition (ed. R. Nelson), Elsevier, p. 927.

Davidson, A.P. (2012) Clinical Approach to Abnormal Pregnancy, in *BSAVA Manual of Canine and Feline Reproduction and Neonatology*, 2nd edition (ed. G. England), BSAVA, pp. 115–120.

Authors: Autumn P. Davidson DVM, MS, DACVIM (Internal Medicine), Janice Cain DVM, DACVIM (Internal Medicine), Melissa Goodman DVM

chapter 53

Pregnancy Ketosis

DEFINITION

- Pregnancy ketosis is a metabolic disorder that occurs in late-stage gestation in which a lack of carbohydrates leads to increased lipid metabolism and ketosis.
- Occurs most commonly in bitches carrying large litters that have become anorectic or are malnourished.

ETIOLOGY/PATHOPHYSIOLOGY

- During late gestation, a sudden increase in energy demands due to rapid fetal growth and milk production leads to a depletion of carbohydrates that are used to produce glucose.
- Pregnant bitches have a decreased ability to produce glucose via gluconeogenesis, glycogenolysis, and lipolysis, and also have a blunted hormonal response to hypoglycemia.
- Bitches with a relative carbohydrate deficiency will increase lipid metabolism in an attempt to meet energy demands.
- Acidic ketone bodies are formed as a byproduct of lipid metabolism.

Systems Affected

- Rapid fat mobilization will often overwhelm the liver's capacity for lipid metabolism and lead to hepatic lipidosis and impaired liver function.

SIGNALMENT/HISTORY

- Late gestation bitches on inadequate nutrition or those who cannot eat enough carbohydrates to meet their energy demands.

Risk Factors

- Bitches carrying large numbers of pups are predisposed; smaller breeds more commonly affected (Fig. 53.1).
- Yorkshire Terriers and Labrador Retrievers may be predisposed.

Blackwell's Five-Minute Veterinary Consult Clinical Companion: Small Animal Endocrinology and Reproduction, First Edition. Edited by Deborah S. Greco and Autumn P. Davidson. © 2017 John Wiley & Sons, Inc. Published 2017 by John Wiley & Sons, Inc. Companion Website: www.fiveminutevet.com/endocrinology

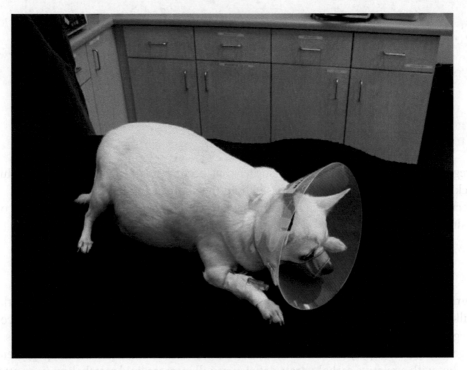

■ **Fig. 53.1.** Small breed bitch with a large litter typical of pregnancy ketosis. This bitch was not fed dog food.

CLINICAL FEATURES

- Anorexia.
- Depression.
- Lethargy.
- Vomiting or diarrhea.
- Sweet-smelling (ketotic) breath.

DIFFERENTIAL DIAGNOSIS

- Pyometra.
- Diabetic ketoacidosis.

DIAGNOSTICS

- Based on the presence of urine ketones in the absence of hyperglycemia or glucosuria.
- Some bitches with pregnancy ketosis may be hypoglycemic.

THERAPEUTICS

- If the condition is recognized early in the course of the disease, supplemental nutrition may be enough. Force-feeding or feeding via an esophageal tube may be necessary in extreme cases.
- If bitches are severely ill, it may be necessary to terminate the pregnancy so that energy demands are reduced and the dam's life is spared.
- Medical abortion can be performed if the bitch is not stable enough for anesthesia and surgery. Ovariectomy or ovariohysterectomy should be performed before the next estrous cycle as the condition will likely recur if pregnancy results and husbandry is not improved.
- Ovariohysterectomy.

Surgical Considerations

- If a bitch with pregnancy toxemia requires surgery for cesarean section or ovariohysterectomy, analgesics and anesthetics need to be chosen cautiously as hepatic lipidosis may lead to impaired hepatic metabolism of drugs.

 ## COMMENTS

- Owners should be advised that pregnancy ketosis is a potentially life-threatening condition for the fetuses and the bitch.
- Repeat testing of urine ketones is helpful in monitoring the effect of treatment.
- Increased consumption of carbohydrates and decreased urine ketones in a bitch whose attitude is good signifies progress in treating pregnancy ketosis.

See Also

Cesarean Section: Elective and Emergency
Medical Pregnancy Termination in the Bitch and Queen

Suggested Reading

Johnson, C. (2008) Glucose homeostasis during pregnancy: insulin resistance, ketosis, and hypoglycemia. *Theriogenology*, 70, 1418–1423.
Johnston, S., *et al.* (2001). *Canine and Feline Theriogenology*. Saunders, Philadelphia.
Root Kustritz, M. (2005) Pregnancy diagnosis and abnormalities in the pregnant dog. *Theriogenology*, 64, 755–765.

Author: E. Freya Kruger DVM, DACVIM (Internal Medicine)

Infectious Causes of Pregnancy Loss, Canine:

Toxoplasmosis/Neosporosis, Cryptosporidium, Herpes Virus, Brucellosis, Minute Virus

TOXOPLASMOSIS/NEOSPOROSIS

DEFINITION

- Obligate intracellular coccidian parasite that infects mammals, including humans.
- Synonym: *Toxoplasma gondii*, *Neospora caninum*.

ETIOLOGY/PATHOPHYSIOLOGY

- Clinical disease depends on location and numbers of cysts present.
- Pathogenesis of signs associated with rupture of the host cells as a result of the rapid proliferation of tachyzoites, which then invade other cells.
- Necrosis of the cells and vasculitis result from immune-mediated reactions to the organism.
- Signs depend on the site and extent of organ damage.
- *T. gondii* exists in three infectious stages: sporozoites; tachyzoites; and bradyzoites.
- Transmission can occur through ingestion of infected tissues or ingestion of oocysts in contaminated food or water. Transmission can also occur congenitally, through sexual transmission and *in utero*, transplacentally, if the dam is acutely infected during pregnancy.
- The enteroepithelial life cycle (and thus fecal shedding) only occurs in cats.
- The extraintestinal life cycle occurs in all hosts.
  - After ingestion of the oocysts or tissue cysts, the organism invades the small intestine and spreads to many extraintestinal tissues through blood and lymph, where it causes a focal necrosis. The CNS, muscle, liver, lungs and eyes are commonly affected.
  - The organism localizes in tissues as cysts, resulting in chronic infection. These cysts may rupture, resulting in clinical relapses during immunosuppression.
- Dogs are both intermediate and definitive hosts
- Dogs that ingest cat feces, may act as transport vectors for sporulated oocysts, as they will shed these sporulated oocysts in their feces for 2 days after ingesting them.

Blackwell's Five-Minute Veterinary Consult Clinical Companion: Small Animal Endocrinology and Reproduction, First Edition. Edited by Deborah S. Greco and Autumn P. Davidson. © 2017 John Wiley & Sons, Inc. Published 2017 by John Wiley & Sons, Inc.
Companion Website: www.fiveminutevet.com/endocrinology

- The life cycle of *N. caninum* involves three infectious stages: tachyzoites; tissue cysts (found primarily in the CNS); and oocysts.
  - Tissue cysts and tachyzoites are found intermediate hosts.
  - Transmission suspected to occur through ingestion of shed oocysts, ingestion of infected tissues, and transplacentally.
  - Transplacental transmission may be the predominant route in dogs. A suspect chronic infected bitch will develop parasitemia during gestation, which spreads transplacentally to the fetuses. Successive litters from the same subclinically infected dam may be born infected, although perhaps at a reduced rate. A variable number of puppies – but not all – in a litter have clinical manifestations. Other pups may carry the infection subclinically with reactivation.

Systems Affected

- Genitourinary.
- Neurologic.

SIGNALMENT/HISTORY

Genetics and Breed Predisposition

- All breeds are equally susceptible to toxoplasmosis. German Short-Haired Pointers, Labrador Retrievers, Boxers, Golden Retrievers, Bassett Hounds, and Greyhounds may be more susceptible to neosporosis.

Risk Factors

- Immunosuppression (e.g., from glucocorticoids or antineoplastic drugs) or concomitant illnesses, such as ehrlichiosis and canine distemper.
- Immunosuppression is not consistently found in cases of neosporosis.

CLINICAL FEATURES

- Toxoplasmosis: anorexia, vomiting, diarrhea, weight loss, lethargy, dyspnea, ocular signs, lameness, signs of CNS dysfunction, and abortion.
- Toxoplasmosis:
  - Clinical signs may be localized in respiratory, neuromuscular, or gastrointestinal (GI) systems, or may be caused by general infection.
  - Older dogs – clinical signs usually associated with neural and muscular systems.
  - In young dogs (aged <1 year) with generalized infection, characterized by fever, tonsillitis, dyspnea, diarrhea, and vomiting. Myocardial involvement usually subclinical, although arrhythmias and heart failure may develop in some dogs.

- Only a few reports of ocular lesions in dogs.
- If an infected litter survives, puppies will usually develop symptoms of neurologic, respiratory, and gastrointestinal abnormalities.
- Neosporosis:
    - Early fetal death, mummification, resorption and birth of weak pups.
    - No reports of abortion in dogs have been produced.

DIFFERENTIAL DIAGNOSIS

- *Brucella canis.*
- Canine herpesvirus.

DIAGNOSTICS

Clinical Pathology

- Non-regenerative anemia, neutrophilic leukocytosis, lymphocytosis, monocytosis, and eosinophilia most commonly observed.
- During acute phase of illness, hypoproteinemia, hypoglobulinemia, increased serum alanine aminotransferase (ALT) and aspartate aminotransferase (AST) and creatinine kinase (CK), have been observed.

Fecal Examination

- Dogs do not shed oocytes.

Cytology

- Tachyzoites may be detected in various tissues and body fluids during acute illness.

Radiology

- Lesions in the CNS may be detected by myelography, computed tomography (CT), or magnetic resonance imaging (MRI).

Serologic Testing

- ELISA or IFA: Serologic evidence of recent or active infection consists of high IgM titers, fourfold or greater, increasing or decreasing, IgG titer (after treatment, recovery or both).
- IgG: A fourfold rise in IgG in paired serum samples taken 2–4 weeks apart, is significant and implies active infection. IgG titer may remain positive for years after exposure.

- IgM: A positive IgM titer indicates active infection. The IgM titer will decrease or disappear as the IgG titer rises. If it remains persistently positive, this may suggest a possible false-positive result, reactivation of tissue cysts, or delay in antibody class shift due to immunosuppression.

Real-Time Polymerase Chain Reaction (RT-PCR)

- Performed on tissue or fluids.

Pathological Findings

- Necrosis is the predominant lesion, particularly the brain, lung, liver, and mesenteric lymph nodes.
- Myositis involving the muscles of the limbs.
- Immunoperoxidase staining or electron microscopy can be used to distinguish *T. gondii* from *N. caninum*.

 # THERAPEUTICS

Drug(s) of Choice

- Clindamycin: 10–20 mg/kg PO, q. 12 h for 4 weeks (*T. gondii*); 15–22 mg/kg PO, q. 12 h for 4–8 weeks (*N. caninum*).
- Pyrimethamine (1 mg/kg PO, q. 24 h for 4 weeks) and rapid-acting sulfonamides (20–30 mg/kg PO, q. 24 h for 4 weeks), such as sulfadiazine, sulfamethazine and triple sulfas, is synergistic. (Both organisms); Treatment of choice for N. caninum with neurologic involvement.
- Trimethoprim-sulfonamide: 15–20 mg/kg PO q 12h × 4–8 weeks (*N. caninum*).
- Adult dogs and puppies older than 16 weeks of age respond better to treatment than puppies less than 16 weeks.

Precautions/Interactions

- Sulfonamides – possible bone marrow suppression; consider folinic acid (5.0 mg/day PO or brewer's yeast 100 mg/kg PO/day).
- Trimethoprim-sulfonamide – monitor for keratoconjunctivitis sicca, polyarthritis in appropriate breeds (e.g. Labrador retriever) and hepatitis.
- Clinidamycin – gastroenteritis.

Alternative Drugs

- Pyrimethamine has also been administered in combination with clindamycin or dapsone. Limited clinical and experimental studies have shown synergy with azithromycin–pyrimethamine, clarithromycin–minocycline, clarithromycin or azithromycin with sulfonamides, and atovaquone with pyrimethamine or sulfonamides.

COMMENTS

Client Education

- The zoonotic potential of *N. caninum* is unknown.
- Humans become infected with *T. gondii* by ingesting viable cysts in raw or undercooked meat or shellfish, or by ingesting oocysts shed in the feces of a recently infected cat. In the United States, at least 50% of acquired infections are associated with the ingestion of meat.
- Transplacental infection of the fetus with *T. gondii* occurs via tachyzoite spread when a pregnant woman is infected for the first time.
- Clinical disease in postnatally infected humans is similar to that in other infected intermediate hosts, such as dogs. Usually asymptomatic and self-limiting, or usually persistent for 1 to 12 weeks.

Patient Monitoring

- Monitor CBC and biochemistries.
- Monitor response to therapy; treat beyond clinical improvement.

Prevention/Avoidance

- Avoid exposure to raw or undercooked meat products.
- On farms, dog should not be allowed to feed on offal or aborted materials.
- *N. caninum* can be transmitted repeatedly through subsequent litters and litters of their progeny. No known therapy to prevent transmission from bitch to fetuses exists.
- No current preventative vaccines.

CANINE CRYPTOSPORIDIUM

 DEFINITION

- Protozoan. *Coccidia*-like parasites.

 ETIOLOGY/PATHOPHYSIOLOGY

- Several distinct species with different degrees of infectivity for animals and humans:
  - *C. canis* – dogs, rarely humans.
  - *C. felis* – cats, rarely humans.
  - *C. hominus* – only in humans.
  - *C. parvum* – as species in ruminants and other hosts that will readily infect humans. This species does not appear to occur in dogs and cats.

- Oocysts infectious upon excretion and extremely environmentally resistant.
- Direct fecal–oral transmission with feces of the infected host, contaminated food or water.
- The oocytes excyst in the digestive tract, and the sporozoites penetrate the microvilli of a variety of epithelial cells. In the small intestine, cryptosporidia develop in the microvillus border and displace it, eventually leading to a loss of mature surface epithelium, thus leading to reduced uptake of fluids, electrolytes, and nutrients from the gut lumen.
- Oocysts are generally shed in the feces 3–6 days after infection.
- Minimum infective dose in dogs unknown.

Systems Affected

- Develop in the microvillus border of epithelial cells in the digestive, respiratory, and genitourinary tracts.

SIGNALMENT/HISTORY

- Infection occurs following ingestion of sporulated oocysts from fecal-contaminated environments, food, articles, or water.

Risk Factors

- Most reported cased of cryptosporidiosis in dogs involves young animals.
- Cases in adult dogs are rare.
- Disease may be more severe, prolonged and sometimes life-threatening in immunocompromised hosts.
- Immunosuppression due to canine distemper may exacerbate infections in dogs.
- Co-infection with other protozoans, such as *Giardia* spp., canine parvovirus and intestinal *Isospora* spp. infection may also aggravate clinical signs.

Historic Findings

- Mild chronic diarrhea.
- Weight loss.

CLINICAL FEATURES

- Most cases are subclinical.
- Chronic or intermittent diarrhea, dehydration and wasting are the primary clinical signs.

DIFFERENTIAL DIAGNOSIS

- Other infectious causes of small or large bowel diarrhea.
- Dietary indiscretion.
- Metabolic causes of diarrhea.

DIAGNOSTICS

- The small size of *Cryptosporidium* oocysts makes them difficult to detect.
- Routine fecal flotation – often overlooked; requires the presence of large numbers of oocytes for detection. Sheather's sugar solution is the best flotation medium.
- Acid-fast staining.
- Direct immunoflourescent antibody (IFA) test. Most *Cryptosporidium* spp., cross-react in commercial IFA-based diagnostic tests used to detect *C. parvum*.
- Fecal Elisa
- PCR-based tests – can differentiate between *C. felis*, *C. canis*, *C. parvum*, and *C. hominis*.

Pathological Findings

- Small (usually distal) intestinal lesions demonstrate loss of microvilli, degeneration of host epithelial cells, and atrophy of villi.

THERAPEUTICS

Drug(s) of Choice

- Few drugs are consistently effective against *Cryptosporidium*; optimal duration of therapy unknown.
- Paromomycin: 150 mg/kg SID for 5 days.
- Tylosin: 10–15 mg/kg TID for 14–21 days (cats).
- Azithromycin: 5–10 mg/kg BID for 5–7 days (dogs).
- Nitazoxanide (NTZ): 100 mg BID for 3–5 days for animals aged 24–47 months; 200 mg BID for 5 days in animals aged 4–11 years. The efficacy of NTZ in dogs is not known. Until recently, only approved for use in humans.

Precautions/Interactions

- Nephrotoxicity; Ototoxicity (paromomycin).
- Gastrointestinal side effects, such as vomiting and diarrhea (NTZ).
- Caution in dogs with hematochezia due to increased absorption.

Nursing Care

- Fluids and supportive care.
- Consider antibiotics if secondary bacterial infection suspected.
- Oral rehydration with solutions containing glutamine.

 COMMENTS

Client Education

- There have been very few reports of people infected with *C. canis* and *C. felis*, and most of these infections occurred in immunocompromised individuals; good hygiene (hand washing) indicated and avoidance of contaminated food or water advised.
- *C. canis* relatively host-specific.
- Further critically controlled studies are needed to determine the importance of dogs as source of *Cryptosporidium* infection in humans.

Patient Monitoring

- Persistent infections often denote an underlying cause, such as canine distemper.

Prevention/Avoidance

- Oocysts immediately infectious when passed and capable of surviving in the environment for extended periods.
- Oocysts are resistant to most disinfectants, including routine chlorine concentrations in drinking water and swimming pools.
- Oocysts are susceptible to commercial formulations of 50% ammonia and heat over 70 °C.
- House dogs indoors and feed processed food.
- Clean dog bowls with water >70 °C.

Expected Course and Prognosis

- In immunocompetent and healthy dogs, the infections are usually self-limiting.

HERPESVIRUS

 DEFINITION

- Viral infection of canids that can present one of four possible clinical scenarios: mild to increased respiratory distress from upper airway infection; abortion; vaginitis; and neonatal puppy mortality up to 3 weeks of age.

ETIOLOGY/PATHOPHYSIOLOGY

- Canine herpesvirus (CHV-1) is a virus of the family Herpesviridae.
- Reported to exist in the United States, Canada, Australia, Japan, England, and Germany.

Systems Affected

- CHV-1 has a predilection for lymphoid and neural cells, both of which may become latent infected, but a dog remains a potential shedder if the virus is re-exacerbated due to stress (e.g., pregnancy, corticosteroids, irradiation).
- Optimal temperature for CHV replication is 33–35 °C (i.e., the temperature of the outer genital and upper respiratory tracts, and the normal body temperature of canine neonates).
- Incubation period is 6–10 days.
- The virus replicates in the epithelial cells of the oronasal and pharyngeal mucosa and the regional lymphatics.

SIGNALMENT/HISTORY

Risk Factors

- Exposure of a naive bitch to CHV-1 during the last 3 weeks of gestation.
- Pups during the first 3 weeks of life.
- Transmission to neonates can occur subsequent to contact with infectious vaginal fluids during whelping or with vulvar or oronasal secretions in the post-partum period.
- Infectious contact with CHV-1 from contact with another dog shedding the organism.

Historic Findings

- Late-term abortion of a litter or neonatal deaths within their first few weeks of life.
- Older (>3–5 weeks of age) puppies exposed to CHV-1 may have an unapparent infection, or disease course may be less severe due to their inability to mount a febrile response.
- Concerns about latency and development of later neurologic signs have been proposed but not confirmed in recent literature.

CLINICAL FEATURES

- CHV infection in postnatally infected puppies – usually occurs between 1 and 3 weeks of age. Puppies demonstrate incessant vocalization, dullness, anorexia, poor weight gain, dyspnea, abdominal pain, incoordination, yellow-green diarrhea, serous to hemorrhagic nasal discharge and petechiation of mucous membranes. Erythematous rash consisting of papules or vesicles and subcutaneous edema of ventral abdominal and inguinal region occasionally noted. Puppies can shed large quantities of virus in body secretions for 2–3 weeks after recovery.

- Bitches infected during their last 3 weeks of gestation develop a systemic infection and placentitis, which results in abortion of mummified or dead fetuses, premature or stillborn pups, or weak or runt newborn puppies. Bitch is otherwise typically asymptomatic. Subsequent litters from the bitch are usually normal.
- Mortality rate in litters infected *in utero* or during birth can approach 100%, with deaths occurring during the first few days to a week of life. Exposed surviving older neonates reported to potentially later demonstrate CNS signs including blindness, ataxia, and deafness. Apparent complete recovery has also been reported.
- Healthy recently infected adult dogs of either gender may show signs of mild upper-respiratory tract infection (sneezing, serous oculonasal discharge) for a few days, but are otherwise usually unremarkable.

 ## DIFFERENTIAL DIAGNOSIS

- Acute-onset respiratory signs: canine adenovirus type 2; canine parainfluenza; *Bordetella bronchiseptica*; upper-airway foreign body.
- Reproductive disease. *Brucella canis*; canine distemper virus; neosporosis; toxoplasmosis.
- Neonatal bacterial septicemia. *E. coli, Streptococcus, Staphylococcus* and *Klebsiella* spp. most commonly.

 ## DIAGNOSTICS

- Antemortem testing:
  - Serologic titers – usually based on virus neutralization tests. Neutralizing antibodies increase after infection and can remain high for only 1 or 2 months; low titers may be detected for at least 2 years. Seropositivity indicates exposure, not necessarily active infection, although viral persistence and latent infection might be presumed. Serologic tests not standardized, resulting in variation in results among laboratories.
  - Virus isolation – of aborted fetus and/or placenta; infected neonates – isolated most commonly from adrenal glands, kidneys, lungs, spleen, lymph nodes, and liver. Virus isolation has not been demonstrated later than 2–3 weeks after infection. Older or recovered animals – usually restricted to the oral mucosa, upper respiratory tract, and external genitalia.
  - Real-time (RT) PCR – usually less turnaround time; confirmatory. In infected neonates – isolated from lung or kidney cells. Most reliable means of detecting latent infection in older animals. False-negative results may be observed from different laboratories or with different sampling methodologies and reduced viral load during latency; false-positive results can occur because of high prevalence of clinically healthy dogs that are carriers of the virus.

- Postmortem testing:
  - Virus isolation.
  - Histopathological evaluation – disseminated multifocal ecchymotic hemorrhages in the kidneys, liver, and lungs.
  - RT-PCR on tissues – confirmatory.

Pathological Findings

- Multifocal petechial hemorrhages within the kidneys.
- Infected placenta underdeveloped and congested with grey-to-white foci.
- Intranuclear inclusion bodies difficult to find.
- Can mimic gross pathology of bacterial sepsis.
- Severe nephrosis (proximal renal tubular epithelial necrosis and renal pelvic epithelial apoptosis with swollen vesicular nuclei), diffuse severe hepatic congestion and inflammation with vacuolar hepatopathy (neutrophilic, histiocytic and lymphocytic infiltration with apoptosis), acute severe necrotizing bronchointerstitial pneumonia with pulmonary edema and hemorrhage (terminal bronchiolar hemorrhage and edema with fibrin accumulation, macrophage infiltration necrosis and alveolar disruption), and thymic, lymph node and splenic lympholysis (severe diffuse cortical lympholysis with sinus congestion).

 # THERAPEUTICS

Drug(s) of Choice

- Unrewarding and rarely effective.
- Recovery suspected to be associated with residual cardiac and neurologic damage; not evident in recent reported cases.
- Immune serum from seroconverted dams – reported to be ineffective in infected puppies.
- Acyclovir – antiviral agent. If instituted in a timely manner, may reduce mortality. Poorly absorbed after oral administration and is primarily hepatically metabolized. Dose (20 mg/kg PO, q. 6 h until 3.5 weeks of age) currently extrapolated from that for humans; Alternatively, 7–10 mg total dose PO, q. 6 h until 3.5 weeks of age is advised.
- Lactoferrin – iron-binding protein found in milk and other mammalian secretions. Has been used topically to treat other mucosal viral infections. Could be administered orally on an empirical basis to protect exposed, clinically healthy pups with preoral transmission of virus is suspected or anticipated.

Precautions/Interactions

- Acyclovir – can increase the toxicity of nephrotoxic drugs. Half-life in humans approximately 3 hours. Use in veterinary medicine is not well established and it should be used with caution. Safety and effectiveness in humans less than 2 weeks of age is not established.

Appropriate Health Care

- Factors predisposing a puppy to septicemia – endometritis in the bitch, a prolonged delivery/dystocia, feeding of replacement formulas, the anecdotal use of ampicillin, stress, low birth weight (<350 g), and chilling with body temperature <35.5 °C (95 °F).
- Bactericidal broad-spectrum antibiotics – Ceftiofur sodium is a third-generation cephalosporin which alters intestinal flora minimally and is usually effective against the causative organisms of bacterial sepsis (e.g., *E. coli*, *Streptococcus* spp., *Staphylococcus* spp., and *Klebsiella* spp.).

Nursing Care

- Pooled serum from older adult dogs (22 ml/kg). SC dosing has been anecdotally reported.
- Increasing neonatal body temperature to 101 °F (38.3 °C) with exogenous heat at 45–55% humidity may be beneficial.
- Umbilicus of neonates should be treated with tincture of iodine immediately after birth to reduce contamination and prevent ascent of environmental bacteria into peritoneal cavity.

Diet

- Optimal nutrition with supported nursing, tube feeding or bottle-feeding.

 ## COMMENTS

Client Education

- Permanent nervous, renal, or lymphoid damage can occur in survivors, but normal outcome has been reported.
- Herpesviruses are generally highly species-specific; the dog does not become naturally infected with human strains, and canine organisms do not infect humans.

Prevention/Avoidance

- Isolating the pregnant bitch naive to CHV-1, during pregnancy and for at least 6 weeks post-partum.
- Expose young bitches to older animals prior to pregnancy (because most adult dogs have been exposed to CHV), but definitely not during the last 3 weeks of pregnancy, in the hope of providing an opportunity to seroconvert and develop protective antibodies. Cesarean section or artificial insemination are not justified to reduce spread of infection.
- Documentation of positive CHV-1 serology in a bitch generally indicates adequate maternal antibodies.
- Vaccination.
  - Development has been hampered by the poor immunogenicity characteristic of the herpesvirus vaccines developed for other species such as feline and bovine rhinotracheitis.

- Vaccine in Europe (Eurican Herpes 205) available since 2003. Advised to be administered to the dam twice; first during estrus or early pregnancy, and again 1–2 weeks prior to whelping. No suggestion for an evaluation of the bitch's serologic status prior to vaccination made by the manufacturer. Revaccination (twice) is advised at each pregnancy. No independent, non-proprietary studies exist corroborating this vaccine's efficacy or benefit. The vaccine is not currently available in the United States.

Expected Course and Prognosis

- Subsequent litters of the infected pregnant or post-partum bitch are usually normal, having acquired resultant maternal antibodies.

Synonyms

- Canine herpesvirus type 1 (CHV-1), CHV, dog herpes, neonatal herpes, fading puppy syndrome.

BRUCELLOSIS

 ## DEFINITION

- Contagious infection of dogs, caused by a Gram-negative, intracellular, aerobic coccobacillus bacteria, *Brucella canis*. *Brucella abortus*, *Brucella melitensis* and *Brucella suis* have occasionally caused canine infections, but comparatively rare.
- Characterized by abortion and infertility in females and epididymitis and testicular atrophy in males.

 ## ETIOLOGY/PATHOPHYSIOLOGY

Systems Affected

- *Brucella canis* – an intracellular parasite; has a propensity for growth in lymphatic, placental, and male genital (epididymis and prostate) tissues.
- Hemic/Lymphatic/Immune-Phagocytized *Brucella canis* remains intracellular within lymph nodes and spleen; bone marrow; mononuclear leukocytes of the reticuloendothelial system for months to years. Bacteremia within 1–4 weeks after infection; episodic for months to more than 5 years.
- Other tissues – intervertebral disks, anterior uvea, meninges.
- Bacteria penetrate exposed mucous membranes of oral cavity, conjunctiva, nasal tissue, penis, or vaginal vault.

- Organisms shed through highly contaminated vaginal discharge (following abortion), urine, milk or lactating bitch, semen, prostatic fluid, vaginal fluid during estrus, and lochia of parturition.
- Transplacental, aerosol, direct cutaneous inoculation and fomite-associated transmission can occur.
- Transmission is primarily venereal and oral. Occurs through direct exposure to bodily fluids containing an infectious dose of organism.

 # SIGNALMENT/HISTORY

Risk Factors

- No known genetic predisposition.
- No evidence of breed susceptibility, but increased incidence in Beagles?
- Dogs, infrequently, humans.
- No age preference.
- Most common in sexually mature dogs.
- Both sexes affected.
- Neutered and maiden or virgin dogs can be affected.
- Breeding kennels and pack hounds.
- Contacts with strays in endemic areas.
- Geographic distribution – increased incidence in southernmost states of the USA, Mexico, Central and South America, The People's Republic of China, and Japan. Sporadic reports in Canada and throughout Europe. Australia and New Zealand appear to be free from the disease.

Historic Findings

- Suspect whenever female dogs experience pregnancy loss or reproductive failures or males have genital disease or change in semen quality.
- Affected animals, especially females, may appear healthy or have vague signs of illness.
- Suboptimal athletic performance.
- Lethargy.
- Loss of libido.
- Weight loss.
- Lymphadenopathy – regional (pharyngeal if orally acquired, and pelvic, if venereally acquired).
- Lumbar pain.
- Abortion – commonly at 6–8 weeks after conception, although pregnancy may terminate at any stage (fetal resorption if early in gestation).

 # CLINICAL FEATURES

- Males – swollen scrotal sac, often with scrotal dermatitis; enlarged and firm epididymides, orchitis, azoospermia or poor semen quality.

- Females – failure to conceive; abortion at 45–59 days of gestation (less commonly, can occur as early as day 20 of gestation); birth of stillborn, partially autolyzed or weak pups; persistent highly infective mucopurulent or serosanguinous vulvar discharge for 1–6 weeks post-partum; pattern of successive abortions followed by a normal whelping of live or dead pups.
- Chronic infection – unilateral or bilateral testicular atrophy and infertility; pyospermia develops 3–4 months post-infection; cloudy eyes (anterior uveitis with corneal edema, often unilateral); nephritis; spinal pain (meningoencephalitis); posterior weakness; ataxia.
- Fever – rare.
- Enlarged superficial lymph nodes.
- Lameness.
- Splenomegaly.
- Lumbar pain.

 ## DIFFERENTIAL DIAGNOSIS

- Abortions – maternal, fetal, or placental abnormalities.
- Systemic infections – canine distemper, canine herpesvirus infection, *B. abortus* infection, hemolytic streptococci, *E. coli*, leptospirosis, and toxoplasmosis.
- Inguinal hernias, orchitis, epididymitis, torsion of spermatic cord, testicular neoplasia, abscess, varicocele, hydrocele, hematoma.
- Infertility/poor semen quality/azoospermia – incorrect timing of breeding, subclinical uterine infection, testicular or prostatic disease.
- Diskospondylitis – fungal, actinomycosis, staphylococcal infections, nocardiosis, streptococci, or *Corynebacterium* diphtheroids.

 ## DIAGNOSTICS

CBC/Biochemistry/Urinalysis

- CBC – may show neutrophilic leukocytosis. Degenerate left shifts, monocytosis and/or lymphopenia uncommonly reported.
- Chemistry panel – often normal; hyperglobulinemia and hypoalbuminemia may be present.
- Urinalysis – generally within normal limits.

Serologic Testing

- RSAT (rapid slide agglutination test) – uses *Brucella ovis* as antigen.
- 2-Mercaptoethanol-modified RSAT (ME-TSAT) – semiquantitative; uses *Brucella canis* as antigen.
- Mercaptoethanol Tube Agglutination Test (TAT) – semiquantitative.
- Indirect IFA or ELISA assay. Negative results reliable; unless, dog exposed <2 months; then retest.

- Screening serology (RSAT, TAT, IFA) sensitive but not specific. False-positives are common (due to cross-reacting antibodies to other microorganisms such as *Bordetella*, *Pseudomonas*, *E. coli* and *Moraxella* spp. Any positive result should be sent for a confirmation test (AGID).
- AGID tests – specific, confirmatory; will identify positive dog from 8–12 weeks post-infection until 3–4 years after achieving abacteremia.

Imaging

- Plain radiography – may show evidence of either multifocal of focal diskospondylitis.
- Sonographic findings – may show no abnormalities, or abdominal lymphadenomegaly and splenomegaly may be present. Prostate may demonstrate irregularity hyperechogenicity, and cavitation.

Isolation of Organism

- Blood cultures – definitive; usually 2–4 weeks post-infection; can become abacteremic after 27–64 months, but remain infected.
- Cultures of vaginal fluids, aborted fetuses, placental material, necropsy specimens (especially spleen, prostate and uterus).
- Cultures of semen or urine – not practical.
- RT-PCR-based assays – may be the most sensitive method of testing.
- Cytological analysis of tissue aspirates of spleen or lymph nodes – lymphoid reactivity, occasional increased numbers of plasma cells.
- Semen examination – diminished sperm counts (oligospermia), poor motility (asthenospermia), increased morphologic abnormalities (teratospermia) such as detached sperm heads, proximal and distal cytoplasmic droplets, acrosomal deformities. An absence of sperm in the ejaculate (azoospermia) may also be found.

Pathologic Findings

- Lymphoplasmacytic to lymphohistiocytic follicular hyperplasia in lymphoid tissues, lymphohistiocytic to neutrophilic endophthalmitis, and mild lymphohistiocytic meningitis.
- Mixed lymphohistiocytic inflammatory response in uterus of females, and the testicles, epididymis and spermatic cord, and prostate of male dogs.
- Prostatic and testicular fibrosis may be found.
- Immunohistochemistry may help confirm presence of *Brucella* spp. in placental tissues.

 # THERAPEUTICS

Drug(s) of Choice

- Antibiotics historically unrewarding. May reduce antibody titers, without clearing the infection. Failure and relapses occur.

- Combination therapy with tetracyclines (doxycycline or minocycline 25 mg/kg orally for 4 weeks and dihydrostreptomycin (10–20 mg/kg BID IM or SC for 2 weeks, weeks 1 and 4) or an aminoglycoside (gentamicin 5 mg/kg q. 24 h IM or SC for 14 days, weeks 1 and 4) has been advocated as most successful. Rifampin (5.5 mg/kg PO, q. 24 h) has been added in some cases.
- Enrofloxacin alone (5 mg/kg BID or 10 mg/kg PO, q. 24 h for 4 weeks) has been reported in limited use. Not completely efficacious in eliminating *B. canis*, but maintained fertility and avoided the recurrence of abortions, transmission of the disease to subsequently whelped puppies, and dissemination of the microorganisms during parturition. Most dogs remained culture-positive.
- Combinations of enrofloxacin and doxycycline may be a more effective alternative for dogs unable to tolerate aminoglycoside or rifampin treatment, but studies are lacking.

Precautions/Interactions

- Renal failure from long-term gentamicin use.
- Relapse or additional clinical signs as bacteremia persists.

Alternative Options

- May be reportable disease in certain jurisdictions. Infected dogs and bitches should be removed from breeding programs and quarantined. Eradication in kennel situations has not been successful without removal (culling) of all current or historically affected dogs. In some situations, euthanasia of affected dogs has been advised.

Surgical Considerations

- Ovariohysterectomy/castration – decreases potential for reservoirs of organisms, but does not eradicate infection. Urine shedding can persist.

Prevention

- Annual testing of all breeding stock.
- Testing of all dogs introduced into a kennel. Ideally, two negative screening tests at least 1 month apart, before introduction into a breeding facility.
- Confirmed positive dogs should be isolated (euthanasia may be considered), neutered, treated, and tested monthly (AGID, culture, or reliable PCR assay) until two negative consecutive tests occur, recognizing that occult infection can still be present.
- Private breeders – should require screening tests of all bitches presented for breeding and negative results on confirmatory tests if positive screening test. Stud dogs should be screened appropriately, at least annually, before breeding or semen shipment. Screening of maiden dogs and bitches also recommended.

- Wear gloves during examination or treatment.
- Quarantine required by certain state regulatory agencies if positive test occurs; enforced for minimum of 2 months until negative results reported.
- Vaccination – agglutinating antibodies are not protective in the dog, and immunity likely depends on cell-mediated immunity. Presently, the development of a vaccine is considered undesirable as the *Brucella* vaccines evaluated have only offered moderate protection, and immunized dogs develop antibodies that confound serodiagnosis.

Environmental Control

- Large numbers of organisms shed in the vulvar discharge of bitches 4–6 weeks post-abortion, and in the semen of infected dogs 2–3 months post-infection, with less amounts for years. Urine can serve as a contaminated vehicle with shedding for months to years. Organisms can also be shed in milk.
- Readily inactivated by common disinfectants such as 1% sodium hypochlorite, 70% ethanol, iodine/alcohol solutions, glutaraldehyde, and formaldehyde.

 # COMMENTS

Client Education

- Zoonotic concern – rare; most commonly occurs through contact with semen from an infected dog, vulvar discharge from an infected bitch, aborted fetus or placentas, or direct accidental laboratory exposure.
- Discourage exposure of affected dogs to children, immunocompromised individuals and pregnant women within that household or area.
- Contact with dogs with reproductive problems or their secretions should be avoided; if handled, recommend wearing of gloves, gowns and face protection; hands should be washed thoroughly.
- May be a reportable disease in dog or human in certain jurisdictions.

Patient Monitoring

- Infected for life.
- Neutered dogs should be periodically treated with antibiotics to decrease risk of bacteremia and subsequent shedding.
- May consider euthanasia for any dog that has a confirmed positive test.

Expected Course and Prognosis

- Prognosis poor, guarded at best.
- Dogs remain infected for life.
- No infected dog should be used for breeding, even if treated with antibiotics.

MINUTE VIRUS

 ## DEFINITION

- Infectious disease caused by virus belonging to family Parvoviridae.
- Canine minute virus (CnMV), also known as canine parvovirus type 1 (CPV-1).
- Antigenically unrelated to canine parvovirus type 2 (CPV-2).

 ## ETIOLOGY/PATHOPHYSIOLOGY

- Transmission oral–nasal or transplacental.
- Virus is spread transplacentally when the dam is infected between 25 and 30 days of gestation, and can cause reabsorption or abortion of fetuses. When infected between 30–35 days, puppies may be born with anasarca and myocarditis.
- Pathological lesions in fetuses found in the lungs and small intestine.

Systems Affected

- Genitourinary.

 ## SIGNALMENT/HISTORY

Risk Factors

- Most common between the ages of 1 to 3 weeks.
- Failure of passive transfer.

Historic Findings

- Mild diarrhea most common complaint.

 ## CLINICAL FEATURES

- CnMV has been associated with asymptomatic infectious, respiratory distress, enteric disease, neonatal mortality and reproductive disorders.
- Can cause transplacental infections leading to subclinical disease, embryonic resorption, abortion, birth deformities, or neonatal mortality.
- Outcome in pregnant bitches depends on time of infection during gestation. Infections during first half of gestation may result in embryo death and resorption, whereas stillbirths and the birth of weak pups are more frequently observed in the late stages of gestation.

- Puppies aged 1–3 weeks develop most severe symptoms, such as respiratory distress, inappetance, and diarrhea and in severe cases, may be fatal.
- Littermates that survive illness, usually recover within a few days.

 # DIFFERENTIAL DIAGNOSIS

- Other infectious causes of diarrhea.

 # DIAGNOSTICS

- Immunofluorescence.
- Virus isolation.
- Detection of intranuclear inclusion bodies – samples submitted should include fetal of neonatal tissues such as myocardium, intestine and lungs.
- PCR.

Pathological Findings

- In nursing puppies, postmortem findings include pneumonia, enteritis, myocarditis, and thymic edema and atrophy.
- Histopathologically, eosinophilic intranuclear viral inclusions observed in epithelial cells of intestinal crypts and in myocardiocytes.
- Other histologic changes include hyperplasia of the intestinal crypts, necrosis of the myocardium, interstitial pneumonia, and lymphocyte depletion in the thymus and other lymphoid tissues.

 # THERAPEUTICS

- No effective treatment due to the rapid progression of the disease.
- Mortality can be reduced by providing warm environmental temperatures and adequate nutrients and hydration.

 # COMMENTS

Prevention/Avoidance

- Currently no vaccination available.
- No zoonotic potential.
- Practice good hygiene.

See Also

Infectious Causes of Pregnancy Loss – Feline

Suggested Reading

Cote, E. (2011) *Clinical Veterinary Advisor Dogs and Cats*, 2nd edition. Mosby Inc., USA.

Farstad, W. (2004) Infectious Causes of Pregnancy Loss in Dogs. American College of Theriogenology Annual Conference, pp. 225–230.

Greene, C.E. (2012) *Infectious Diseases of the Dog and Cat*, 4th edition. Elsevier Saunders Inc., St Louis, MO.

Hoskins, J.D. (2001) *Veterinary Pediatrics*, 3rd edition. W.B. Saunders, Philadelphia, PA.

Johnston, S.D., Root Kustritz, M.V., Olson, P.N.S. (2001) *Canine and Feline Theriogenology*. W.B. Saunders, Philadelphia, PA.

England, G., von Heimendahl, A. (2010) *BSVA Manual of Canine and Feline Reproduction and Neonatology*, 2nd edition. BSAVA, Gloucester, England.

Arantes, T.P., Lopes, W.D., Ferreira, R.M., *et al.* (2009) *Toxoplasmosis gondii*: Evidence for the transmission be semen in dogs. *Exp. Parasitol.*, **123** (2), 190–194.

Davidson, A.P. (2013) Canine Herpesvirus Infection, in *Canine and Feline Infectious Diseases* (ed. J.E. Sykes), Elsevier, pp. 166–169.

Davidson, A.P., Sykes, J.E. (2013) Canine Brucellosis, in *Canine and Feline Infectious Diseases* (ed. J.E. Sykes), Elsevier, pp. 512–519.

Author: Benita von Dehn DVM, DACVIM (Internal Medicine)

chapter 55

Infectious Causes of Pregnancy Loss – Feline

DEFINITION

- Pregnancy loss refers to the death of an embryo or fetus.
- The clinical outcome depends upon the stage of pregnancy during which the pregnancy loss occurred.
- Early pregnancy loss will typically result in resorption (could be interpreted as apparent infertility), whilst mid to late pregnancy loss results in abortion, still-birth, mummification, or retention.

ETIOLOGY/PATHOPHYSIOLOGY

- The most common intrauterine bacteria-associated causes of abortion in the queen include *Streptococcus* spp., *Escherichia coli*, *Campylobacter*, and Salmonella.
- Virus-associated pregnancy loss is more frequently associated with feline leukemia virus (FeLV), feline panleukopenia virus (FPV), feline herpes virus (FHV), and feline immunodeficiency virus (FIV).
- Fungal and parasitic causes of pregnancy loss are rare.
- The queen is considered an induced ovulatory, however spontaneous ovulation does occur (without copulation).
- After ovulation and conception, the corpora lutea (CL) maintain serum progesterone concentrations for the first 35 days of gestation, after which time the placenta provides a second progesterone source, both of which are needed to maintain pregnancy to term.
- Maintenance of feline pregnancy requires a serum progesterone concentration great than 2 ng/ml.
- Pregnancy loss in the queen may be directly associated with viral, bacterial, or protozoal infections. It may also occur in association with significant systemic disease by interfering with placental or luteal function.

Blackwell's Five-Minute Veterinary Consult Clinical Companion: Small Animal Endocrinology and Reproduction, First Edition. Edited by Deborah S. Greco and Autumn P. Davidson. © 2017 John Wiley & Sons, Inc. Published 2017 by John Wiley & Sons, Inc.
Companion Website: www.fiveminutevet.com/endocrinology

Systems Affected

- Hemic/Lymphatic/Immune: changes in peripheral hemogram, and leukogram may be noted in association with any viral and bacterial infection, but are most striking with FPV (neutropenia), and FeLV (anemia, thrombocytopenia). Lymph node enlargement may be noted in neonates in association with *Streptococcus*.
- Nervous: behavioral alteration may be noted in neonates with FPV-associated cerebellar hypoplasia. It may also be noted in queen or neonates with severe toxoplasmosis with intra-cranial involvement.
- Reproductive: vaginal discharge, stillbirth, abortion, lactation in response to decreasing serum progesterone concentrations; early pregnancy loss/resorption frequently presents as an increased interestrous interval (IEI).

 # SIGNALMENT/HISTORY

Pregnancy Loss

- Presentation typically <6 years of age due to average breeding age of queens.
- Early pregnancy loss/resorption may presents for evaluation of subfertility, or prolonged IEIs as early pregnancy may not be detected.
- Late pregnancy loss typically presents due to clinical signs of abortion (vaginal discharge, expulsion of fetus), and/or systemic manifestations of the disease in the queen.

Risk Factors

- Poor husbandry, nutrition, including maintenance of carrier cats in the breeding population (FeLV, FIV, bacterial isolates).
- Lack of vaccination (FPV).
- Lack of prior exposure (FHV).
- Young age (<2 years) – *Streptococcus*.

Historic Findings

- Subfertility in a breeding population, or individual female.
- Prior litter losses, poor neonate survival, low birth weight.

 # CLINICAL FEATURES

Bacterial Infections

Brucellosis

- Cats are not susceptible to infection with *Brucella*.

Streptococcus spp.

- Lancefield Group G β hemolytic streptococci are considered commensal vaginal flora in the queen.
- Sporadic disease (metritis, placentitis, abortion and neonatal septicemia) may be seen with exposure in a younger immune-naive population.
- During pregnancy the vaginal bacterial load increases in younger queens, resulting in a higher post natal loss due to neonatal septicemia; infection is transmitted from the birth canal.
- There is an age-associated ability to clear the carrier state by mid-gestation; prevalence decreases with age.

Escherichia coli

- One of the most frequently isolated bacteria from the healthy urogenital tract in the queen.
- Is not a common cause of abortion.
- Reproductive tract infections are opportunistic, caused by strains within the gastrointestinal tract.

Salmonella

- *In-utero* infection may be associated with abortion or stillbirth.
- Prolonged involution may be noted.

Viral Infections

Feline Herpesvirus (FHV)

- FHV-1 is associated with severe upper respiratory tract disease.
- Abortion is noted with other herpesvirus infections, abortion in queens infected with FHV-1 is related to systemic disease rather than a direct impact on the reproductive tract.
- α herpesvirus infection is associated with abortion, intrauterine fetal death and maceration; coagulation necrosis of the placenta is a feature.

Feline Panleukopenia Virus (FPV)

- FPV is a member of the parvovirus family, with fecal-oral transmission.
- In the pregnant queen, the fetus is a target tissue due to its high mitotic activity.
- Infection during early pregnancy will result in subfertility, and resorption; infections mid-pregnancy are typically associated with abortion or fetal mummification.
- The classic FPLV cerebellar hypoplasia manifesting clinically as tremors, and incoordination, is associated with late pregnancy infections and fetal nervous tissue invasion.
- Kittens infected in the first 10 days may also be affected.

Feline Immunodeficiency Virus (FIV)

- FIV is a lentivirus that may be transmitted horizontally at the time of insemination or through bite wounds, and vertically transplacentally, or via colostrums.

- Subfertility, arrested fetal development, abortion, stillbirth, and low birth weight are common findings.
- Infection rates in kittens from infected queens is high, although it is important to remember when screening that during the first 16 weeks kittens may test positive due to maternally derived antibody.

Feline Leukemia Virus (FeLV)

- FeLV is a retrovirus that is shed in large amounts in saliva; transplacental infection, and neonate grooming, represent the main form of vertical transmission.
- Mammary colonization is possible; lactation represents an alternate method of transmission.
- Fetal resorption, abortion, and a high percentage of neonatal death are clinical features.

Protozoal Infections

Toxoplasma gondii

- Queens are generally asymptomatic.
- Immunosuppression and FIV status are known risk factors for susceptibility and more severe clinical disease.
- Trans-placental infection may result in stillbirths and/or early neonate death.

 DIFFERENTIAL DIAGNOSIS

Maternal Health

- Poor nutrition, or underlying chronic disease may result in significant morbidity to the queen, with pregnancy loss.
- Full evaluation of husbandry practices, and baseline health data for the queen should be established; reproductive history should be evaluated not only for the queen but also for the tom cat(s) used, and their respective colonies.

Trauma

- May occur during efforts to assist delivery, or as a result of maternal behavior.
- Physical examination of the queen and fetus/neonate typically provide supportive evidence.

Failure to Conceive

- Teratospermia is common in the domestic cat, and ovulation is possible without conception.
- Without physical examination and imaging, it is difficult to distinguish early pregnancy loss from failure to conceive.

Dystocia

- As the queen is an induced ovulator, accurate prediction of parturition is difficult unless time with the tomcat is limited and documented.
- Dystocia may result in still birth, and this must be distinguished from other infectious causes.
- Trans-abdominal uterine monitoring is clinically useful to evaluate for uterine activity and signs of fetal distress in the peri-parturient period.

 # DIAGNOSTICS

- A key component to any evaluation of pregnancy loss includes a full reproductive history, physical examination, and diagnostics of the queen *and* evaluation of the placenta and embryo/fetus where available.

CBC/Biochemistry/Urinalysis

- The queen should be evaluated for neutropenia consistent with FPV, anemia consistent with FeLV, leukocytosis (inflammation and/or bacterial focus).
- Biochemistry should be evaluated for evidence of organ dysfunction, in particular hypocholesterolemia and/or low proteins consistent with malnutrition/malabsorption/malassimilation.

Serum Hormone Evaluation

- A serum progesterone concentration >2 ng/ml in the queen is consistent with adequate luteal and/or placental function.

Serum Antibody and Antigen Evaluation

- The queen and tom cat should be FIV antibody and FeLV antigen screened.
- Any surviving kittens should be FeLV antigen screened.
- *Toxoplasma gondii* IgG and IgM titers should be submitted as clinically indicated.

Aerobic Culture

- Aerobic culture of the placenta, lung, and liver (pooled) should be submitted to screen for bacterial pathogens.
- The most commonly isolated pathogens are readily cultured with standard protocols.

PCR

- Samples of fetal lung and liver should be submitted for *Salmonella* spp. screening.
- Tissue samples of the kidneys, in addition to whole blood, should be collected and stored refrigerated in a sterile manner for viral PCR testing; abortion PCR panels with culture are now commercially available.

Imaging

- Abdominal ultrasound should be performed to evaluate uterine content, and heart rate in remaining fetuses.
- A healthy fetus should have a heart rate >180 bpm.

Clinical/Anatomic Pathology Evaluation

- The aborted fetus should be evaluated and gross and post-mortem findings recorded, with particular attention to the heart, lungs, liver, and kidneys.
- Intracranial evaluation is important to evaluate trauma.
- Representative samples of the lung, liver, kidney, and thymus should be placed in formalin for further histologic evaluation.
- If the placenta is available, the gross appearance should be noted, a sample collected for PCR/culture, and an impression smear of the chorioallantois collected for evaluation of inflammatory cells. A sample should be preserved in formalin for histopathology.
- For those cases involving cesarean section, uterine biopsies (placental site and endometrium) are advised.

 THERAPEUTICS

- The evaluation of pregnancy loss is typically a retrospective evaluation.
- If infectious disease is identified as a causal agent, appropriate husbandry and management change is advised to prevent repeat occurrence and prepare for subsequent pregnancies.
- For those cases of bacterial causes, treatment should be based on culture and sensitivities where appropriate.
- Further breeding of queens identified as positive for either FeLV or FIV is not advised.

Drug(s) of Choice

- Treatment for bacterial causes of infection should be based on the sensitivity results of the isolated organism.
- Prophylactic antimicrobial use at the time of subsequent breeding may be considered; however, its use is controversial; no evidence-based studies support this and the promotion of resistant organisms is likely.

Precautions/Interactions

- Standard vaccination protocols, quarantine procedures, and monitoring of general queen and tom cat health status is paramount to ensure breeding success.

COMMENTS

Prevention/Avoidance

- The most effective management system to prevent infectious causes of pregnancy loss in the queen include rigorous health maintenance of both the queen and tom, routine annual screening for underlying health problems, retrovirus status, and excellent nutrition.
- Queens should be maintained in a closed-colony environment, and new additions to the colony quarantined.

Expected Course and Prognosis

- With the exception of FeLV- and FIV-positive cases, provided that underlying causes of infectious abortion are identified and resolved, a return to fertility is expected.

Abbreviations

bpm = beats per minute
CL   = corpora lutea
FeLV = feline leukemia virus
FHV = feline herpesvirus
FIV   = feline immune-deficiency virus
FPV = feline panleukopenia virus
HR   = heart rate
IgG   = immunoglobulin G
IgM   = immunoglobulin M
PCR = polymerase chain reaction

See Also

Infectious Causes of Pregnancy Loss – Canine

Suggested Reading

Lamm, C.G., Njaa, B.L. (2012) Clinical approach to abortion, stillbirth, and neonatal death in dogs and cats. *Vet. Clin. North Am. Small Anim. Pract.*, **42** (3), 501–513.
Decaro, N., Carmichael, L.E., Buonavoglia, C. (2012) Viral reproductive pathogens of dogs and cats. *Vet. Clin. North Am. Small Anim. Pract.*, **42** (3), 583–598.
Graham, E.M., Taylor, D.J. (2012) Bacterial reproductive pathogens of cats and dogs. *Vet. Clin. North Am. Small Anim. Pract.*, **42** (3), 561–582.

Author: Sophie A. Grundy BVSc, MACVSc, DACVIM (Internal Medicine)

chapter 56

Priapism and Paraphimosis

DEFINITION

- Priapism is a persistent erection lasting longer than 4 hours, without sexual stimulation. Priapism is classified as either non-ischemic (arterial, high flow) or ischemic (veno-occlusive, low flow) (Fig. 56.1).
- Paraphimosis occurs when the penis cannot be ensheathed back into the prepuce. The penis may be erect (as with semen collection) or edematous/swollen (Fig. 56.2).

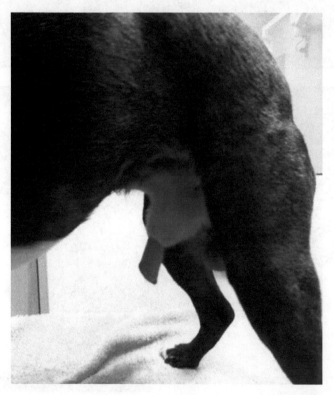

■ **Fig. 56.1.** Priapism in a Boston Terrier with syringohydromyelia and a meningomyelocoele in the lumbar spine.

Blackwell's Five-Minute Veterinary Consult Clinical Companion: Small Animal Endocrinology and Reproduction, First Edition. Edited by Deborah S. Greco and Autumn P. Davidson. © 2017 John Wiley & Sons, Inc. Published 2017 by John Wiley & Sons, Inc. Companion Website: www.fiveminutevet.com/endocrinology

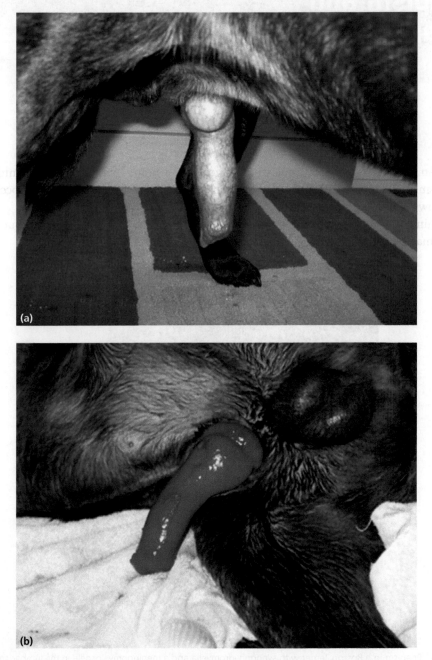

■ **Fig. 56.2.** (a) Paraphimosis as a normal consequence of semen collection. Occuring immediately post ejaculation, this is responsible for the copulatory lock in dogs. (b) Problematic post-ejaculatory paraphimosis in an 11-month-old Cane Corso Mastiff which persisted 4 hours after breeding. The preputial opening was too small and prevented detumescence.

ETIOLOGY/PATHOPHYSIOLOGY

- Non-ischemic priapism results from increased arterial inflow through the corpus cavernosa. Non-ischemic priapism is often caused by trauma, but also may be caused by neurological conditions, vasoactive drugs, or it may be idiopathic. Neurological causes include distemper, spinal injury and meningomyelocoele with syringohydromyelia. Dysnergic neurostimulation of inflow and outflow blood vessels in the penis is thought to prolong vascular or smooth muscle spasms. Dysregulation may occur at the level of the penis, or at other regulatory areas of the penis, including the central or peripheral nervous system. The pelvic nerve mediates the canine erection. The pelvic nerve arises from the 1st and 2nd sacral nerves, and is composed of parasympathetic fibers. Pelvic nerve stimulation increases penile blood pressure, dilates penile arteries, and partially inhibits venous drainage, resulting in an erection. The pudendal nerve, arising from S1–S3 stimulates contraction of the extrinsic penile muscles. Sympathetic chain fibers inhibit erection by increasing arterial resistance, decreasing corpus cavernosal pressure, and decreasing venous resistance. Sympathetic inhibition of erection is mediated by the α1-adrenergic system. Phenothiazine drugs, such as acepromazine, are α-adrenergic antagonists and can cause priapism in people, cats, and horses (Fig. 56.3). The retractor penis muscle in

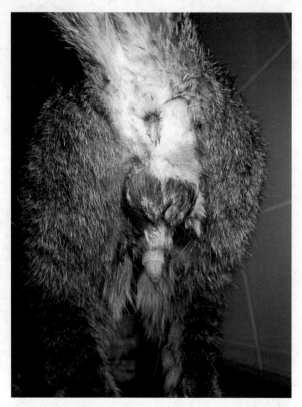

■ **Fig. 56.3.** Priapism in a 4-year-old male Savannah cat resulting from over-dosage with acepromazine.

horses is solely under the control of α-adrenergic fibers, and is considered a major factor for priapism in stallions.

■ Ischemic priapism is caused by venous congestion to the penis and increased blood viscosity. A traumatic cause is most common. It was associated in a cat with feline infectious peritonitis (FIP). In humans, hematological dyscrasias, hemodialysis, vasoactive drugs, anesthesia, neoplasia and neurological conditions can cause ischemic priapism. Both, ischemic and non-ischemic priapism are rarely reported in dogs and cats.

■ Paraphimosis can result from an inadequate length of the prepuce, trauma, weakened preputial muscles, or from a too-small preputial orifice as compared to the size of the penis during detumescence. The preputial opening can fold inwards during detumescence and entrap the tip of the penis, inducing severe edema (Fig. 56.4). A shortened prepuce with infolding at the opening can induce chronic changes, induce excoriation, and result in desiccation of the tip of the penis, usually in a neutered dog (Fig. 56.5).

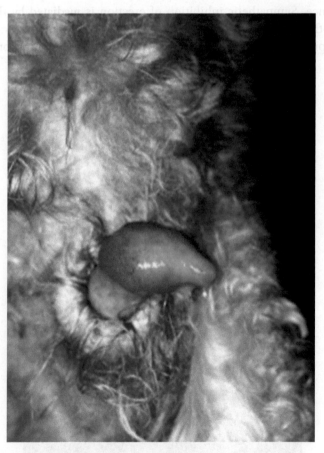

■ **Fig. 56.4.** Paraphimosis secondary to inward rolling of the preputial skin during detumescence following semen collection. Distal penile edema occurs within minutes after ejaculation.

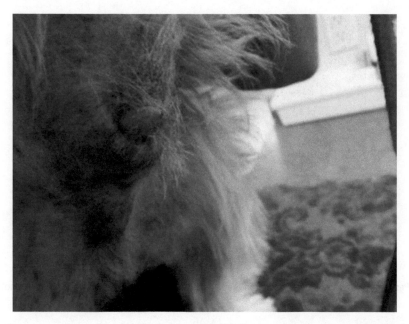

■ **Fig. 56.5.** Chronic paraphimosis in a Miniature Schnauzer. The distal prepuce has become inverted, the distal penis desiccated. Self-trauma perpetuated this problem.

Systems Affected

- Reproductive.
- Nervous.
- Hemic.

 ## SIGNALMENT/HISTORY AND CLINICAL FEATURES

- Male dogs and cats are affected by priapism and paraphimosis. There is no known age pre-dilection. Siamese cats are over-represented compared to other breeds of cats. No known breed predisposition is present in dogs.
- Ischemic priapism is typically painful, with a rigid penile shaft and soft glans. Non-ischemic priapism is not painful with a partially rigid penis. With paraphimosis the penis may be swollen/edematous from extrusion, but is not erect from sexual stimulation, except in the immediate post-ejaculatory period.

 ## DIFFERENTIAL DIAGNOSIS

- Priapism can be easily confused with paraphimosis, especially if erection causes the cranial portion of the penis to be extruded. Neoplasia of the penis can lead to either condition and should be ruled out (Fig. 56.6).

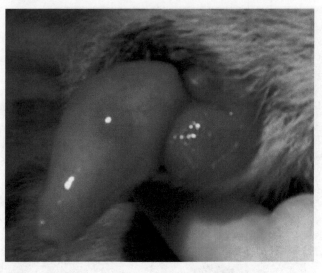

■ **Fig. 56.6.** Penile neoplasia resulting in paraphimosis. The penis was palpably enlarged, but priapism not present.

 ## DIAGNOSTICS

■ A physical examination of the penis for trauma (rupture of the tunica albuginea) or masses should be performed (Fig. 56.7). Ultrasound of the perineum and the entire penile shaft is indicated to evaluate for anatomic abnormalities such as neoplasia, fracture of the os penis, hematoma formation and thromboemboli, and to evaluate the penile blood supply. Priapism can be readily confirmed with ultrasound (Fig. 56.8a,b). A retrograde urethrogram can be used to rule out urethral obstruction that can occur with neoplasia of the penis.

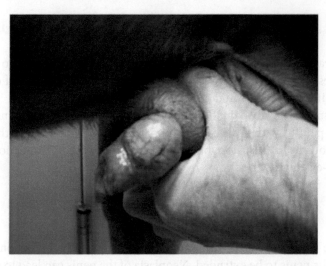

■ **Fig. 56.7.** Rupture of the tunica albuginea secondary to trauma. The penis was palpably enlarged, but priapism was not present.

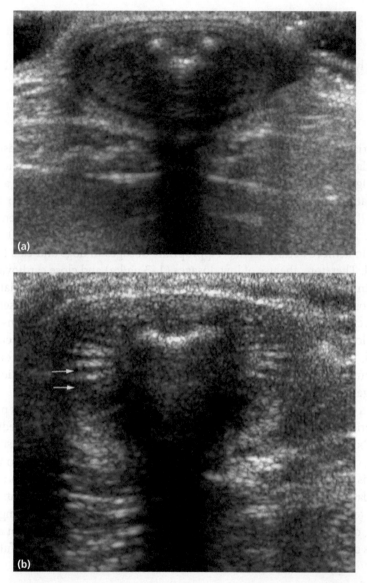

■ **Fig. 56.8.** (a) Transverse ultrasound image of a normal, non-erect canine penis. (b) Transverse image of canine priapism. The vessels in the corpus cavernosum are engorged (indicated by arrows). Ultrasound images courtesy of T.W. Baker.

■ Corpus cavernosum blood gas evaluation can differentiate between ischemic and non-ischemic priapism. Ischemic priapism typically has dark blood with a pH <7.25, a PO_2 <30 mmHg and a PCO_2 >60 mmHg. Non-ischemic priapism typically has bright-red blood with a pH >7.4, a PO_2 >90 mmHg and a PCO_2 <40 mmHg.

THERAPEUTICS

■ If an underlying cause for priapism or paraphimosis is identified it should be treated as indicated.

Priapism

■ Ischemic priapism is considered an emergency in people due to a rapid onset of hypoxia and tissue damage. In ischemic priapism, aspiration of blood from the corpus cavernosum ± saline irrigation is recommended. Under heavy sedation or anesthesia, aspiration and saline irrigation can relieve pain, flush out deoxygenated blood, and can lead to detumescence. If erection persists, the intracavernous injection of an α-adrenergic sympathomimetic agent such as phenylephrine diluted with saline to 100– 500 µg/ml can be performed to achieve detumescence. Appropriate dosages in dogs and cats have not been determined. Therefore, the use of low dosages (1–3 µg/kg) and close cardiovascular monitoring are important. Lubrication of the penis limits tissue damage associated with prolonged exposure and excoriation. An Elizabethan collar can help prevent self-mutilation. If detumescence is not achieved, surgery may be indicated. Bilateral incisions in the tunica albuginea, longa glandis or the corpus cavernosa have been made to evacuate accumulated blood, followed by saline irrigation. If significant tissue damage has occurred, then penile amputation and perineal urethrostomy may be indicated. Antibiotic therapy and pain management should be used as clinically indicated.
■ Aspiration is considered of diagnostic benefit in non-ischemic priapism, but is not considered of therapeutic benefit. Saline irrigation and injection of vasoconstrictive medication is not considered beneficial in non-ischemic priapism. Non-ischemic priapism can resolve spontaneously. Thus, conservative therapy and protecting penile integrity with lubrication ± an Elizabethan collar is recommended. Several medications are of potential benefit, although very little controlled data exists regarding the efficacy of systemic drug therapy. Gabapentin 5–30 mg/kg PO, q. 8 h, terbutaline 0.1–0.2 mg/kg PO, q. 12 h, or pseudoephedrine 1.5 mg/kg (1 mg/kg in cats) PO, q. 8–12 h should be tried in dogs and cats. If detumescence is not achieved after several days of treatment with one drug, switching to another may be successful.

Paraphimosis

■ Treatment of paraphimosis includes saline irrigation as the penis is placed back into the prepuce. Lubrication of the penis is helpful to protect the penile integrity and to help with placement. Heavy sedation or anesthesia can be required. Diuretics and hypertonic solutions are not of significant benefit in decreasing penile swelling. Temporary purse-string sutures can be helpful in some cases, but interference with urination must be avoided. Surgical correction, usually preputial opening revision, of any underlying anatomic abnormalities may be necessary if the penis cannot be ensheathed in the prepuce or the problem recurs repeatedly, or becomes chronic (Fig. 56.9). Antibiotic therapy and pain management should be used as clinically indicated.

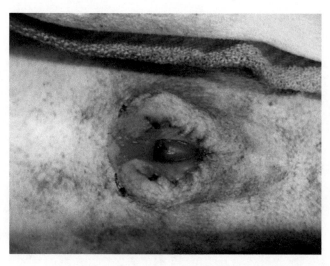

■ **Fig. 56.9.** Preputial revision, seen postoperatively, in a dog with chronic historical paraphimosis (as seen in Fig. 56.5).

Suggested Reading

Lavely, J.A. (2009) Priapism in dogs. *Topics Comp. Anim. Med.*, **24**, 49–54.

Montague, D.K., Jarow, J., Broderick, G.A., *et al.* (2003) American Urological Association guideline to the management of priapism. *J. Urol.*, **170**, 1318–1324.

Orima, H., Tsutsui, T., Waki, T., *et al.* (1989) Surgical treatment of priapism observed in a dog and a cat. *Nippon Juigaku Zasshi*, **51**, 1227–1229.

Yuan, J., DeSouza, R., Westney, L., *et al.* (2008) Insights of priapism mechanism and rationale treatment for recurrent priapism. *Asian J. Androl.*, **1**, 88–101.

Author: James Lavely DVM, DACVIM (Neurology)

Primary Hyperaldosteronism in Cats

chapter 57

DEFINITION

- Primary hyperaldosteronism (PHA) or low-renin hyperaldosteronism is an adrenocortical disorder characterized by excessive, autonomous secretion of aldosterone leading to systemic hypertension and/or hypokalemia.
- This disorder is also referred to as Conn's syndrome. In cats, inappropriate aldosterone secretion is caused by either unilateral or bilateral neoplasia or bilateral nodular hyperplasia of the adrenal zona glomerulosa.

ETIOLOGY/PATHOPHYSIOLOGY

- The principal function of aldosterone is the regulation of systemic blood pressure and extracellular fluid volume in response to changes in renal blood flow and electrolytes. Aldosterone production in the zona glomerulosa of the adrenal cortex is regulated by the rennin–angiotensin–aldosterone system (RAAS) and extracellular potassium concentrations.
  - In cats with PHA, excess aldosterone causes hypertension, and an increased urinary loss of potassium may result in profound hypokalemia.
  - Disorders that cause a reduction in effective blood volume activate the RAAS, which in turn persistently stimulates aldosterone synthesis. Examples include heart failure, edema or ascites secondary to hypoproteinemia, and intrarenal ischemia from chronic kidney disease (CKD).
  - This pathophysiological response to hypovolemia/ischemia is called secondary hyperaldosteronism or high-renin hyperaldosteronism.
  - Hypokalemic nephropathy refers to a subset of cats with CKD and secondary hyperaldosteronism that develop hypokalemia. In contrast, PHA is due to autonomous hypersecretion of aldosterone by neoplastic or non-neoplastic zona glomerulosa tissue (i.e., bilateral nodular hyperplasia).
  - Aldosterone secretion in PHA is associated with suppressed plasma renin activity, and is often termed low-renin hyperaldosteronism.

Blackwell's Five-Minute Veterinary Consult Clinical Companion: Small Animal Endocrinology and Reproduction, First Edition. Edited by Deborah S. Greco and Autumn P. Davidson. © 2017 John Wiley & Sons, Inc. Published 2017 by John Wiley & Sons, Inc.
Companion Website: www.fiveminutevet.com/endocrinology

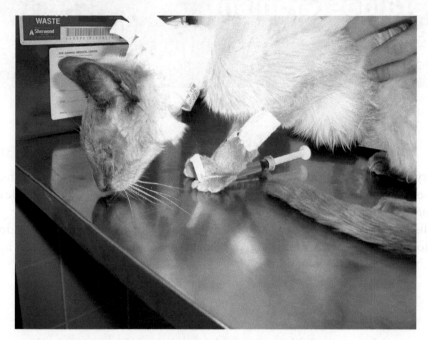

■ **Fig. 57.1.** Cat with primary hyperaldosteronism exhibiting cervical ventroflexion.

 # SIGNALMENT/HISTORY

- Only 49 cases of presumed or confirmed feline PHA have ever been reported.
- Affected cats were presented with a median age of 13 years (range 5–20 years).
- There is no apparent sex or breed predilection.

Historic Findings

- Loss of vision.
- PU/PD.
- Anorexia.
- Weight loss.
- Depression.
- Inability to jump.

Physical Examination

- Mydriasis.
- Hyphema.
- Retinal detachment.
- Intraocular hemorrhages.
- Muscle weakness – episodic or acute.

- Plantigrade stance of the hind limbs.
- Cervical ventroflexion.
- Lateral recumbency.
- Collapse.
- Pendulous abdomen.

Laboratory Abnormalities

- Hypokalemia (<3.5 mEq/l).
- Arterial hypertension (>170/100 mmHg).
- Elevated blood urea nitrogen (BUN) and creatinine.
- Elevated creatine kinase (CK).
- Hyperglycemia (less common).
- Hypophosphatemia (less common).
- Plasma aldosterone concentration (PAC) is increased.
- Plasma renin activity (PRA) is below or within the reference interval.

Screening Tests for PHA in Cats

- The ratio between the PAC and PRA, termed the aldosterone-to-renin ratio (ARR), has been widely accepted as the screening test of choice for PHA in cats.
- The combination of a high-normal or elevated PAC and a low PRA indicates persistent aldosterone synthesis in the presence of little or no stimulation by the rennin–angiotensin system.
- Cats with idiopathic bilateral nodular hyperplasia of the zona glomerulosa will have a PAC that may only be slightly elevated or within the upper limit of the reference range.
- In addition, the potassium concentration should also be considered when evaluating the PAC. In the presence of hypokalemia, even a mildly elevated aldosterone level can be regarded as inappropriately elevated.
- The Ohio State University (OSU) Reference Laboratory is one of the few laboratories that measures renin activity commercially for cats. A 2-ml frozen plasma blood sample is required for PRA determination. To preserve the enzymatic activity of renin, the sample must be cooled immediately and shipped on dry ice by overnight mail.
- In addition, it is suggested that a control sample from a healthy cat be included because reference values for PRA have not been established for cats at this laboratory.
- Basal urine aldosterone-to-creatinine ratio may be measured; however, if it is normal, a suppression test may be needed to document autonomous secretion of aldosterone.

Confirmatory Tests for PHA in Cats

- The suppression test with the greatest utility in cats is the fludrocortisone suppression test.
  - Fludrocortisone is administered at a dose of 0.05 mg/kg q. 12 h for 4 days.
  - A basal UACR $<7.5 \times 10^{-9}$ excludes PHA, while a value of $>45.9 \times 10^{-9}$ confirms it. Values between 7.5×10^{-9} and 45.9×10^{-9} indicate suppression by <50% and also confirm the diagnosis of PHA.

- Spirolactone and potassium-wasting diuretics be discontinued for at least 4 weeks.
- If the result of the ARR is inconclusive, other potentially interfering agents, such as beta-blockers, amlodipine, angiotensin-converting enzyme inhibitors (ACEIs) and angiotensin receptor blockers (ARBs) should be discontinued for 2 weeks if possible. Discontinuing these antihypertensive agents carries a risk of loss of control arterial pressure and further end-organ damage.

 # DIAGNOSTICS

- Diagnostic imaging techniques such as ultrasonography, magnetic resonance imaging (MRI), and computed tomography (CT) are used to identify adrenal abnormalities and, in the case of neoplasia, to evaluate possible extension into the caudal vena cava and the presence of distant metastasis.
- However, there are several limitations with regard to diagnostic imagery and its ability to determine an optimal treatment strategy for PHA. Functional neoplasms of the zona glomerulosa may not be large to be clinically relevant and may even be below the detection limit of ultrasonography, CT, or MRI.
- On the other hand, non-functional adrenocortical neoplasms may be readily visible with ultrasonography, CT or MRI, but may not cause clinical signs.

 # THERAPEUTICS

Surgery

- Unilateral adrenalectomy is the treatment of choice for confirmed unilateral PHA.
- Preoperative and perioperative hypokalemia should be controlled as well as possible by oral and intravenous supplementation.
- Perioperative complications have been reported, including intra-abdominal hemorrhage, thromboembolism, acute renal failure, and sepsis.

Medical Therapy

- Potassium supplementation.
- ARBs such as spironolactone. The initial dose is 2 mg/kg twice daily, increased as needed to control hypokalemia. A dose in excess of 4 mg/kg may cause anorexia, vomiting, and diarrhea.
- Persistent arterial hypertension is often treated successfully with the calcium channel blocker amlodipine, at an initial dose of 0.1 mg/kg once daily.
- In PHA due to bilateral adrenal hyperplasia, normokalemia can be sustained for long intervals with spironolactone alone or combined with low doses of potassium.

Prognosis

- After complete removal of a non-metastasized aldosterone-producing tumor, the prognosis is excellent.
- Cats that survive the immediate postoperative period continue to be clinically asymptomatic for one to several years.

Suggested Reading

Galac, S., Reusch, C.E., Kooistra, H.S., Rijnberk, A. (2010) Adrenals, in *Clinical Endocrinology of Dogs and Cats*, 2nd edition (eds A. Rijnberk, H.S. Kooistra), Schlütersche, Hannover, pp. 93–154.

Djajadiningrat-Laanen, S.C., Galac, S., Boroffka, S.A.E.B., Naan, E., IJzer, J., Kooistra, H.S. (2013) Evaluation of the oral fludrocortisone suppression test for diagnosing primary hyperaldosteronism in cats. *J. Vet. Intern. Med.*, **27**, 1493–1499.

Willi, B., Kook, P.H., Quante, S., Boretti, F., Sieber-Ruckstuhl, N.S., Grest, P., *et al.* (2012) Primary hyperaldosteronism in cats. *Schweiz. Arch. Tierheilkd.*, **154**, 529–537.

Djajadiningrat-Laanen, S.C., Galac, S., Cammelbeeck, S.E., van Laar, K.J., Boer, P., Kooistra, H.S. (2008) Urinary aldosterone to creatinine ratio in cats before and after suppression with salt or fludrocortisone acetate. *J. Vet. Intern. Med.*, **22**, 1283–1288.

Ash, R.A., Harvey, A.M., Tasker, S. (2005) Primary hyperaldosteronism in the cat: a series of 13 cases. *J. Feline Med. Surg.*, **7**, 173–182.

Lo, A.J., Holt, D.E., Brown, D.C., Schlicksup, M.D., Orsher, R.J., Agnello, K.A. (2014) Treatment of aldosterone-secreting adrenocortical tumors in cats by unilateral adrenalectomy: 10 cases (2002–2012). *J. Vet. Intern. Med.*, **28**, 137–143.

Author: Rhett Nichols DVM, ACVIM (Internal Medicine)

chapter 58

Canine Prostate Disease:

Benign Prostatic Hyperplasia, Cystic Benign Prostatic Hyperplasia, Prostatitis

DEFINITION

- Relatively common in sexually intact mature male dogs.
- Typically involves some degree of gland enlargement and overlapping clinical signs.
- Benign prostatic hypertrophy (BPH) is a spontaneous disease of aging intact males involving both hyperplasia and hypertrophy at the cellular level.
- Cystic BPH (CBPH) occurs when intraparenchymal fluid filled cysts develop in association with hyperplasia.
- Prostatitis (IP) is an inflammatory process, usually with a bacterial component, and often secondary to BPH. It may be acute or chronic.

ETIOLOGY/PATHOPHYSIOLOGY

- With age, the canine testes secrete increasing levels of estradiol, which alters the androgen:estrogen ratio.
- This endocrine change enhances increased levels of prostatic dihydrotestosterone, a testosterone metabolite via the enzyme 5-α-reductase, which mediates prostatic hyperplastic growth; enlargement is eccentric and not concentric making urethral compression less likely.
- This glandular hyperplasia frequently leads to the formation of cystic structures within the prostatic parenchyma.
- BPH is accompanied by increased vascularity and sterile inflammation.
- This alteration of the normal architecture of the prostate gland predisposes to bacterial colonization by interfering with normal defense mechanisms and by providing an environment that supports bacterial growth.
- Bacterial route of entry is usually via the urethra, although hematogenous spread is possible.
- Fungal prostatitis is rare.
- Other prostatic diseases may lead to prostatitis, such as squamous metaplasia, neoplasia, paraprostatic cysts.

Blackwell's Five-Minute Veterinary Consult Clinical Companion: Small Animal Endocrinology and Reproduction, First Edition. Edited by Deborah S. Greco and Autumn P. Davidson. © 2017 John Wiley & Sons, Inc. Published 2017 by John Wiley & Sons, Inc. Companion Website: www.fiveminutevet.com/endocrinology

Systems Affected

- Gastrointestinal
    - Enlarged gland may cause tenesmus and decreased diameter of stool.
    - Acute bacterial prostatitis can result in vomiting.
- Musculoskeletal
    - Pain/discomfort can result in a stilted, hindlimb lameness.
- Renal/urologic
    - Inflammatory debris can affect bladder.
    - Bacteria may extend into renal/urinary tract and testes.
- Reproductive
    - Affected dogs may be reluctant or unable to breed/ejaculate.
    - Alterations in prostatic fluid may lead to medical infertility.

 # SIGNALMENT/HISTORY

- Intact males of all breeds are affected.
- A higher prevalence has been reported in Doberman Pinschers and German Shepherd dogs.
- The author has also noted an increased incidence in Rhodesian Ridgebacks and Portuguese Water Dogs.
- There is no known genetic basis, although breed predisposition suggests there may be an inherited component to clinical disease.
- Mean affected age is 5–7 years, with a range of 1 year to more than 16 years.
- Clinical signs
    - Often no signs noted (BPH, CBPH).
    - Hemorrhagic preputial discharge not associated with urination, hemospermia, hematuria (BPH, CBPH), stranguria (IP).
    - Pain during breeding/semen collection (IP).
    - Tenesmus and/or ribbon-like stool.
    - With acute bacterial infection, can see fever, lethargy, pain, stilted gait, vomiting.

Risk Factors

- Non-neutered males.
- Exposure to estrogens (exogenous, Sertoli cell tumor, etc.) predisposes to squamous metaplasia.
- Impaired immunity will contribute to bacterial prostatitis.
- Bacterial cystitis can contribute high numbers of bacteria.

Historic Findings

- Blood in ejaculate as an incidental finding (BPH, CBPH).
- Hemorrhagic preputial discharge not associated with urination with no sign of clinical illness (BPH, CBPH).

- Frequently occurs after exposure to bitches in season causing sexual stimulation (BPH, CBPH).
- Occasionally straining to defecate or urinate.
- Systemic signs (febrile, depressed, etc.) seen with acute bacterial disease.

 ## CLINICAL FEATURES

- Routine physical examination is usually normal.
- Can see serosanguinous discharge from tip of penis.
- Combined rectal and abdominal palpation will allow palpation of the prostate, to evaluate for size, shape, symmetry, evidence of pain:
  - Uncomplicated BPH and CBPH will show varying degrees of enlargement, usually symmetrical, smooth, non-painful.
  - Cysts may alter symmetry and shape.
  - Bacterial prostatitis/severe inflammation will often be painful.
- With acute bacterial prostatitis may have signs of systemic disease (fever, etc.).

 ## DIFFERENTIAL DIAGNOSIS

- Other causes of prostatic enlargement include prostatic retention cysts, paraprostatic masses or cysts, neoplasia, prostatic abscess.
- Other causes of tenesmus include large intestinal disease, GI masses, foreign bodies.
- Other causes of urinary tract disease; urolithiasis, urinary bladder neoplasia, urinary bladder polyp.
- Other causes of pain and lameness; polyarthritis, diskospondylitis.
- Coagulopathy.

 ## DIAGNOSTICS

- Prostatic radiography
  - Survey radiographs help identify prostatic enlargement.
  - Contrast radiography may help characterize prostate size and shape, identify the location of cystic structures.
- Prostatic ultrasonography
  - Excellent and useful diagnostic tool but operator-dependent.
    - □ BPH characterized by increased parenchymal echogenicity with 'wagon wheel' appearance (Fig. 58.1).
    - □ CBPH characterized by parenchymal cysts containing hypoechoic fluid (Fig. 58.2).
    - □ IP characterized by both hypoechoic and hyperechoic non-homogenous parenchyma (Fig. 58.3).

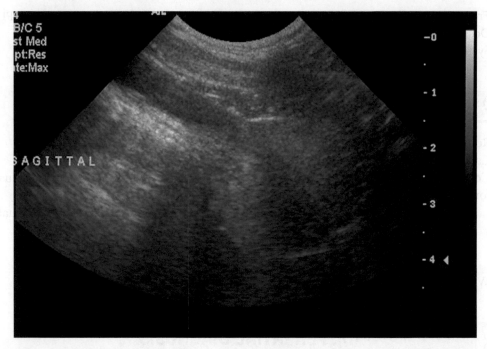

■ **Fig. 58.1.** Benign prostatic hyperplasia. 'Wagon wheel' appearance of parenchyma, moderate echogenicity. Image courtesy of T.W. Baker.

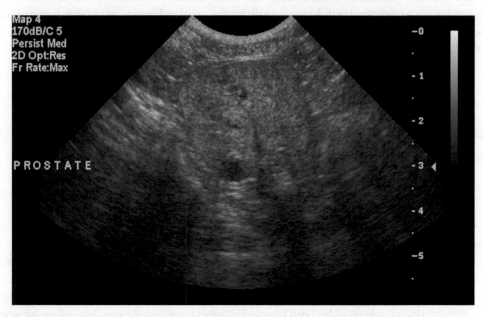

■ **Fig. 58.2.** Cystic benign prostatic hyperplasia. Variable hypoechoic cystic structures are evident in the parenchyma. Image courtesy of T.W. Baker.

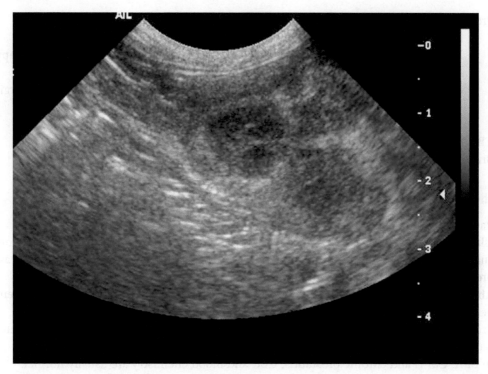

■ **Fig. 58.3.** Prostatitis. Non-homogenous, echogenic parenchyma with echogenic cystic structures (abscessation). Image courtesy of T.W. Baker.

    ☐ Ultrasonographic changes can be non-specific necessitating tissue sampling; all three conditions can occur together.
- Allows accurate measurements of length, width and depth of gland to be determined and followed over time.
- Allows visualization of internal architecture, abnormal fluid-filled cavities, stromal and parenchymal abnormalities.
- Allows guidance when performing fine-needle aspiration or percutaneous biopsy.
■ Prostatic fluid evaluation
- Ideal sample for cytology and microbial culture and sensitivity testing; limited by the ability to collect semen if the dog is painful; normal urethral flora must be differentiated.
- Obtained as third fraction during semen collection.
■ Prostatic wash/massage
- Useful when ejaculation cannot be obtained, to use for cytology and bacteriology.
- More likely to obtain neoplastic cells than in ejaculated sample.
■ Prostatic fine-needle aspiration
- Typically performed using transabdominal ultrasound guidance with sedation.
- Collect fluid and tissue for cytologic evaluation and culture and sensitivity testing.
- Also useful to drain fluid from cystic lesions.
- Can be contraindicated if abscess is suspected to avoid seeding abdomen with bacteria.

- Prostatic biopsy
  - Most accurate diagnostic tool via histopathology.
  - Indicated when less-invasive tests are non-diagnostic or response to initial therapy has been poor.
  - Obtained via ultrasound-guided percutaneous approach under sedation, or via surgical laparotomy.
  - Rarely necessary as other diagnostic methods are usually adequate.
- CBC/biochemistry panel/urinalysis.
- *Brucella canis* testing.

Pathological Findings

- Radiography may show prostatic enlargement.
- Ultrasonography will show prostatic enlargement, focal to multifocal areas of hyperechoic and/or hypoechoic tissue with inflammation/hyperplasia/neoplasia, anechoic cystic areas, prostatic capsular edema, and sublumbar lymphadenopathy.
- Abnormal prostatic fluid will contain large numbers of red blood cells indicating recent hemorrhage and/or leukocytes indicating inflammation.
- Prostatic fluid cultures should be quantitative in nature, to differentiate significant bacterial growth from the normal flora of the distal urethra.
- In BPH, CBPH and chronic prostatitis, CBC and blood chemistry are usually normal.
- In acute prostatitis, an increased WBC count with a left shift may be seen.
- Urinalysis results may be normal or show similar changes as seen on prostatic fluid analysis.

 THERAPEUTICS

- Since BPH/cystic BPH/prostatitis are hormonally influenced via testosterone, the main objective of treatment is to remove this hormonal influence.
- Surgical castration is the treatment of choice.
  - The prostate will begin to decrease in size within one week after castration, with complete involution within 4 months.
- Medical management is indicated in valuable breeding dogs, or in dogs that are not good surgical/anesthetic candidates.
  - Finasteride is currently the drug of choice for medical management. This 5-α-reductase inhibitor blocks the conversion of testosterone to dihydrotestosterone, which is responsible for BPH.
  - An initial dosage of 0.1–0.5 mg/kg PO, q. 24 h until repeat ultrasonography and prostatic fluid evaluation are normal.
  - Dosing frequency may then be slowly decreased to the lowest that controls clinical signs.
  - Treatment may be stopped for 5 days prior to breeding or semen collection to allow normal prostatic fluid volume.
  - Dogs may be maintained on finasteride indefinitely, but should be re-evaluated periodically with dosing changed as necessary.

- Bacterial prostatitis should be treated with appropriate antimicrobials, based on culture and sensitivity testing.
- In chronic infectious prostatitis, pH of the prostatic fluid should be considered when choosing an antibiotic to allow better penetration into the prostatic stroma, and therapy should be continued for 4–6 weeks.
- Surgical drainage and marsupialization can be indicated in chronic prostatitis with abscessation.

COMMENTS

Expected Course and Prognosis for BPH and CBPH

- Medical management is highly successful, safe and effective, but requires ongoing treatment and management.
- Castration is highly effective and essentially curative.

Expected Course and Prognosis for IP

- Guarded prognosis without aggressive antimicrobial therapy and follow-up.

See Also

TVT
Sertoli cell tumors
Prostatic adenocarcinoma
Prostatic transitional cell neoplasia

Suggested Reading

Smith, J. (2008) Canine prostatic disease: A review of anatomy, pathology, diagnosis, and treatment. *Theriogenology*, **70**, 375–383.

Sirinarumitr, K., Johnston, S.D., Kustritz, M.R., *et al.* (2001) Effects of finasteride on size of the prostate gland and semen quality in dogs with benign prostatic hypertrophy. *J. Am. Vet. Med. Assoc.*, **218** (8), 1275–1280.

Cohen, S.M., Taber, K.H., Malatesta, P.F., *et al.* (1991) Magnetic resonance imaging of the efficacy of specific inhibition of 5-alpha-reductase in canine spontaneous benign prostatic hyperplasia. *Magnet. Reson. Med.*, **21**, 55–70.

Purswell, B.J., Parker, N.A., Forrester, S.D. (2000) Prostatic diseases in dogs: A review. *Vet. Med.*, **95** (4), 315–321.

Gormley, G.J., Stoner, E., Bruskewitz, R.C., *et al.* (1992) The effect of finasteride in men with benign prostatic hyperplasia. *N. Engl. J. Med.*, **327** (17), 1185–1191.

Author: Melissa Goodman DVM

chapter 59

Reproductive Malignancies

CANINE TRANSMISSIBLE VENEREAL TUMOR (TVT)

DEFINITION

- Sexually transmitted disease of dogs.
- Increased prevalence in areas with temperate climates and urban environments with many free-roaming dogs.
- Enzootic in the Southern United States. Other enzootic regions outside of the United States include Central and South America, the Middle East, southeastern Europe, and certain regions in Africa.

ETIOLOGY/PATHOPHYSIOLOGY

- Round cell tumor thought to be of histiocytic origin.
- Transmitted directly from dog to dog, with coitus being the typical mode of transmission.
- Transmission occurs by exfoliation and then implantation of tumor cells within tissue.
- Transplantation of tumor cells can occur during coitus, through natural canine behaviors of sniffing and licking, and through damaged mucosal surfaces.

Systems Affected

- Reproductive – main systemic affected due to transmission of disease by coitus.
- Renal/urologic – can be affected as a consequence of penile or vaginal masses.
- Respiratory – nasal involvement can occur through sniffing of the mass in an affected animal and subsequent transplantation.
- Gastrointestinal – the oral cavity can be affected due to licking of the mass and then transplantation.

Blackwell's Five-Minute Veterinary Consult Clinical Companion: Small Animal Endocrinology and Reproduction, First Edition. Edited by Deborah S. Greco and Autumn P. Davidson. © 2017 John Wiley & Sons, Inc. Published 2017 by John Wiley & Sons, Inc.
Companion Website: www.fiveminutevet.com/endocrinology

SIGNALMENT/HISTORY

- Typically occurs in young sexually intact dogs of either gender.
- History usually involves a dog living in an endemic area or traveling to such an area.
- Dogs tend to have a history of free-roaming or contact with other dogs.
- No breed predispositions, but does occur more commonly in mixed-breed dogs.

Risk Factors

- Sexually intact dogs that are free-roaming and living in endemic areas.

CLINICAL FEATURES

- Latency period for tumor development can range from 2–6 months.
- Can undergo spontaneous remission and this will occur within 3 months following implantation.
- Spontaneous regression does not occur in immunodeficient dogs or young puppies.
- More likely to metastasize in immunodeficient dogs or young puppies.
- Classic appearance is a cauliflower-like friable mass.
- Commonly affects the external genitalia.
  - Male dogs: base of glans penis; requires retraction of penile sheath for identification.
  - Female dogs: caudally in the vagina or vestibule.
- Affected dogs usually have signs of discomfort (licking excessively) or hemorrhagic or serosanguinous discharge.
- Rarely metastasizes, but reported sites include regional lymph nodes, skin, brain, eyes, bone, kidney, and orbit.

DIFFERENTIAL DIAGNOSIS

- Other neoplasias of the genitalia such as squamous cell carcinoma, transitional cell carcinoma, leiomyomas, leiomyosarcomas, lymphoma, and mast cell tumors.
- Vaginal hyperplasia.
- Vulvovaginal or preputial foreign body.

DIAGNOSTICS

- A presumptive diagnosis can be made based on signalment, history, geographic location, and location of the mass. Adoption from an endemic area should raise the index of suspicion.
- General staging diagnostics recommended, though metastatic rate is low.
- Staging diagnostics include regional lymph node aspirates, thoracic radiographs, and abdominal ultrasound, basic blood work (CBC, chemistry panel), and a urinalysis.

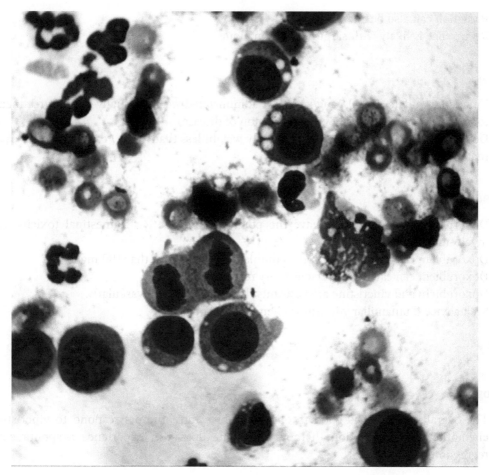

■ **Fig. 59.1.** Fine-needle aspirate cytology of canine venereal tumor. Note mitotic figure in center of field. Image courtesy of Dr Jane Sykes.

- A paraneoplastic erythrocytosis has been reported in a limited number of dogs.
- Diagnosis can be made by cytology or histopathology.
- On cytology, features include round to oval cells with abundant pale blue cytoplasm, prominent nucleoli, and numerous clear cytoplasmic vacuoles (Fig. 59.1).
- Histopathology can be used for confirmation of the diagnosis and immunohistochemistry can be used for diagnosing TVT involving unusual locations (usually from metastasis).

 THERAPEUTICS

- May spontaneously regress, though treatment recommended since this can be unreliable.
- Regression of the tumor is unlikely if it has been present for 6 months or longer.
- Medical therapy with vincristine offers a 90–95% complete response rate.

- Radiation can also be curative.
- Recurrence is likely with surgical excision alone.

Drugs

- Vincristine sulfate (0.5–0.7 mg/m^2) IV is administered weekly, usually for 2–6 treatments total (give two treatments beyond resolution of disease).
- Doxorubicin (30 mg/m^2 or 1 mg/kg if body weight less than 10 kg) can be used for cases that are resistant to vincristine.

Precautions

- Doxorubicin and vincristine have the potential to cause gastrointestinal toxicity and myelosuppression.
- Doxorubicin can be cardiotoxic at a cumulative dose greater than180 mg/m^2.
- Doxorubicin can cause a hypersensitivity reaction.
- Doxorubicin and vincristine are vesicants if administered perivascularly.
- Seek advice if unfamiliar with these chemotherapeutics.

 COMMENTS

Prognosis

- The overall prognosis is good to excellent since most tumors respond to vincristine chemotherapy or radiation therapy, and some dogs will experience a spontaneous regression.

Prevention

- Neuter intact dogs.
- Prevent dogs from roaming free.

Abbreviation

TVT = transmissible venereal tumor.

Suggested Reading

Withrow, S.J., Vail, D.M. (2007) *Withrow and MacEwen's Small Animal Clinical Oncology*, 4th edition. Saunders Elsevier, St Louis, pp. 799–804.

Mukaratirwa, S., Gruys, E. (2003) Canine transmissible venereal tumour: cytogenetic origin, immunophenoytpe, and immunobiology: a review. *Vet. Q.*, **25**, 101–111.

Das Utpal, Das Arup Kumar (2000) Review of canine transmissible venereal sarcoma. *Vet. Res. Commun.*, **24**, 545–556.

SERTOLI CELL TUMORS

 ## DEFINITION

- Derived from the sustentacular cells of Sertoli.
- Third most common testicular tumor in dogs (preceded by interstitial cell tumors and seminomas).
- Cryptorchidism is a risk factor, with 54% of Sertoli cell tumors occurring in intact cryptorchid male dogs.
- Metastasis is uncommon.

 ## ETIOLOGY/PATHOPHYSIOLOGY

Systems Affected

- Hemic/lymphatic/immune – secondary to hyperestrogenism which can cause pancytopenia.
- Reproductive – testicular organ is primary tissue affected and hyperestrogenism can cause changes to other reproductive organs.
- Skin/exocrine – hyperestrogenism can cause bilaterally symmetric alopecia and hyperpigmentation.

 ## SIGNALMENT/HISTORY

- Occurs in intact older male dogs, rarely cats.

Risk Factors

- Cryptorchid testes have a higher incidence of developing Sertoli cell tumors.

 ## CLINICAL FEATURES

- Regional or distant metastasis occurs in less than 15% of cases.
- If metastasis does occur, this tends to involve the regional lymph nodes and then liver, lungs, kidney, spleen, adrenal glands, pancreas, skin, eyes, and central nervous system.
- Clinical signs can be variable and associated with the primary tumor, metastasis, or paraneoplastic syndromes.
- A testicular mass can be found upon palpation or an enlarged testicle may be present.
- The contralateral testicle may be atrophied.
- Semen quality can decline in unilateral cryptorchids.
- In cryptorchid dogs, there can be a mass effect in the abdominal cavity or inguinal space.
- Testicular torsion can occur secondary to enlargement from neoplastic transformation; these cases present as an acute abdomen.

- Signs of feminization can occur, such as bilaterally symmetric alopecia and hyperpigmentation, pendulous prepuce, gynecomastia, galactorrhea, and atrophy of the penis.
- Hyperestrogenism can have severe hematologic consequences including blood dyscrasias and bone marrow hypoplasia that can present as pancytopenia.
- Squamous metaplasia of the prostate can occur.

DIFFERENTIAL DIAGNOSIS

- Other testicular neoplasia such as interstitial cell tumors and seminomas.
- Benign testicular diseases such as orchitis, epididymitis, and testicular torsion.
- Other neoplasia or granuloma as a differential for abdominal or inguinal space masses.

DIAGNOSTICS

- Fine-needle aspiration and cytology may allow for a presumptive diagnosis, but histopathology is required for definitive diagnosis.
- CBC findings can include anemia, leukopenia, and thrombocytopenia secondary to hyperestrogenism.
- Some dogs with signs of hyperestrogenism can have elevated levels of estradiol-17β.
- Staging diagnostics including thoracic radiographs and abdominal ultrasound are recommended, since many dogs affected are geriatric.
- Abdominal ultrasound can be helpful to identify an abdominal mass or mass within the inguinal space for cryptorchid dogs, and can allow for the evaluation of regional lymph nodes.
- Ultrasound of the testicles may allow for differentiation between neoplastic and non-neoplastic testicular disorders and permit guided fine-needle aspiration (Fig. 59.2).
- Cytology of preputial mucosa can show estrogen effect: cornification of mucosal epithelial cells (Fig. 59.3).

THERAPEUTICS

- The treatment of choice is orchiectomy with scrotal ablation.
- Supportive care is necessary for cases with hyperestrogenism and associated pancytopenia.
  - This includes blood products and antibiotics.
  - Therapy may be required for weeks before signs of regeneration occur.

COMMENTS

Prognosis

- Good prognosis for most cases.
- Guarded prognosis for cases with pancytopenia secondary to hyperestrogenism.

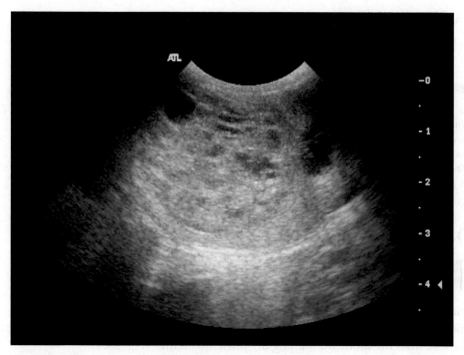

■ **Fig. 59.2.** Intratesticular Sertoli cell tumor. Image courtesy of T.W. Baker.

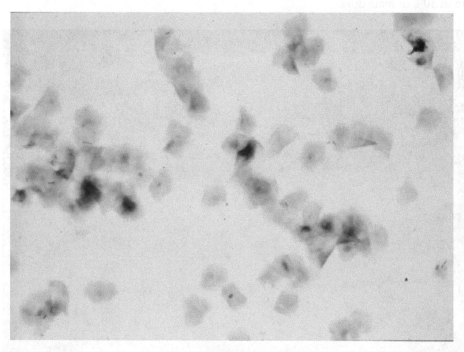

■ **Fig. 59.3.** Preputial cytology showing estrogen effect on the mucosal epithelial cells. Note angular cytoplasmic margins, pyknotic or absent nuclei.

See Also

Hyperestrogenism (estrogen toxicity)

Suggested Reading

Grieco, V., Riccardi, E., Greppi, G.F., *et al.* (2008) Canine testicular tumours: a study on 232 dogs. *J. Comp. Pathol.*, **138**, 86–89.

Withrow, S.J., Vail, D.M. (2007) *Withrow and MacEwen's Small Animal Clinical Oncology*, 4th edition. Saunders Elsevier, St Louis, pp. 637–641.

Sherding, R.G., Wilson, G.P., III, Kociba, G.J. (1981) Bone marrow hypoplasia in eight dogs with Sertoli cell tumor. *J. Am. Vet. Med. Assoc.*, **178**, 497–501.

PROSTATIC TRANSITIONAL CELL CARCINOMA (TCC)

 DEFINITION

- Epithelial malignancy that originates from the transitional epithelium.
- Prostatic TCC can be an extension of TCC of the urinary bladder into the prostate, or can originate from the urothelium lining the prostatic urethra (Fig. 59.4).
- TCC most commonly affects the urinary bladder, but has been reported to affect the prostate in 30% of male dogs.

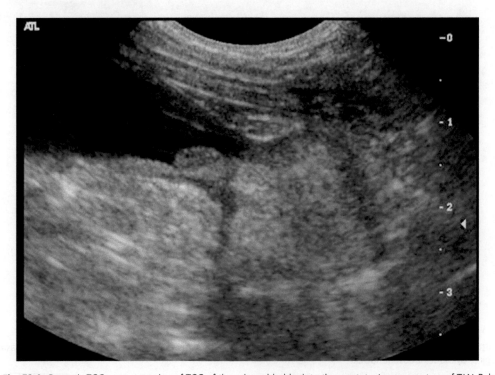

■ **Fig. 59.4.** Prostatic TCC as an extension of TCC of the urinary bladder into the prostate. Image courtesy of T.W. Baker.

- Lymph node metastases are present in 16% of dogs at diagnosis, and distant pulmonary metastases are present in 14% at diagnosis. Infrequently metastasizes to bone.
- Uncommon in cats.

ETIOLOGY/PATHOPHYSIOLOGY

- The etiology is likely multifactorial and is largely unknown. Certain risk factors have been identified that play a role in the development of this cancer.

Systems Affected

- Renal/urologic – compression or invasion of the urethra is common and eventually can result in urethral obstruction and associated post-renal azotemia.
- Nervous – local invasion of prostatic TCC into lumbar vertebrae and nerve roots.
- Gastrointestinal – tenesmus due to compression of the rectum by the enlarged neoplastic prostate and sublumbar lymphadenopathy.
- Musculoskeletal – bone metastasis occurs uncommonly. Paraneoplastic hypertrophic osteopathy has been reported with TCC.

SIGNALMENT/HISTORY

Signalment

- Scottish Terriers, Shetland Sheepdogs, Beagles, Wirehaired Fox Terriers, and West Highland White Terriers are the most commonly affected breeds by TCC.
- Middle-aged to older dogs with a reported mean age of 11 years.

Risk Factors

- Several risk factors have been identified in dogs.
- Exposure to topical insecticides and herbicides.
- Exposure to marshes that have been sprayed for mosquito control.
- Obesity.
- Breed – Scottish Terriers have an 18-fold increased risk of developing TCC compared to mix-breed dogs. Other commonly affected breeds include Shetland Sheepdogs, Beagles, Wirehaired Fox Terriers, and West Highland White Terriers.
- Possibly cyclophosphamide administration.
- Topical products containing fipronil are not associated with an increased risk of TCC.

Historic Findings

- The most common historical findings are lower urinary tract signs such as stranguria, dysuria, pollakiuria, and hematuria.
- Tenesmus or constipation.

- Lumbar pain and gait abnormalities including ataxia can be associated with local invasion of prostatic adenocarcinoma into the lumbar vertebrae.

 # CLINICAL FEATURES

- Rectal palpation – the prostate gland can be enlarged, asymmetric, firm, and immobile. Occasionally there can be pain upon palpation. Sublumbar lymphadenopathy can also be digitally palpated.
- Abdominal palpation can reveal a caudal abdominal mass effect. Abdominal palpation may also reveal and enlarged urinary bladder secondary to urethral obstruction.
- Pelvic limb ataxia and paralysis.

 # DIFFERENTIAL DIAGNOSIS

- Other prostatic neoplasms, including adenocarcinoma or squamous cell carcinoma.
- Other less common types of prostatic neoplasia include fibrosarcoma, leiomyosarcoma, hemangiosarcoma, and lymphoma.
- Benign prostatic diseases including benign prostatic hyperplasia, prostatitis, and prostatic cysts.

 # DIAGNOSTICS

- Complete staging diagnostics are recommended in all patients suspected of having prostatic TCC.
- CBC – often normal.
- Serum biochemistry – post-renal azotemia secondary to urethral obstruction.
- Urinalysis – pyuria, hematuria, bacteriuria. Examination of urine sediment can allow for diagnosis in 30% of cases. Note that reactive, non-neoplastic, transitional cells can appear similar to neoplastic transitional cells.
- Urine culture is recommended in all patients to evaluate for a secondary urinary tract infection. There is a possible risk of tumor seeding along the needle tract when obtaining a urine sample by cystocentesis.
- Thoracic radiographs – metastatic pattern can be variable in some cases and the radiograph appearance includes nodular interstitial opacity, diffuse unstructured interstitial opacity, or alveolar infiltrates.
- Abdominal radiography – can be useful if abdominal ultrasonography is not available, but unlikely to show a mass within the urinary bladder if present. Prostatomegaly with mineralization and prostatic enlargement as well as sublumbar lymphadenopathy can be visualized.
- Abdominal ultrasound – useful to evaluate for prostatic enlargement, prostatic mineralization, involvement of the urinary bladder, and sublumbar lymphadenopathy. If urethral obstruction is present, there may be evidence of hydroureter and hydronephrosis (Fig. 59.5a,b). Used as the main modality to assess response to therapy, but not always

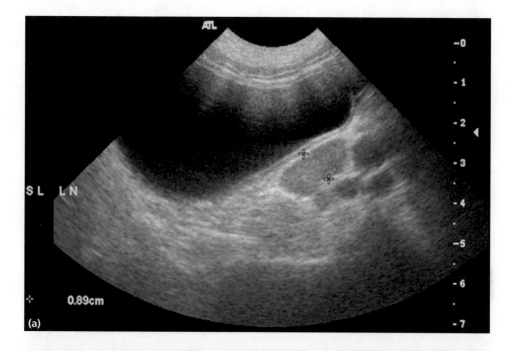

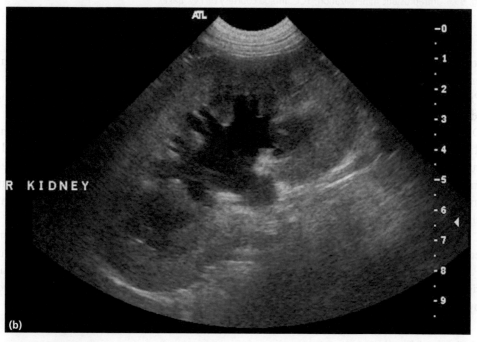

■ **Fig. 59.5.** (a) Sublumbar lymphadenomegaly associated with prostatic neoplasia. (b) Hydroureter and hydrone-phrosis associated with prostatic TCC causing obstruction of the distal ipsilateral ureter. Images courtesy of T.W. Baker.

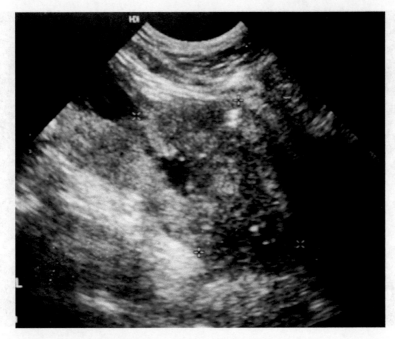

■ **Fig. 59.6.** Intraprostatic mineralization, TCC. Image courtesy of T.W. Baker.

reliable for monitoring urinary bladder masses due to changes in urinary bladder volume and changes in ultrasonography operator.
- Prostate mineralization (based on ultrasonographic or radiographic assessment) in neutered dogs is highly suggestive of prostatic neoplasia (Fig. 59.6).
- Definitive diagnosis requires histopathologic examination of affected tissues and can help differentiate between prostatic adenocarcinoma. Tissue samples are usually obtained by surgical biopsy. Care must be taken when performing surgical biopsy because tumor seeding can occur with tumor manipulation. Precautions that should be taken include changing of gloves and surgical instruments when handling the tumor and copious flushing should be employed.
- Cystoscopy with biopsy can be helpful if tumor extension into the urinary bladder is present. Brush cytology is a sampling method that may yield a diagnosis during this procedure.
- Prostatic aspirate using ultrasound-guidance for cytologic evaluation. There is a possible risk of tumor seeding along the needle tract with this procedure and is therefore avoided by some clinicians.

Pathological Findings

- The majority of tumors are papillary infiltrative and of intermediate to high grade. Carcinoma *in situ* is rare in dogs.

THERAPEUTICS

- Prostatectomy is associated with a high complication rate, but can be considered for local disease confined within the prostatic capsule. TCCs are highly exfoliative, and tumor seeding is a concern with surgical intervention. Care must be taken to change gloves and surgical instruments and to lavage the abdomen after surgery.
- Palliative radiation to relieve clinical symptoms and improve quality of life.
- Urethral stenting to relieve urethral obstruction. Complications can include incontinence, recurrence of obstruction, and stent dislodgement.

Drugs

- NSAIDs
    - Dogs treated with NSAIDs survived significantly longer than dogs that did not receive NSAIDs for prostatic carcinomas.
    - Piroxicam (0.3 mg/kg PO, q. 24 h with food) is the primary NSAID used for TCC, with a response rate of 18%.
    - Deracoxib (3 mg/kg PO, q. 24 h) is an alternative to piroxicam, with a response rate of 17%.
    - Consider use concurrent gastric protectants such as famotidine.
    - Chemotherapy for local and metastatic disease can result in clinical responses.
- Several protocols exist and most include the use of piroxicam:
    - Mitoxantrone (5 mg/m^2 IV, q. 3 weeks) combined with piroxicam has a response rate of 35%.
    - Carboplatin (300 mg/m^2 IV, q. 3–4 weeks) combined with piroxicam has a response rate of 38%.
    - Vinblastine (2.0–2.5 mg/m^2 IV, q. 2 weeks) used alone has a response rate of 36%.
    - Gemcitabine (800 mg/m^2 IV, q. 1 week over 30–60 minutes) in combination with piroxicam has a response rate of 26%.
    - Cisplatin (50–60 mg/m^2 q. 3–4 weeks IV) has been used historically with a response rate of 20% when used alone. Combination of cisplatin with piroxicam is not recommended due to the risk of nephrotoxicity.
- Stool softeners if tenesmus is present.
- Other oral analgesics may be necessary for pain especially if there is evidence of skeletal metastasis or extension of the tumor into the lumbar region.

Precautions

- Seek advice if unfamiliar with these chemotherapeutics.
- Monitor all patients receiving chemotherapy for myelosuppression.
- Cisplatin should never be administered to cats due to fatal pulmonary edema.
- Cisplatin needs to be administered with saline diuresis due to the risk of nephrotoxicity.

- Carboplatin is excreted renally and precaution must be taken in patients with pre-existing renal disease.
- Do not administer NSAIDs to patients with gastrointestinal ulcers and renal insufficiency.

 COMMENTS

- Prognosis guarded for most patients.
- Most dogs will eventually develop urethral obstruction.

Abbreviations

TCC   = transitional cell carcinoma.
NSAID = Non-steroidal anti-inflammatory drug.

See Also

BPH, CBPH and Prostatitis

Suggested Reading

Arnold, E.J., Childress, M.O., Fourez, L.M., *et al.* (211) Clinical trial of vinblastine in dogs with transitional cell carcinoma of the urinary bladder. *J. Vet. Intern. Med.*, **125**, 1385–1390.

McMillan, S.K., Boria, P., Moore, G.E., *et al.* (2011) Antitumor effects of deracoxib treatment in 26 dogs with transitional cell carcinoma of the urinary bladder. *J. Am. Vet. Med. Assoc.*, **239**, 1084–1089.

Marconato, L., Zini, E., Linder, D., *et al.* (2011) Toxic effects and antitumor response of gemcitabine in combination with piroxicam treatment in dogs with transitional cell carcinoma of the urinary bladder. *J. Am. Vet. Med. Assoc.*, **238**, 1004–1010.

Withrow, S.J., Vail, D.M. (2007) *Withrow and MacEwen's Small Animal Clinical Oncology*, 4th edition. Saunders Elsevier, St Louis, pp. 649–657.

Mutsaers, A.J., Widmer, W.R., Knapp, D.W. (2003) Canine transitional cell carcinoma. *J. Vet. Intern. Med.*, **17**, 136–144.

PROSTATIC ADENOCARCINOMA

 DEFINITION

- Malignant glandular epithelial neoplasm of the canine prostate gland.
- Uncommon canine malignancy having a low prevalence of 0.2–0.6% based on necropsy studies.
- Extremely rare in cats.
- Occurs in both sexually intact and castrated dogs.
- Locally invasive and metastatic tumor with metastasis occurring to regional lymph nodes, lungs, and skeleton.

ETIOLOGY/PATHOPHYSIOLOGY

- Etiology is largely unknown in dogs.
- Most canine prostatic adenocarcinomas do not express androgen receptors and therefore, do not seem to be influenced by androgens. This is also supported by the fact that castration appears to be a risk factor for the development of this neoplasm.

Systems Affected

- Renal/urologic – compression or invasion of the urethra occurs by neoplastic prostatic enlargement.
- Nervous – local invasion of the neoplastic prostate into lumbar vertebrae and nerve roots.
- Musculoskeletal – axial skeletal metastasis occur in 24–42% of patients.
- Gastrointestinal – tenesmus secondary to compression of the rectum by the enlarged neoplastic prostate and sublumbar lymphadenopathy.
- Respiratory – compromise due to pulmonary metastasis.

 ## SIGNALMENT/HISTORY

- Most commonly presents in medium- to large-breed dogs with an average age of 10 years.
- Usually presents in castrated male dogs.

Risk Factors

- Castration early in life may be a risk factor for the development of canine prostate cancer.

Historic Findings

- Lower urinary tract signs such as stranguria and dysuria.
- Hematuria may be present.
- Tenesmus with the presence of ribbon-like stools due to either enlargement of the prostate gland or sublumbar lymph nodes.
- Lumbar pain and gait abnormalities including due to local tumor invasion into the lumbar vertebrae.

 ## CLINICAL FEATURES

- On rectal palpation, the prostate gland can feel enlarged, asymmetric, firm, and immobile. Occasionally there can be pain upon palpation. Sublumbar lymphadenopathy can also be felt upon rectal palpation.
- Abdominal palpation may be painful and may reflect a caudal abdominal mass effect. Abdominal palpation may also reveal an enlarged urinary bladder secondary to urethral obstruction.

- Pelvic limb ataxia and paralysis.
- Lumbar pain or other sites of bone pain of the axial skeleton.
- Thin body condition.
- Dyspnea, respiratory distress.

 ## DIFFERENTIAL DIAGNOSIS

- Other prostatic neoplasms, especially transitional cell carcinoma, or squamous cell carcinoma.
- Other less common types of neoplasia of the prostate that have been reported include fibrosarcoma, leiomyosarcoma, hemangiosarcoma, and lymphoma.
- Benign prostatic hyperplasia.
- Prostatitis.
- Prostatic cysts.

 ## DIAGNOSTICS

- Complete staging diagnostics are recommended in all patients suspected of having prostatic adenocarcinoma.
- CBC – anemia, leukocytosis.
- Serum biochemistry panel – elevated ALP, rarely hypercalcemia, post-renal azotemia secondary to urethral obstruction.
- Urinalysis – pyuria and hematuria. Bacteriuria can be present due to secondary urinary tract infection. Malignant epithelial cells can be present upon evaluation of fresh free-catch samples.
- Urine culture recommended in all patients due to secondary urinary tract infections. There is a possible risk of tumor seeding along needle tract when performing cystocentesis.
- Thoracic radiographs – evaluate for pulmonary metastasis which can appear as a nodular or interstitial pattern. Sternal lymphadenopathy can be present.
- Abdominal radiography – can be useful if abdominal ultrasonography is not available. Prostatomegaly with mineralization and prostatic enlargement. Sublumbar lymphadenopathy. Lytic bone lesions of the pelvis or lumbar vertebrae.
- Abdominal ultrasound – prostatic enlargement, prostatic mineralization, sublumbar lymphadenopathy. If urethral obstruction is present, there may be evidence of hydroureter and hydronephrosis.
- Prostate mineralization (based on ultrasonographic or radiographic assessment) in neutered dogs is highly suggestive of prostatic neoplasia.
- Prostatic aspirate using ultrasound guidance. There is a possible risk of tumor seeding along needle tract with this procedure; hence, this technique is avoided by some clinicians.
- Prostatic biopsy usually performed surgically. Ultimately, histopathologic assessment is required to differentiate prostatic adenocarcinoma from prostatic transitional cell carcinoma.

Pathological Findings

- Prostatic adenocarcinoma is thought to originate from the glandular portion of the prostate. This is in contrast to prostatic transitional cell carcinoma, which originates from the urothelium that lines the prostatic urethra.

 THERAPEUTICS

- Prostatectomy is associated with a high complication rate, but it can be considered for local disease confined within the prostatic capsule.
- Palliative radiation to relieve clinical symptoms and improve quality of life.
- Urethral stenting to relieve urethral obstruction. Complications can include incontinence, recurrence of obstruction, and stent dislodgement.

Drugs

- NSAIDs are important for their role in therapy for prostatic adenocarcinoma and for pain relief. Dogs treated with NSAIDs survived significantly longer than dogs that do not receive NSAIDs for prostatic carcinomas.
- Chemotherapy for local or metastatic disease can result in clinical responses. Agents used include carboplatin, cisplatin, gemcitabine, or doxorubicin.
- Other oral analgesics that can be combined with an NSAID safely should be used for pain relief.
- Stool softeners if tenesmus is present.
- Intravenous bisphosphonates such as pamidronate may help relieve pain if skeletal metastases are present.
- Gastric protectants should be used as indicated in patients on NSAIDs.

 COMMENTS

- Prognosis guarded and poor if skeletal metastasis is present.
- Most dogs eventually develop disseminated disease or urethral obstruction.

Abbreviations

NSAID = Non-steroidal anti-inflammatory drug.

See Also

BPH, CBPH and Prostatitis

Suggested Reading

LeRoy, B.E., Northrup, N. (2009) Prostate cancer in dogs: comparative and clinical aspects. *Vet. J.*, **180**, 149–162.

Bradbury, C.A., Westropp, J.L., Pollard, R.E. (2009) Relationship between prostatomegaly, prostatic mineralization, and cytologic diagnosis. *Vet. Rad. Ultrasound*, **50**, 167–171.

Withrow, S.J., Vail, D.M. (2007) *Withrow and MacEwen's Small Animal Clinical Oncology*, 4th edition. Saunders Elsevier, St Louis, pp. 641–646.

Weisse, C., Berent, A.C., Todd, K., *et al.* (2006) Evaluation of palliative stenting for management of malignant urethral obstruction in dogs. *J. Am. Vet. Med. Assoc.*, **229**, 226–234.

Sorenmo, K.U., Goldschmidt, M.H., Shofer, F.S., *et al.* (2004) Evaluation of cyclooxygenase-1 and cyclooxygenase-2 expression and the effect of cyclooxygenase inhibitors in canine prostatic carcinoma. *Vet. Comp. Oncol.*, **2**, 13–23.

Authors: Danielle O'Brien DVM, DACVIM (Oncology), Carlos Rodriguez DVM, PhD, DACVIM (Oncology)

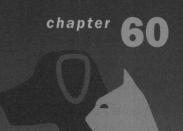

Canine Semen Abnormalities – Orchitis/Epididymitis

chapter 60

DEFINITION

- Orchitis is inflammation of the testis or testes, while epididymitis is inflammation of the epididymis or epididymides.
- Conditions may be seen separately, together or with extension through the vaginal tunic to the scrotum.
- Semen abnormalities found with orchitis and/or epididymitis are seen in the second fraction, and include the presence of bacteria or other causative agents, inflammatory cells (including polymorphonuclear cells and macrophages with engulfed sperm), red blood cells, and lymphocytes.

SIGNALMENT/HISTORY

- Dogs of any age, but more often younger postpubertal dogs. Signs include:
  - Unilateral or bilateral swelling of the scrotum.
  - May be acute onset or found chronically.
  - Systemic illness acutely with pyrexia, lethargy, scrotal edema, hind limb lameness.
  - Painful scrotum.
  - Semen grossly abnormal in color or viscosity.
  - Infertility.
  - Testicular and/or epididymal asymmetry.
  - Firm, fibrotic, often irregularly shaped testes and/or epididymides on palpation.
  - Acutely difficult to palpate scrotal contents.
  - Semen and spermatozoal abnormalities found during routine breeding soundness evaluation.

CLINICAL FEATURE

Congenital

- None described.

Blackwell's Five-Minute Veterinary Consult Clinical Companion: Small Animal Endocrinology and Reproduction,
First Edition. Edited by Deborah S. Greco and Autumn P. Davidson. © 2017 John Wiley & Sons, Inc.
Published 2017 by John Wiley & Sons, Inc.
Companion Website: www.fiveminutevet.com/endocrinology

Acquired

- Trauma – bite wounds, vehicular trauma.
- Sequel to hematocele or hydrocele.
- Specific infections of the reproductive tract – Brucellosis; Leishmaniasis.
- Opportunistic organisms – *E. coli*, *Proteus vulgaris*, *Staphylococcus* spp., *Streptococcus* spp., *Mycoplasma* spp., Ureaplasma, Blastomyces.
- Ascending infection from prostate/bladder/urethra.
- Intratesticular injections of zinc gluconate/L-arginine.

DIFFERENTIAL DIAGNOSIS

- Excessive numbers of kinked or coiled tails may be iatrogenic artifacts caused by the eosin-nigrosin stain; re-examine the sample under phase-contrast microscopy after dilution with formalin phosphate-buffered saline solution, or use other stain available in clinic, especially any modified Wright Giemsa stain (e.g., Diff-Quik® or Protocol™).

DIAGNOSTICS

Other Laboratory Tests

- CBC and biochemical profile to assess severity of illness, especially in acute cases.
- Ultrasound of scrotum and contents.
- Cytology and aerobic and anaerobic culture of ejaculate (especially second fraction) or, if unattainable, ultrasound-guided aspirate of affected area(s) of testis(es), epididymis(ides), scrotal contents.
- Brucellosis – rapid slide agglutination test – used as a screening test (D-Tec® CB, Zoetis); recommend re-check of dogs with positive slide test with agar gel immunodiffusion test (Cornell University Diagnostic Laboratory) or bacterial culture of whole blood or lymph node aspirate or PCR or semen or whole blood.

Imaging

Ultrasonography to diagnose/differentiate causes of scrotal content asymmetry including ultrasound-guided aspirate in acute or biopsy in chronic cases.

Diagnostic Procedures

- Bright-field microscopic evaluation of stained dry-mount slide of semen (see Differential Diagnosis, above).
- Common sperm abnormalities would include heads without tails, defects of head, midpiece and tail, oligozoospermia, and asthenozoospermia.
- Acrosome staining (see Spermatozoal Abnormalities).

- In semen or directed aspirate, look for polymorphonuclear cells, macrophages ± engulfed sperm, lymphocytes, round cells – possibly immature sperm or lymphocytes.

Pathologic Findings

- After acute episode, testicular biopsy seeking continued inflammation or infection or blockages due to sperm granuloma(s) and/or fibrosis.
- Testicular atrophy and/or enlarged epididymis require repeated sperm and ultrasound assessments at monthly intervals, and may lead one to perform a unilateral orchiectomy.

 THERAPEUTICS

- Depends on the cause and severity of infection/inflammation – bacteria treated usually according to sensitivity for minimum 6 weeks while recognizing poor penetration by penicillins, cephalosporins and aminoglycosides.
- Intravenous fluids and supportive care in severe infections.
- *Brucella* cases – bilateral orchiectomy and a minimum 8 weeks of enrofloxacin with monthly RSAT tests; continuing antibiotic for one month past being negative on two successive tests; placement in a home without young children or elderly or immunocompromised individuals; continued six monthly testing after enrofloxacin is discontinued.
- Leishmania cases will usually not survive as the disease is usually severe and also zoonotic.
- Unilateral closed orchiectomy for unilateral severe orchitis or epididymitis.
- Sexual rest for penetrating wounds of the scrotum.
- Remove any environmental issues that could lead to scrotal trauma, scrotal dermatitis, self-mutilation (consider Elizabethan collar).
- Use NSAIDs as necessary for the animal's comfort.

Contraindications

- If enlargement of testis or epididymis is slow to resolve or animal remains obviously systemically ill for more than a few days, consider closed unilateral orchiectomy.

Patient Monitoring

- Depending on cause, semen evaluation should be performed 65–80 days after resolution of clinical signs, or after unilateral orchiectomy.
- If unilateral orchiectomy is performed on a dog that is peripubertal, sperm numbers may greatly improve after treatment, but this is less likely in mature dogs.

Prevention/Avoidance

- Address concurrent prostatic disease, access to traumatic encounters such as aggressive intact male dogs.
- Palpate scrotal contents daily.

Suggested Reading

Johnston, S.D., Root Kustritz, M.V., Olson, P.N.S. (2001) Disorders of the canine testes and epididymis, in *Canine and Feline Theriogenology*, W.B. Saunders Co., Philadelphia, pp. 312–332.

Davidson, A.P., von Dehn, B.J. Schlafer, D.J. (2015) Adult onset lymphoplasmacytic orchitis in a labrador retriever stud dog. *Topics Comp. Anim. Med.*, 04/2015; **30** (1). DOI:10.1053/j.tcam.2015.03.003

Hesser, A.C., Davidson, A.P. (2015) Spermatocele in a South African Boerboel Dog. *Topics Comp. Anim. Med.*, 03/2015; **30**(1). DOI:10.1053/j.tcam.2015.03.001

Author: Cathy J. Gartley DVM, DVSc, DACT

chapter 61

Semen Peritonitis

DEFINITION

- Peritonitis secondary to intra-abdominal semen deposition.

ETIOLOGY/PATHOPHYSIOLOGY

- This is an uncommon cause of an acute abdomen and peritonitis which occurs secondary to the intra-abdominal deposition of semen. Reactive peritonitis results from foreign protein antigens in the prostatic portion of semen, with the potential for vaginal flora causing secondary bacterial contamination of the peritoneal space. Affected bitches can develop the systemic inflammatory response syndrome (SIRS), the body's response to circulating inflammatory mediators. Intra-abdominal deposition of semen can occur if semen leaks out of the fallopian tube(s) during natural breeding, or if perforation of the vagina or cervix occurs during artificial insemination, or via accidental copulation with a tie in a recently ovariohysterectomized estrual bitch.

Systems Affected

- Reproductive.
- Cardiovascular.
- Hemic/Lymphatic/Immune.

SIGNALMENT/HISTORY

Risk Factors

- Recent natural or artificial breeding of an estrual bitch.
- An unsupervised estrual bitch which may have had access to a male.

Blackwell's Five-Minute Veterinary Consult Clinical Companion: Small Animal Endocrinology and Reproduction, First Edition. Edited by Deborah S. Greco and Autumn P. Davidson. © 2017 John Wiley & Sons, Inc. Published 2017 by John Wiley & Sons, Inc.
Companion Website: www.fiveminutevet.com/endocrinology

- Ovariohysterectomy performed when bitch is in proestrus/estrus; possible access to a male dog; less than 14 days post operative period. Less than 10 days post ovariohysterectomy performed when the bitch is in proestrus/estrus, with possible access by a male.

Historic Findings

- Estrus.
- Acute onset of lethargy.
- Marked and progressive abdominal pain.
- Recently bred or inseminated.
- Proestrus or estrus at the time of recent ovariohysterectomy.

 ## CLINICAL FEATURES

- An acute onset of abdominal pain, ± sanguinous vaginal discharge, lethargy, fever, tachycardia, free abdominal fluid, shock.

 ## DIFFERENTIAL DIAGNOSIS

- Pyometra, uterine rupture, uterine torsion, uroabdomen, other causes of acute abdomen outside of the genitourinary tract.

 ## DIAGNOSTICS

- Physical examination and abdominal ultrasound to differentiate from other causes of acute abdomen, and to identify and sample free abdominal fluid.
- Abdominal fluid glucose to peripheral blood glucose differential to identify septic peritoneal fluid.
- CBC, serum chemistries, PT/PTT, careful cytologic evaluation of peritoneal fluid.
- Vaginal cytology to confirm estrus.

Pathological Findings

- Intra-abdominal suppurative inflammation.
- Free abdominal fluid.
- Leukocytosis, sometimes degenerative.
- Prolongation of prothrombin time and partial thromboplastin time are possible.
- Vaginal cytology consistent with estrus (>70% superficial epithelial cells).
- Sperm cells could be evident in the vaginal cytology or in cytology of vaginal discharge.
- Inflammatory peritoneal fluid cytology with sperm cells sometimes present (Fig. 61.1).
- Neutrophilic phagocytosis of sperm cells possible (Fig. 61.2).

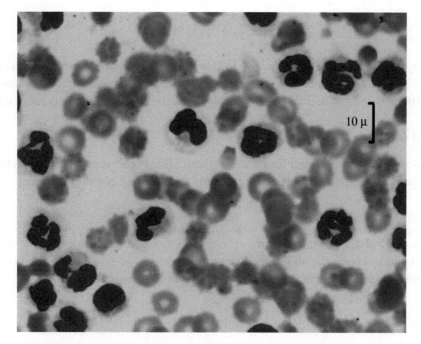

■ **Fig. 61.1.** Peritoneal fluid cytology showing sperm cell head and toxic neutrophils.

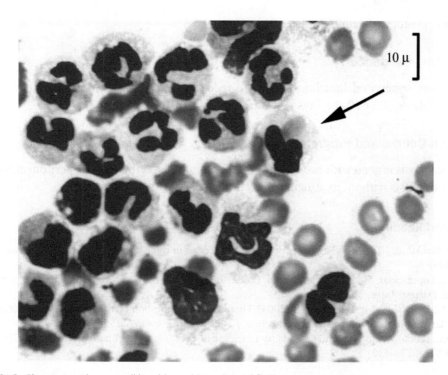

■ **Fig. 61.2.** Phagocytosed sperm cell head (arrow) in peritoneal fluid.

THERAPEUTICS

- Surgical exploration with peritoneal lavage to reduce the inflammation associated with the intra-peritoneal deposition of semen is the treatment of choice. Because of the risk of secondary bacterial infection, an abdominal fluid culture sample should be obtained prior to peritoneal lavage.

Drug(s) of Choice

- Intravenous fluids as indicated for peritonitis and SIRS, broad-spectrum bactericidal antibiotics, pain medication as indicated, preferably narcotic and not non-steroidal.

Surgical Considerations

- This is a surgical disease and requires an exploratory laparotomy to assess the reproductive tract and to lavage the abdomen. Ovariohysterectomy is usually indicated if a rent is not identified in the genitourinary tract, or it cannot be repaired.

COMMENTS

Patient Monitoring

- Routine postoperative monitoring.

Prevention/Avoidance

- Prevent unsupervised breedings, separate recently ovariohysterectomized bitches from intact male dogs for 10–14 days post surgery.

Expected Course and Prognosis

- The prognosis is good with prompt surgical exploration and therapeutic peritoneal lavage.
- Poor prognosis without treatment for peritonitis.

Suggested Reading

Held, J.P., Blackford, J.T. (1984) Vaginal perforation after coitus in three mares. *J. Am. Vet. Med. Assoc.*, **185**, 533–534.

Yaniz, J.L., Lopez-Bejar, M., Santolaria, P., *et al.* (2002) Intraperitoneal insemination in mammals: a review. *Reprod. Domest. Anim.*, **35**, 75–80.

Slater, L.A., Davidson, A.P., Dahlinger, J. (2004) Theriogenology question of the month. Acute peritonitis secondary to intra-abdominal semen deposition. *J. Am. Vet. Med. Assoc.*, **225** (10), 1535–1537.

Morey, D.L. (2006) Acute peritonitis secondary to traumatic breeding in the bitch. *J. Vet. Emerg. Crit. Care Soc.*, **16** (2), 128–130.

Author: Laura Slater DVM

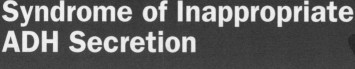
Syndrome of Inappropriate ADH Secretion

DEFINITION

- The syndrome of inappropriate antidiuretic hormone secretion (SIADH) is characterized by persistent production of arginine vasopressin (AVP) despite decreased plasma osmolality.

ETIOLOGY/PATHOPHYSIOLOGY

- SIADH is caused by inappropriate secretion of AVP. This, combined with unrestricted water intake, results in excessive renal tubular reabsorption of water, extracellular volume expansion, and hyponatremia.

Systems Affected

- Endocrine/renal/metabolic.

Incidence/Prevalence

- Rare.

SIGNALMENT/HISTORY

Species

- Dogs and cats.

Mean Age and Range

- Any age.

Blackwell's Five-Minute Veterinary Consult Clinical Companion: Small Animal Endocrinology and Reproduction, First Edition. Edited by Deborah S. Greco and Autumn P. Davidson. © 2017 John Wiley & Sons, Inc. Published 2017 by John Wiley & Sons, Inc.
Companion Website: www.fiveminutevet.com/endocrinology

Signs

- The clinical features of SIADH are related to severity of the hyponatremia (usually <125 mEq/L) and the rate at which the serum sodium concentration is lowered.
  - The principal signs are neurologic, such as weakness, lethargy, tremor, seizures, and coma.
  - Polyuria and polydipsia has been is noted in some cases.
  - Many animals, especially those being treated for central diabetes insipidus (CDI) with excessive dosages of synthetic AVP (DDAVP), are asymptomatic.

 ## CLINICAL FEATURES

- Idiopathic.
- Drug reaction.
- Encephalitis.
- Hydrocephalus.
- Brain tumor.
- Sequelae to hypophysectomy for pituitary-dependent Cushing's disease.
- Has been associated with *Dirofilaria immitus* infestation and low-sodium diet.
- Excessive administration of DDAVP in dogs properly diagnosed and misdiagnosed with CDI.

 ## DIFFERENTIAL DIAGNOSIS

- The diagnosis of SIADH begins with the exclusion of other causes of hyponatremia such as:
  - Hypoadrenocorticism.
  - Hypothyroidism.
  - Recent diuretic use.
  - Pseudohypernatremia secondary to extreme hyperproteinemia or hyperlipidemia.
  - Hospital-acquired fluid imbalance.

 ## DIAGNOSTICS

CBC/Biochemistry/Urinalysis

- CBC is often unremarkable.
- Serum biochemistry shows marked hyponatremia, and calculated or measured osmolality is low.
- Urinalysis results may be variable. Urine specific gravity may be low but >1.010 in animals with polyuria. However, urine specific gravity and osmolality is invariably higher than plasma values. Urine and plasma osmolality should be measured concurrently to allow the correct interpretation of results.

Other Laboratory Tests

- Plasma ADH concentration (not practical or readily available).
- CSF analysis if neurologic disease is suspected.
- ACTH response test.
- Thyroid function testing.
- Heartworm test.

Imaging

- MRI or CT scan if a brain tumor is suspected.
- Chest radiographs to rule out neoplasia or heartworm disease.

Criteria for Diagnosing SIADH

- A diagnosis of SIADH is based on the following criteria:
  - Exclusion of other causes of hyponatremia (see Differential diagnosis).
  - Serum or plasma hypoosmolality (P_{osm} <280 mOsm/kg).
  - Inappropriately concentrated urine (>100 mOsm/kg), although usually >P_{osm}.
  - Natriuresis (>30 mEq/l) despite hyponatremia.
  - Correction of hyponatremia with fluid restriction.

 THERAPEUTICS

Appropriate Health Care

- If SIADH secondary to drug therapy is suspected, the medication should be immediately discontinued.
- Therapy for asymptomatic SIADH is moderate water restriction.
- Symptomatic hyponatremia may require more aggressive management. This can be accomplished by judicious administration of hypertonic saline (3–5%). The aim of treatment is to resolve clinical signs by slowly increasing the serum sodium concentration to 125 mEq/l over 6–8 hours. The increase in sodium concentration should be carefully monitored, and should not exceed 0.5 mEq/l/h.

Medications

Drugs

- In human medicine, a number of drugs are available for the treatment of SIADH. Receptor-specific AVP antagonists block the action of AVP in the renal tubule and thus promote water excretion. To date, there has been only limited use of these drugs in the treatment of SIADH in veterinary medicine. These agents are referred to as V2 receptor antagonists.

Patient Monitoring

- Monitoring advice and frequency of re-check office visits is based on the underlying cause.
- In general, treatment is adjusted according to the patient's clinical signs and serum sodium concentration.
- Laboratory tests such as PCV, total solids, and serum sodium are useful for monitoring hydration status, and can help determine the optimal dose of DDAVP and frequency of dosing for animals being treated for CDI.

Possible Complications

- Anticipate recurrence of hyponatremia and complications associated with the primary cause of the syndrome (e.g., brain tumor).

Expected Course and Prognosis

- The condition is usually permanent unless caused by a drug reaction.
- The prognosis is dependent on the underlying cause. For example, if the cause is idiopathic, the prognosis is good. If the cause is a brain tumor, the prognosis is guarded to poor.

See Also

Hyponatremia

Abbreviations

ADH = antidiuretic hormone
AVP = arginine vasopressin
CDI = central diabetes insipidus
CT = computed tomography
DDAVP = l-desamino-8-d-arginine vasopressin
MRI = magnetic resonance imaging
PCV = packed cell volume
P$_{osm}$ = plasma osmolality
SIADH = syndrome of inappropriate antidiuretic hormone secretion

Suggested Reading

Feldman, E.C., Nelson, R.W. (2006) *Canine and Feline Endocrinology and Reproduction*, 3rd edition. WB Saunders, Philadelphia.
Mooney, C.T., Peterson, M.E. (2012) *BSAVA Manual of Canine and Feline Endocrinology*, 4th edition. British Small Animal Veterinary Association, Gloucester.
Rijnberk, A., Koostra, H.A. (2010) *Clinical Endocrinology of Dogs and Cats*, 2nd edition. Schlutersche Verlagsgesellschaft, Hanover.

Author: Rhett Nichols DVM, ACVIM (Internal Medicine)

chapter 63

Uterine Inertia

DEFINITION

- Uterine inertia is described in two contexts:
  - Primary uterine inertia – Complete failure to initiate first-stage labor.
  - Secondary uterine inertia – Lack of strength or frequency or both in an existing labor pattern, making the labor pattern ineffective at fetal delivery.

ETIOLOGY/PATHOPHYSIOLOGY

- Primary Uterine Inertia – cause is not clearly defined. Hypotheses include lack of hormone stimulus, overstretched uterus. Major risk is fetal compromise related to lack of placentation from prolonged gestation.
- Secondary Uterine Inertia – exhausted myometrium, hypocalcemia, hypoglycemia, dehydration. Secondary inertia can occur at any point during whelping/queening. Failure to move from first stage to second stage, as well as extreme delay between fetal deliveries, are both examples of secondary inertia. Assessment for fetal malposition should be ruled out before the diagnosis of inertia is made, as an obstructive dystocia may be the primary diagnosis.

SIGNALMENT/HISTORY

Primary Uterine Inertia

- Can be completely asymptomatic. Could be suspect in gestations that are more than about 67 days post LH surge, or up to 67 days after the last breeding with an un-timed breeding. In monitored whelpings (*n* = 15 000) the incidence of primary inertia was less than 1%. In the monitored group most bitches established a labor pattern, but were unable to move into second-stage labor without medical management. Temperature changes (hypothermia) were not a reliable indication for the presence of labor or the documentation of

Blackwell's Five-Minute Veterinary Consult Clinical Companion: Small Animal Endocrinology and Reproduction,
First Edition. Edited by Deborah S. Greco and Autumn P. Davidson. © 2017 John Wiley & Sons, Inc.
Published 2017 by John Wiley & Sons, Inc.
Companion Website: www.fiveminutevet.com/endocrinology

primary inertia. Symptoms of parturition were also not a reliable source for diagnosis, as bitches or queens may be symptomatic 48 hours prior to the onset of an actual labor pattern of contractions. Documentation of inertia is best accomplished using tocodynamometry specifically designed for use in animals (Fig. 63.1a,b).

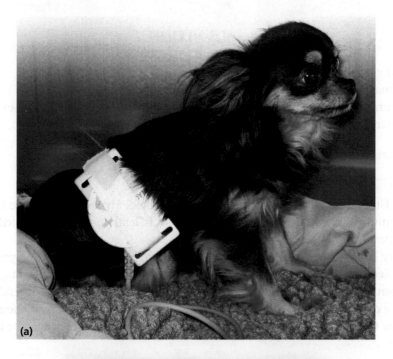

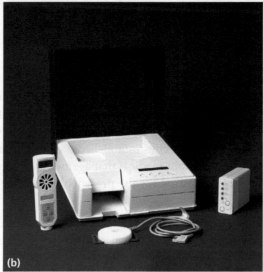

■ **Fig. 63.1.** (a) A Chihuahua bitch fitted with sensor for a tocodynamometry session. (b) Tocodynamometry unit: modem, recorder and sensor, and hand-held Doppler probe.

Secondary Uterine Inertia

- Occurs after the animal has established a 'labor pattern' of contractions. These patterns vary greatly within species and within breeds, but the presence of an organized pattern of contractions, as documented by either expert palpation or by a tocodynamometer, is the only method to ascertain that the animal is in labor – that is, experiencing myometrial contractions that are progressing in frequency and strength (Fig. 63.2). Normal pregnancies will typically exhibit one to three contractions per hour for the last 7 days of gestation. This frequency of contractions is considered normal (Fig. 63.3). The diagnosis of secondary inertia is most commonly made during parturition when delays in fetal deliveries occur. However, in monitored whelpings/queenings it is not unusual for secondary inertia to develop after 10 hours of active labor *prior to* actual fetal deliveries. The largest risk of secondary inertia is that the occurrence of placental detachments will increase as the prolonged contracting myometrium will shear off the placental sites. In whelpings that are not monitored with tocodynamometry the animal may present with symptoms of labor that have not progressed to stage 2 or a span of time from last fetal delivery of >2 hours, excessive straining, and/or uteroverdin. If the animal is not being monitored with tocodynamometry it may be difficult for the practitioner to differentiate a dystocia from inertia, as excessive abdominal straining may be the result of a lack of strength to the uterine contractions rather than a malpositioned fetus.

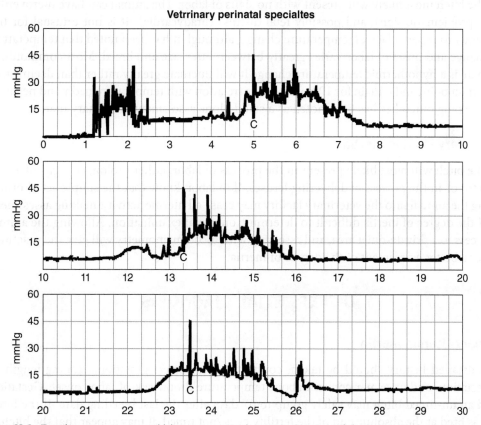

■ Fig. 63.2. Tocodynamometry; normal labor pattern. Y-axis, contraction strength in mmHg; X-axis, time in minutes (contraction duration).

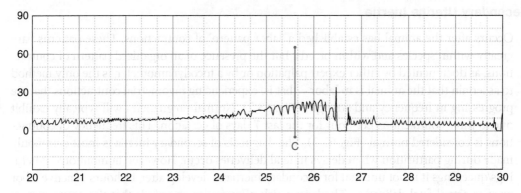

■ **Fig. 63.3.** Tocodynamometry; normal single contraction during 8th gestational week. Y-axis, contraction strength in mmHg; X-axis, time in minutes (contraction duration).

CLINICAL FEATURES

Primary Uterine Inertia

- The bitch most likely will present with no signs of labor. The animal can have uteroverdin (a problematic sign), and possibly fetal distress (bradycardia). It is not unusual for the owner to report a lack of temperature change, although it has been noted that temperature change and onset of labor varies greatly between litter size and breed. Most commonly, if there is a hypothermic temperature change it will fluctuate greatly rather than decline to a certain point and remain for 12 hours. No correlation with temperature nadir and negative whelping outcomes has been noted as a stand-alone assessment of primary inertia.

Secondary Uterine Inertia

- The bitch will most likely present in the process of labor; either prolonged signs of active labor or in the process of delivering fetuses. If in labor, know that the simple act of bringing the animal into the veterinary facility may cease all uterine activity, making assessment of the degree of inertia difficult to determine on visual examination. Allowing the animal access to a private-quiet area, and assessing with tocodynamometry will give the practitioner a better assessment of the degree of inertia.

DIFFERENTIAL DIAGNOSIS

Primary Uterine Inertia

- A detailed history should be taken, confirming the correct gestational timing-length of gestation, and/or owner concern about temperature drops/lack of labor onset. Gestation in an un-timed bitch may safely go up to 67 days after the last breeding date. If the bitch was bred at the absolute end of the fertility cycle/not timed, it may appear that the bitch is over-due, especially with multiple breeding dates. Conception may occur 3–4 days AFTER the last breeding date. The overwhelming tendency of breeders to breed early/frequently in the heat cycle without any progesterone timing can make determining actual due dates difficult. Serum progesterone levels <2 ng/ml indicate that the animal should whelp in the next 24–36 hours, and can be helpful in the diagnosis of primary inertia.

Secondary Uterine Inertia

- A detailed history should be taken, confirming the described onset of labor or actual documented onset by tocodynamometry. Normal length of first-stage labor when using tocodynamometry is 8–12 hours, outlying 16–18 hours for some breeds. This is the length of time that has been documented as normal, using tocodynamometry, prior to the delivery of the first fetus, barring the presence of fetal distress. Ask the owner about the use of uterotonics; Red Raspberry, Caulophyllum, Oxytocin, Calcium (PO or injectable). Arbitrary use of any of these substances, especially early in the labor, can cause a metabolic dystocia. This author STRONGLY discourages the use of Red Raspberry and Caulophyllum as their effect can be very difficult to regulate and they can have deleterious effects on fetal well-being. Other uterotonic medications, if not used correctly, may cause uterine tetany rather than treat inertia. Differential diagnosis of atony versus a normal labor pattern is best accomplished by the use of a tocodynamometer. External uterine monitoring is the most accurate way to assess for the presence/absence of an adequate labor pattern versus the presence of inertia (Fig. 63.4). After active labor is established, progesterone assessments are of little benefit.

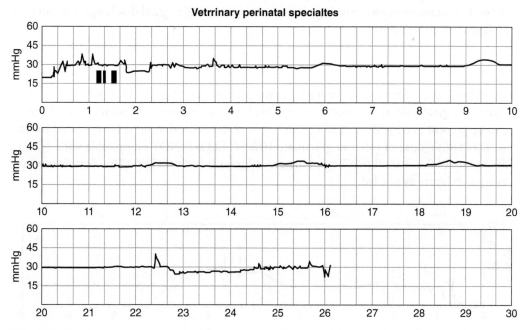

Fig. 63.4. Tocodynamometry; uterine inertia. Y-axis, contraction strength in mmHg; X-axis, time in minutes (contraction duration).

THERAPEUTICS

Primary Uterine Inertia

- If the animal is indeed past dates assess for the presence of viable fetuses (ultrasound). Examine serum progesterone levels, but be aware that there are breeds such as Mastiffs than can run a very low baseline progesterone level normally and may not be experiencing primary inertia. If any evidence of fetal compromise and the gestation is considered 'term' an immediate C-section is suggested. Generally, medical management of true primary inertia with a viable litter is not successful; operative intervention is encouraged. If the litter is not viable, a discussion can be instituted to allow the animal to try and deliver the demised fetuses rather than go through the risk/expense of a C-section.

Secondary Uterine Inertia

- Medical management with uterotonic agents is a good option as long as fetal well-being is documented, or the owner is aware that there may be fetal compromise if fetal well-being is not assessed. Optimally, documentation of the degree of inertia is a first priority, using a tocodynamometer. Subsequent management (medical or surgical) should be based on information from the tocodynamometer and documented objective response to medications or the presence of fetal distress (Fig. 63.5). If tocodynamometry is not available, the practitioner may need to base a positive response to uterotonic medications by evaluating subjective signs; increased panting/restlessness, increasing vaginal discharge, presentation of fetus, expulsive efforts.

Medical Management

- Oxytocin is the primary drug for inertia management; however, the effectiveness of oxytocin can be greatly decreased without available (cellular) calcium. A 'calcium-based' inertia can be present even with normal serum levels of ionized calcium. It is suggested to start with a loading dose of calcium gluconate 10% SC (23% is NOT compatible with SC use) at the rate of 0.5–1.0 ml per 5 kg of maternal (gravid) body weight. This dose is repeated every 4–6 hours as needed.

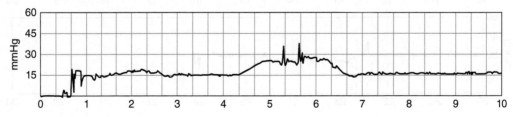

■ **Fig. 63.5.** Tocodynamometry; improved labor pattern in bitch with inertia (as in Fig. 63.4) following medical management. Y-axis, contraction strength in mmHg; X-axis, time in minutes (contraction duration).

Oxytocin

- Optimal management of inertia is accomplished by titrating oxytocin doses to improve the labor pattern, using objective assessments from a uterine tocodynamometer. If tocodynamometry is not available, begin initial management with 0.5–1 unit of oxytocin (Note: UNITS not ml) SQ or IM. Note that successful oxytocin dosing is not based on maternal weight. If no response in 30 minutes (after IM dose) or 45 minutes (after SQ dose), increase dose by 1 unit from first dose, and administer IM. If no increase in labor activity is noted, repeat oxytocin again, doubling the last dose and administering the dose IM. Intravenous administration is not recommended unless concurrent tocodynamometry is available, as uterine tetany can be very rapid with IV doses of oxytocin.
- Once adequate contractions are established it is expected that subsequent doses of oxytocin, sometime in small incremental increases of 0.5–1 unit, will be needed to maintain an effective labor pattern. Micro doses of oxytocin have been shown to be much more effective and safer for both the bitch/queen as well as the fetuses. Larger doses of oxytocin will initially cause uterine tetany, preventing forward movement of the fetuses, and eventually saturating the oxytocin receptors in the myometrium, causing a complete inertia.
- If tocodynamometry is not available, medical management should be accompanied by serial fetal heart rate monitoring. If fetal deceleration occurs after the administration of oxytocin, further medical management is contraindicated.

Hydration/Hypoglycemia

- Dehydration and hypoglycemia will contribute to secondary inertia. Bitches may be inappetent for days and with the increased metabolic requirements of both pregnancy and labor, optimal fluid/glucose levels may not be present for both the bitch and fetuses. Hydration with IV fluids, containing balanced electrolytes and dextrose, may contribute greatly to a more rapid resolution of inertias, and resolution of mild fetal distress.

 COMMENTS

- Primary inertia is very commonly misdiagnosed. Contributing to this diagnosis is the over-anxious owner who is constantly bombarded by incorrect information on the internet, or who has a "…dog show to go to this weekend" and "…simply wants them delivered". It is the practitioner's responsibility to assess both the animal's readiness for labor and/or if the animal is actually overdue. Other signs used to evaluate whether a bitch is at or past term gestation include the presence/absence of a flaccid vulvovaginal area, the presence/absence of mammary development with expressible colostrum in at least the caudal four mammary glands, and the presence of normal fetal heart rates. With favorable parameters it may be advisable to wait and continue to monitor the pregnancy for another 12–24 hours, during which time a progesterone level can be assessed for further information. With any date calculation errors, fetuses that are too premature to survive present a large risk for early surgical intervention.

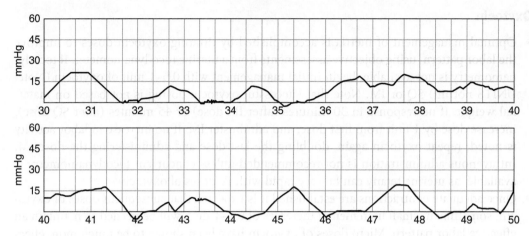

■ **Fig. 63.6.** Tocodynamometry; uterine hypercontractility. Y-axis, contraction strength in mmHg; X-axis, time in minutes (contraction duration).

■ Secondary inertia can be very difficult to evaluate without the use of tocodynamometry. 'Guessing' at adequate oxytocin doses can cause a hyperstimulation of the existing contraction pattern. Excessive oxytocin can make what was a normal labor pattern now a dystocia because of hyperstimulation of the uterus (Fig. 63.6).

See Also

Dystocia
Cesarean Section Elective or Emergency

Suggested Reading

Davidson, A.P. (2012) Reproductive causes of hypocalcemia. *Topics Compan. Anim. Med.*, **27** (4), 165–6.
Davidson, A.P. (2011) Primary uterine inertia in four Labrador bitches. *J. Am. Anim. Hosp. Assoc.*, **47** (2), 83–88.
Davidson, A.P. (2003) Obstetrical monitoring in dogs. *Vet. Med.*, **June**, 508–516.
Copley, K. (2009) Parturition Management 15,000 Whelpings Later; and Outcome-based analysis. Clinical Theriogenology Proceedings of the Society for Theriogenology, American College of Theriogenologists, Albuquerque, New Mexico.
Hollinshead, F.K., *et al.* (2007) Serum Calcium and Parathyroid Concentrations in the Whelping Bitch. Proceedings of the 32nd WSVA Congress, Sidney, Australia.

Author: Karen Copley RNC BSN

chapter 64

Evaluation of Ovulation with Ultrasound

INDICATIONS

- The detection of the day of ovulation is the most important factor to determine the optimal breeding time.
- Ultrasound is one of the best ways to detect ovulation and identify the most fertile period, but it has limitations on its use (multiple examinations, operator expertise).
- The mains indications are:
  - Choosing the best time for artificial insemination with chilled or frozen semen.
  - Estimation of the number of follicles.
  - Detection of ovulation versus follicular maturation failure.
  - Optimize treatment options in cases with pathology (e.g., guided aspiration of ovarian cysts).

EQUIPMENT

- A quality ultrasound machine is needed
- Frequency of probes:
  - 7.5 MHz is ideal in most bitches.
  - 10–12 MHz if small bitches or queen.
  - Sectorial probes are easier to handle.

PROCEDURE

- Shave the area around the 3rd or 4th lumbar spaces, just caudal to the kidneys (the right ovary is more cranial than the left ovary).
- Sedation is generally not needed.
- Positioning the bitch or queen (Figs 64.1 and 64.2):
  - Standing position
  - Dorso-lateral (more comfortable with use of cushions)

Blackwell's Five-Minute Veterinary Consult Clinical Companion: Small Animal Endocrinology and Reproduction, First Edition. Edited by Deborah S. Greco and Autumn P. Davidson. © 2017 John Wiley & Sons, Inc. Published 2017 by John Wiley & Sons, Inc.
Companion Website: www.fiveminutevet.com/endocrinology

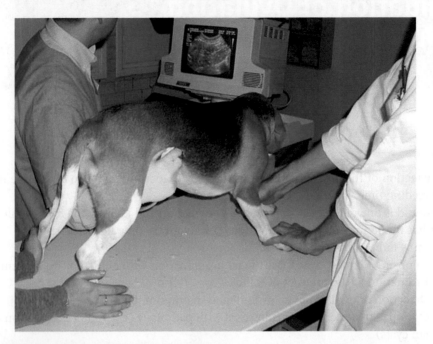

■ **Fig. 64.1.** Ultrasound of the bitch in a standing position.

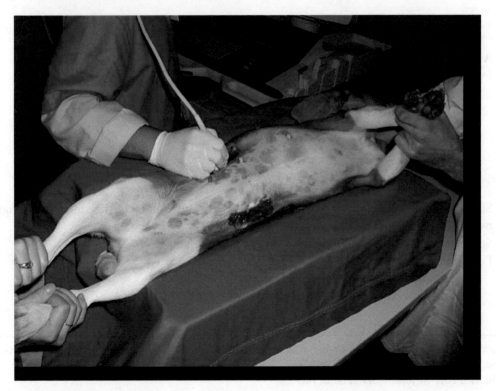

■ **Fig. 64.2.** Ultrasound of the bitch in a dorsal position.

Location of the Ovaries

- Very superficial.
- Find the caudal part of the ispsilateral kidney.
- Move the probe a few centimeters behind the kidney (longitudinal/sagittal view is better).
- If necessary change the positioning of the bitch.
- Compared with the kidney, the localization of the ovaries can be:
  - medio-caudal;
  - caudo-lateral; or
  - ventral.

At the Start of Pro-Estrus

- Ovaries are often localized more ventrally
- The outline becomes easy to identify:
  - Ovarian size: 1.5 cm × 1.0 cm
- Follicles are numerous and have a thin wall:
  - Follicular size: 2–5 mm.
  - Rapid increase in size at the end of proestrus.

Pre-Ovulatory Period (Fig. 64.3)

- Ovarian size is increased to about 3.0 cm × 1.5 cm.
- Follicles:
  - Lower number than in pro-estrus (selection).
  - Rapid increase from around the 7th day of heat.

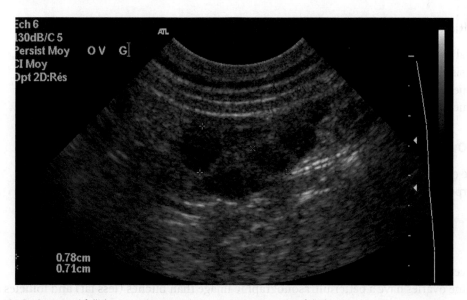

■ **Fig. 64.3.** Ovary and follicles just prior to ovulation; cursors measuring follicle size.

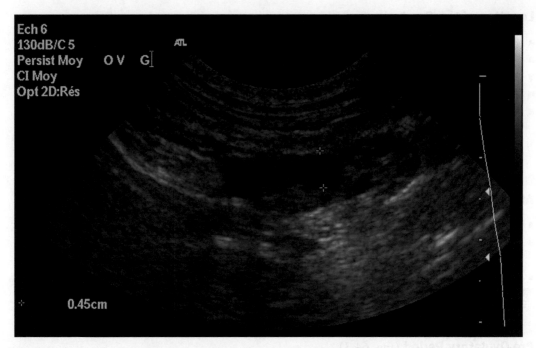

■ **Fig. 64.4.** Ovary and follicles at time of ovulation; cursors mark collapsing follicle.

- Maximal size just before ovulation (6 mm to 1.0 cm).
- Follicular wall is thick (1 mm): probably due to the pre-ovulatory luteinization.

Ovulation (Figs 64.4 and 64.5)

- Total or partial disappearance of follicular cavities.
- Persistence of intra-ovarian small structures.
- Some non-ovulated follicles may persist.
- Some free fluid originating from the follicles regressing can be find around the ovary.

Post-Ovulatory Period (Fig. 64.6)

- The ovaries have an irregular outline.
- Corpora lutea appear with thicker wall and an hypoechoic center.

 COMMENTS

- Queens need a quiet environment.
- Feline ovaries have a better ultrasonographic image than bitches (less fat) and follicles are smaller in size (0.25–0.35 cm).

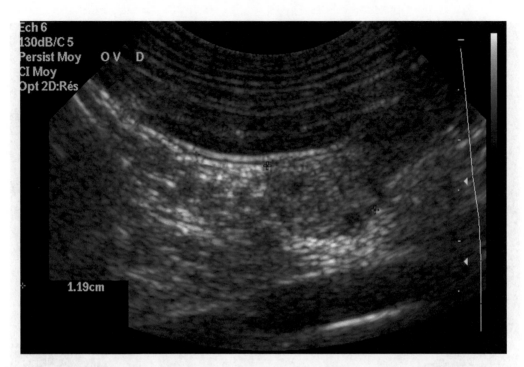

■ **Fig. 64.5.** Ovary immediately post ovulation; (+) marking ovarian height at cranial pole.

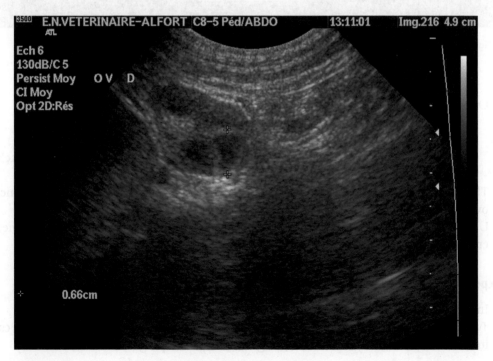

■ **Fig. 64.6.** Ovary with corpora lutea marked by cursors.

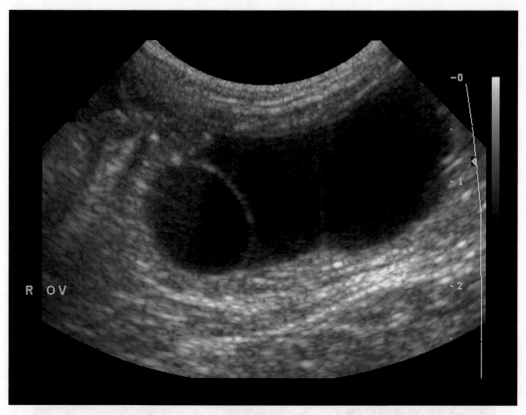

■ **Fig. 64.7.** Ovary with hypoechoic follicular cyst (cranial pole).

■ Ovulation can be especially difficult to detect in some cases:
  • Obese animal
  • Poor skin or coat quality, unshaven (e.g., Shar Peis, Chow-Chows).
  • Pre-ovulatory follicles are similar to early corpora lutea; knowledge of the bitch's vaginal cytology or serum progesterone is important.
■ The time of ovulation between the left and the right ovary has no significant difference; ovulation is completed in a maximum of 24 hours in both ovaries.
■ Ultrasound studies for ovarian pathology such as follicular or luteal cysts can complement endocrine evaluation (Fig. 64.7).

Expected Course and Prognosis

■ Improve fertile breedings.
■ Twice-daily ovarian ultrasound scans are best, but even performed once daily, it can increase the precision of ovulation timing compared with progesterone assays alone.

Suggested Reading

Concannon, P.W. (2000) Canine Pregnancy: predicting parturition and timing of events of gestation. Available at: www.ivis.org.

England, G., Concannon, P.W. (2002) Determination of the optimal breeding time in the bitch: basic considerations. Available at: www.ivis.org.

Hase, M., *et al.* (2000) Plasma LH and progesterone levels before and after ovulation and observation of ovarian follicles by ultrasonographic diagnosis system in dogs. *J. Vet. Med. Sci.*, **62** (3), 243–248.

Marseloo, N., Fontbonne, A., Bassu, G., *et al.* (2004) Comparison of ovarian ultrasonography with hormonal parameters for the determination of the time of ovulation in bitches. 5th International Symposium on Canine and Feline Reproduction, Sao Paulo, Brazil.

Rivière, S., Marseloo, N., Noël, F., *et al.* Comparison of ovulation estimated by ovarian ultrasonography with vaginal smears, hormonal parameters, sexual behavior and reproductive performances in beagle bitches. Fourth EVSSAR Congress, Barcelona, Spain.

Author: Giovana Bassu DVM, DECAR

Ultrasonographic Gestational Aging in the Bitch and Queen

Chapter 65

INDICATIONS

- Gestational aging can be obtained by ultrasonographic measurement of extra fetal and fetal structures, even when the day of breeding or the day of ovulation are unknown.
- Ultrasonographic gestational aging is possible from week 4 to 9 of gestation.
- An accurate prediction of delivery date from gestational aging is of critical importance to provide a prompt assistance to parturition, to properly manage a prolonged gestation, and to plan an elective cesarean section.
- Normal gestation is assumed to be 64–66 days from the LH surge in the bitch, and 65 days from the LH surge induced in the queen.

EQUIPMENT

- Ultrasonographic machine, B-mode scanning, equipped with a micro-convex or linear probe, frequency 5–13 MHz, depending on the bitch/queen size.

PROCEDURES

- Depending on the gestational age, different parameters can be measured.
- The most suitable ultrasonographic parameters for accurate gestational aging are: the inner chorionic cavity (ICC) in early pregnancy (4–5 weeks of gestation) and the biparietal diameter (BP) in advanced pregnancy (5–9 weeks of gestation).
- Regardless of the parameter considered, taking more than one measurement for the same structure in multiple fetuses during the examination, and calculating the overall mean value, improves accuracy.
- For some parameters different formulas are needed depending on the size of the bitch:
  - Small size 4–10 kg.
  - Medium size 11–30 kg.
  - Large size over 30 kg.

Blackwell's Five-Minute Veterinary Consult Clinical Companion: Small Animal Endocrinology and Reproduction, First Edition. Edited by Deborah S. Greco and Autumn P. Davidson. © 2017 John Wiley & Sons, Inc. Published 2017 by John Wiley & Sons, Inc.
Companion Website: www.fiveminutevet.com/endocrinology

- The parameters measured may be expressed in centimeters (cm) or millimeters (mm), depending on the formula applied.
- The gestational aging obtained by the application of the equations proposed may be expressed as:
  - Days before parturition (DBP) – negative number.
  - Days of gestation (DG) – positive number.

Early Pregnancy

- ICC: Mean of two orthogonal inner diameters obtained on a transverse section of the embryonic vesicle (from one side of the trophoblastic decidual reaction to the other) (Fig. 65.1):
  - Small-size bitches: DBP = (ICC, in mm – 68.68)/1.53.
  - Medium-size bitches: DBP = (ICC, in mm – 82.13)/1.8.
  - Queens: DBP = (ICC, in mm – 62.03)/1.1.
- Crown–rump length (CRL): Distance between the most rostral point of the fetal crown to the caudal edge of the perineum (Fig. 65.2):
  - Bitches: DG = (3 × CRL, in cm) + 27.
  - Queens: DG = (2.0087 × CRL, in mm) – 31.43.
- Other parameters, such as placental thickness and placental length, have been proposed for the determination of gestational age; however, the accuracy obtained is low.

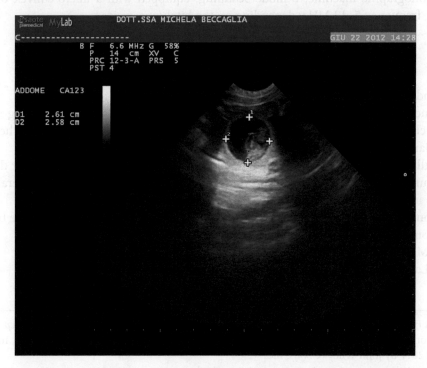

■ **Fig. 65.1.** Inner chorionic cavity (gestational sac diameter) measurements shown in dorsoventral (1) and lateromedial (2).

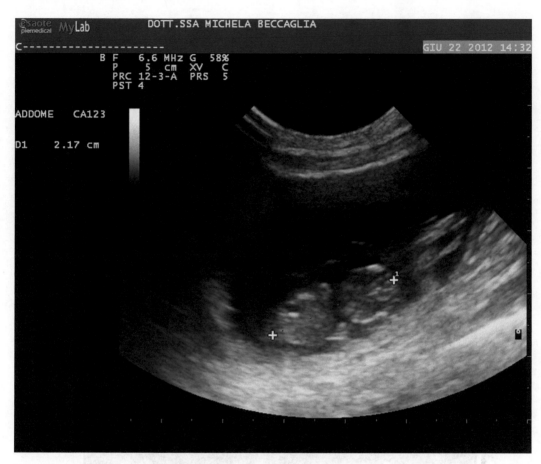

■ **Fig. 65.2.** Cursors shown measuring the CRL of a fetus.

Advanced Pregnancy

■ BP: distance between the two parietal bones that, in the correct scan need to be parallel, obtained on the longitudinal section of the fetal head (Fig. 65.3):
- Small-size bitches: DBP = (BP, in mm − 25.11)/0.61.
- Medium-size bitches: DBP = (BP, in mm − 29.18)/0.7.
- Queens: DBP = (BP, in mm − 23.39)/0.47.

■ BD: Mean of the two diameters made at 90° angles in the transverse plane at the level of fetal liver and stomach (Fig. 65.4):
- Bitches: DG = (7 × BD, in cm) + 29.
- Queens: DG = (11 × BD, in cm) + 21.

■ Other parameters, such as heart and head diameter, have been proposed for the determination of gestational age; however, the accuracy obtained is low or the formula proposed is difficult to apply (exponential, logarithmic calculation).

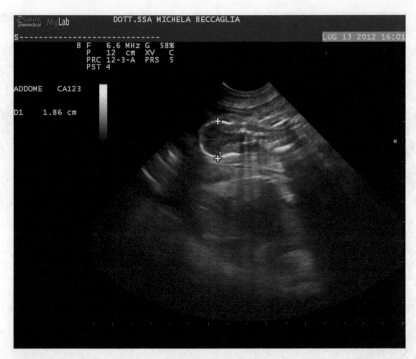

■ **Fig. 65.3.** Cursors shown measuring the BP diameter of a fetal skull.

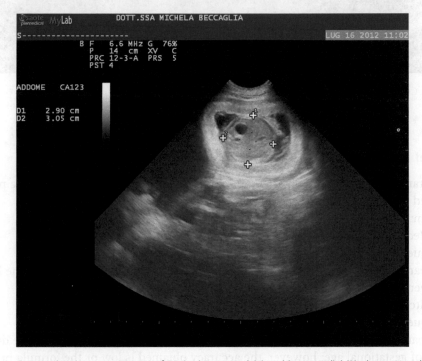

■ **Fig. 65.4.** Cursors showing measurement of BD in dorsoventral (1) and lateromedial (2) planes. Note hypoechoic oval structure (stomach) and hepatic parenchyma localizing site for measurement.

COMMENTS

Expected Results and Difficulties

ICC

- Accuracy (±1 day) of the prediction of parturition is approximately 77% in small-size and medium-size bitches, and 75% in queens.
- The accuracy of gestational aging through ICC measurement is not affected by litter size or fetal sex ratio (in terms of prevalence of males/females in the litter).
- High accuracy is obtained at weeks 4 and 5 of pregnancy, whereas after the 5th week of gestation the elongation of ICC leads to a more difficult measurement of structure and a lower accuracy.
- In bitches up to 40 kg body weight the medium-size dog formula can be applied to obtain a reasonably accurate prediction of parturition.

CRL

- The CRL is highly correlated with gestational age, and can be best visualized until approximately 25 days before parturition.
- After 45 days of gestation, flexion of the fetus, both laterally and dorso-ventrally, hinder CRL measurement. Moreover, the overlapping of other fetuses and fetal length that exceeds the size of the sector image field make this measurement increasingly difficult to obtain.

BP

- Accuracy (±1 day) of prediction of delivery is 75%, 63%, and 64% in small-size bitches, medium-size bitches, and queen, respectively; accuracy at ±2 days, is 88%, 81%, and 86%, respectively.
- Accuracy is not affected by the fetal sex ratio, but a higher accuracy is obtained in a normal litter size (number of newborns within one standard deviation of the mean: small-size bitches, 2–6 pups; medium-size bitches, 5–9 pups).
- Accuracy (±1 day) based on BP measurement is significantly higher at weeks 5 and 6 of pregnancy than after the 6th week, whereas with accuracy ±2 days of the prediction is high up to the 8th week of gestation.
- Close to term, the overlapping of multiple fetuses in the same ultrasonographic image field renders the measurement of BP more difficult and thus less accurate.
- Difficulties in performing ultrasonographic gestational aging in toy and giant dogs are reported; specific formulas or correction factors for these categories of animal need to be studied.

Abbreviations

ICC = inner chorionic cavity
OUD = outer uterine diameter

BP = biparietal diameter
CRL = crown-rump length
BD = body diameter
LH = luteinizing hormone
DBP = days before parturition
DG = days of gestation

See Also

Caesarean Section Elective and Emergency
Dystocia

Suggested Reading

Beccaglia, M., Luvoni, G.C. (2012) Prediction of parturition in dogs and cats: accuracy at different gestational ages. *Reprod. Domest. Anim.*, 47 (Suppl. 6), 1–3.

Luvoni, G.C., Beccaglia, M. (2006) The prediction of parturition date in canine pregnancy. *Reprod. Domest. Anim.*, 41, 27–32.

Mattoon, J.S., Nyland, T.G. (2002) Ovaries and Uterus, in *Small Animal Diagnostic Ultrasound*, 2nd edition (eds T.G. Nylan, J.S. Mattoon), Saunders, Philadelphia, pp. 231–249.

Michel, E., Spörri, M., Ohlerth, S., *et al.* (2011) Prediction of parturition date in the bitch and queen. *Reprod. Domest. Anim.*, 46, 926–932.

Author: Michela Beccaglia DVM, PhD, DECAR

Chapter 66

Unusual Thyroid Disorders (Feline Hypothyroidism, Canine Hyperthyroidism)

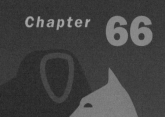

DEFINITION

Feline hypothyroidism – low to non-existent circulating levels of serum thyroxine caused by failure of the thyroid gland to secrete hormone, or failure of the pituitary gland to secrete thyroid-stimulating hormone.

Canine hyperthyroidism – high circulating levels of serum thyroxine caused by a thyroid tumor (usually adenoma), or by feeding of exogenous thyroid tissue (treats, food).

ETIOLOGY/PATHOPHYSIOLOGY

Feline Hypothyroidism

- Acquired hypothyroidism is most commonly associated with radioactive iodine therapy, surgery or medical treatment for hyperthyroidism. Rarely, lymphocytic (autoimmune) thyroiditis similar to that seen in dogs with hypothyroidism is observed.
- Congenital hypothyroidism in cats is more common than acquired and may be caused by aplasia or hypoplasia of the thyroid gland, thyroid ectopia, dyshormonogenesis, maternal goitrogen ingestion, maternal radioactive iodine treatment, iodine deficiency (endemic goiter), hypopituitarism, isolated thyrotropin deficiency, hypothalamic disease, or isolated TRH deficiency.

Canine Hyperthyroidism

- Thyroid tumor (rare, usually adenoma).
- Exogenous thyroid tissue in food or treats (usually raw).

Blackwell's Five-Minute Veterinary Consult Clinical Companion: Small Animal Endocrinology and Reproduction, First Edition. Edited by Deborah S. Greco and Autumn P. Davidson. © 2017 John Wiley & Sons, Inc. Published 2017 by John Wiley & Sons, Inc.
Companion Website: www.fiveminutevet.com/endocrinology

SIGNALMENT/HISTORY

- Congenital feline hypothyroidism is seen in young animals usually less than 1 year of age.
- Acquired feline hypothyroidism is seen in older cats (more than 8 years of age) treated for hyperthyroidism.
- Immune-mediated hypothyroidism is seen in young to middle-age cats.

Risk Factors

- Feline hypothyroidism – radioactive or surgical treatment for hyperthyroidism.
- Canine hyperthyroidism – feeding of treats or pet foods containing thyroid tissue.

CLINICAL FEATURES

Feline

- Disproportionate dwarfism (see Fig. 66.1).
- Large birth weight.
- Weakness.
- Mental dullness.

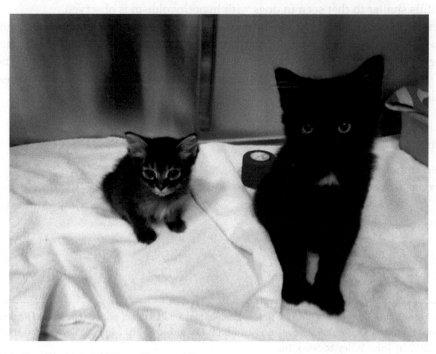

■ **Fig. 66.1.** Hypothyroid dwarf kitten with normal littermate.

- Hypotonia.
- Delayed dental eruption.
- Lethargy.
- Inappetence.
- Constipation.
- Dermatopathy.

Canine

- Polydipsia/polyuria.
- Hyperexcitability.
- Polyphagia.
- Behavior changes.

Physical Examination Findings

Feline
- Hypothermia.
- Abdominal distension.
- Macroglossia.
- Midface hypoplasia, broad nose, and a large protruding tongue.
- Effusions of the body cavities (myxedematous fluid accumulation).
- Retained puppy haircoat.
- Thinning of the haircoat.
- Ataxia.

Canine
- Hyperactivity.
- Tachycardia.
- Seizures.

 # DIFFERENTIAL DIAGNOSIS

Feline

- Congenital hypothyroidism
- Pituitary dwarfism
  - PSS
- Congenital renal disease
  - FIP
- Acquired hypothyroidism

Canine

- Other causes of polyuria/polydypsia (PU/PD), such as Cushing's disease, diabetes inspidus (DI), etc.
- Other causes of liver enzyme elevation (hepatopathy, etc.).
- Other causes of hyper excitability (pheochromocytoma).

 DIAGNOSTICS

Minimum Data Base

Feline
- Mild normocytic normochromic anemia.
- Hypercholesterolemia, hypercalcemia.

Canine
- Polycythemia (increased PCV).
- Increased liver enzymes.

Radiographs
- Feline congenital hypothyroidism – Epiphyseal dysgenesis.

Thyroid Hormone Measurement

Feline hypothyroidism
- Low normal or low TT4 and or FT4 for the age of the kitten.
- Normal kittens aged 5–6 weeks, have serum total thyroxine (TT4) two- to threefold higher than normal adults.
- Low FT4 in a cat.
- Endogenous cTSH – high.

Canine hyperthyroidism
- High TT4 and FT4.
- Low endogenous cTSH.

Pathological Findings

Feline
- Goiter – enlarged thyroid gland filled with colloid.
- Lymphocytic thyroiditis.
- Congenital aplasia.

Canine
- Thyroid adenoma.

THERAPEUTICS

Drug(s) of Choice

- Levothyroxine 0.1 mg per cat once or twice (kittens) daily.

Precautions/Interactions

- Avoid generic levothyroxine.

Alternative Drugs

- Not applicable.

Diet

- Canine – discontinue diet or treats containing thyroid tissue.

Surgical Considerations

- Not applicable.

COMMENTS

Client Education

Feline
- Life-long therapy will be required in congenital and autoimmune hypothyroidism.
- 50% of cats with acquired hypothyroidism will revert to normal within 6 months to a year.

Canine
- Feed commercial pet food and treats from major manufacturers.

Patient Monitoring

- Growth should normalize in congenital cases.
- Every month initially and then every 6 months.

Prevention/Avoidance

Feline
- Avoid goitrogens.
- Adjust radioactive iodine dosage and tailor to individual patient.

Canine

- Avoid raw or homemade treats and pet food.

Possible Complications

- Feline – iatrogenic hyperthyroidism.

Expected Course and Prognosis

- Feline – excellent with thyroid hormone replacement.

Synonyms

- Cretinism (congenital hypothyroidism).
- Hamburger toxicosis (hyperthyroidism from meat).

Abbreviations

TT4 = thyroxine.
FT4 = free thyroxine.
cTSH = canine thyroid-stimulating hormone.

See Also

Canine hypothyroidism
Feline hyperthyroidism

Suggested Reading

Greco, D.S. (2006) Diagnosis of congenital and adult-onset hypothyroidism in cats. *Clin. Tech. Small Anim. Pract.*, **21** (1), 40–44.

Köhler, B., Stengel, C., Neiger, R. (2012) Dietary hyperthyroidism in dogs. *J. Small Anim. Pract.*, **53**, 182–184.

Author: Deborah S. Greco DVM, PhD, DACVIM

Chapter 67

Vulvovaginal Malformations

DEFINITION

- Altered vulvovaginal anatomy due to congenital or acquired conditions.

ETIOLOGY/PATHOPHYSIOLOGY

Congenital

- Congenital vulvar and vaginal malformations are associated with errors during embryological development. These developmental abnormalities arise from: (i) incomplete fusion of the Müllerian ducts (elongated vertical vaginal septum, double vagina); (ii) incomplete perforation of the hymen (circumferential vaginovestibular strictures, discrete vaginal septae); and (iii) imperfect joining of the vaginal folds to the genital swelling (vestibulovulvar strictures or hypoplasia). Other reported abnormalities include recessed vulvas and os clitoridis.

Acquired

- Vulvovaginal malformations are common sequelae to many primary and secondary vulvovaginal and urogenital conditions. These can include: vaginal trauma (mating injuries, dystocia trauma, traumatic insult); exogenous estrogen exposure (human transdermal estrogen-based therapeutic products will result in vulval enlargement with or without serosanguinous discharge); neoplasia (leiomyomas and leiomyosarcomas are the two most common benign and malignant vaginal tumors reported, respectively); vaginal hyperplasia; vaginal prolapse. Other reported acquired causes include: transmissible venereal tumors, rectovaginal fistulas, foreign bodies, and polyps. Primary or secondary vaginitis can cause vulval enlargement and associated vaginal discharge.

Blackwell's Five-Minute Veterinary Consult Clinical Companion: Small Animal Endocrinology and Reproduction, First Edition. Edited by Deborah S. Greco and Autumn P. Davidson. © 2017 John Wiley & Sons, Inc. Published 2017 by John Wiley & Sons, Inc. Companion Website: www.fiveminutevet.com/endocrinology

Systems Affected

- Reproductive – interference with natural mating, artificial insemination and whelping. Frequently associated with a concurrent vaginitis.
- Urinary – may have concurrent ascending urinary tract infection or incontinence.
- Skin/Exocrine – perivulvar dermatitis secondary to vaginal discharge, urinary incontinence or persistent licking.

Incidence/Prevalence

- Incidence is unknown, as no clinical signs may be apparent in many patients unless used for breeding. Vaginal septa and circumferential strictures are the most commonly reported abnormalities; vaginal septa incidence reported as 0.03%. A slight narrowing at the vestibulovaginal junction is normal.

 # SIGNALMENT/HISTORY

Species

- Dogs and cats.

Breed Predilections

- No specific breeds, but a hereditary component may exist for congenital vulvar and vaginal malformations associated with errors during embryological development. Reported incidence of os clitoridis is 3% in American Cocker Spaniel, and 2% in German Shorthair Pointers.

Mean Age and Range

- Vaginal septa 2.4 years; vestibulovaginal strictures 4.6 years. Many of these conditions are asymptomatic, and only present when an owner begins breeding an intact affected bitch for the first time. Congenital lesions typically present in young dogs. Acquired lesions can present at any age in post-pubertal dogs. Neoplastic conditions have a mean age of presentation of 10 years.

 # CLINICAL FEATURES

Historic Findings

- A history of chronic vaginitis (including chronic discharge, chronic licking of vulva and attracting male dogs), inability to breed naturally or refuses natural mating, urinary incontinence, chronic urinary tract infection, dystocia, infertility, ambiguous external genitalia, perivulvar dermatitis.

Physical Examination Findings

- Serosanguinous to mucopurulent vaginal discharge; perivular dermatitis; hypoplastic vulva; or normal external physical findings.

Causes and Risk Factors

- Congenital.
- Inflammatory.
- Hormonal.
- Traumatic.
- Neoplastic.
- Unknown hereditary component.

 # DIFFERENTIAL DIAGNOSIS

- Intersex condition – differentiated by karyotype analysis.
- Vaginitis – differentiated by vaginal cytology, vaginal culture and cytology, vaginoscopy and positive contrast vaginography.
- Urinary tract infection – differentiated by vaginal cytology and urinary sample collected by cystocentesis.
- Pyometra – differentiated by CBC, biochemistry, ultrasonography and radiographic examination.
- Exogenous estrogen – vaginal cytology and client history.

 # DIAGNOSTICS

Diagnostic Procedures

- The order of the vaginal diagnostics is important. Vaginal culture and sensitivity testing should be performed first, as the other techniques will lead to possible contamination of the vagina, resulting in potentially erroneous culture and sensitivity results.

Vaginal Culture and Sensitivity

- Vaginal culture is not diagnostic for any of the congenital conditions. Culture results most frequently observed are *E. coli*, *Streptococcus* spp. and *Staphylococcus intermedius*, which can be normal flora of both the caudal and cranial vagina. A vaginal culture rarely yields heavy growth of a single organism; however, such a result may be indicative of a pathogenic organism. Procedure preferably performed with a guarded culturette.

Vaginal Cytology

- Vaginal cytology may be indicative of a low-grade vaginitis. Cytology may contain parabasal cells, neutrophils (low to large numbers, both regular and degenerate neutrophils), bacteria (both free and phagocytosed), and mucoid debris. Vaginal cornification (superficial and anu-clear cells) is representative of elevated serum estrogen (endogenous or exogenous source), and their presence should be sufficient to categorize the stage of estrus (Fig. 67.1). The presence of low numbers of neutrophils is normal except during late pro-estrus and all of estrus. Vaginal cytology is not diagnostic for any of the congenital conditions. Transmissible venereal tumor cells are round, with a large nucleus:cytoplasm ratio, and chromatin clumping; numerous nucleoli and mitotic figures are commonly seen (Fig. 67.2). Cells do not readily exfoliate with other types of vaginal neoplasia.

Digital Vaginal Examination

- A lubricated gloved finger will frequently locate septa and strictures, as they are most frequently located at the vestibulovaginal junction, just cranial to the urethral papilla. This can be a painful procedure and should be performed under sedation or general anesthesia, especially in non-estrous or small-breed females.

Vaginal Speculum

- Vaginal speculum or otoscope examination is not as sensitive as digital palpation, as most otoscopes are narrower than a finger. Insertion of the speculum may pass tissue bands and give a false-negative interpretation of vaginal strictures, or even hymenal remnants. Also, in large breeds it is possible that vaginal abnormalities cannot be reached or visualized by palpation and speculum examination.

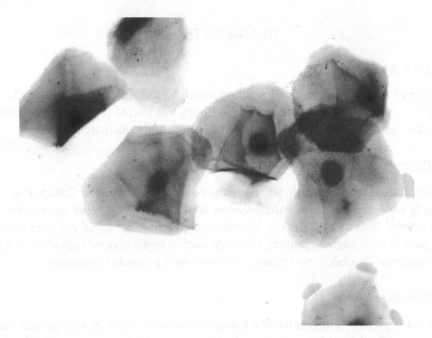

■ **Fig. 67.1.** Superficial vaginal epithelial cells typical of estrogen influence.

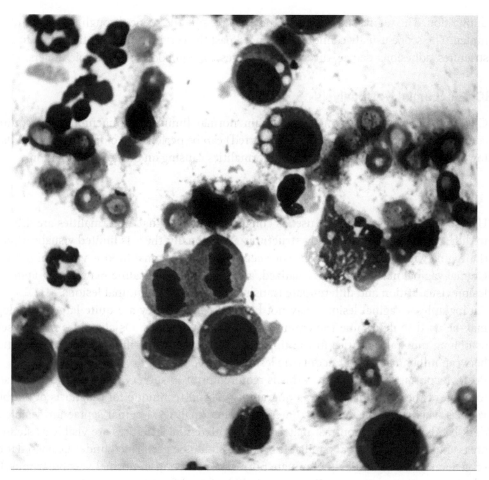

■ **Fig. 67.2.** Vaginal cytology, transmissible venereal turmor.

Vaginoscopy

■ Visualization of the vagina is possible using rigid or flexible cystoscopes. Recommended sizes include 2.7-mm diameter scope, 18 cm long with a 14.5 Fr outer sheath for dogs weighing less than 10 kg. For larger-sized dogs, a 4-mm diameter cystoscope, 32 cm long with a 17 Fr outer sheath should be sufficient. It is recommended that vaginoscopy is performed under general anesthesia. The dog may be positioned in dorsal, lateral or sternal recumbency. Sterile techniques should be practiced including, minimizing fecal contamination, sterile gloves and sterile lubricants. The vagina can be distended with sterile, warm isotonic saline or lactated Ringers solution. Similar to palpation and speculum examination, abnormalities can be missed as they are commonly located just cranial to the urethral papilla. The vestibulovaginal junction should be a smooth, continuous, symmetrical opening, and a smaller minimally distensible opening would suggest a vestibulovaginal stricture. The presence of two or more openings would suggest a diagnosis of vaginal septa or vaginal duplication. The vagina should be examined by passing the scope through the center of the lumen. The scope usually cannot be advanced past the cervix. Abnormalities noted include strictures, adhesions, septae, diverticulae, masses, foreign bodies and ectopic ureters.

CBC/Biochemistry/Urinalysis

- CBC and biochemistry are usually within normal limits for congenital and acquired conditions. Urinalysis (cystocentesis preferred) can be performed to diagnose a secondary lower urinary tract infection, due to abnormalities causing an outflow obstruction.

Imaging

- Ultrasound – this is of limited use, as congenital vulvovaginal abnormalities are difficult to differentiate from surrounding structures. Additionally, there is limited visualization of the vagina within the bony pelvis. The accumulation of vaginal fluid is visible, if present. Cranial vaginal masses can be visualized, and the infusion of saline may further augment lesion visualization and differentiate transluminal from extraluminal lesions.
- Radiography – vaginal lesions may not be visible unless they are quite large. Radiology may be used to determine the cranial extent of large masses. Os clitorides may present as oblong mineral opacities in the tip of the ventral vulva. Radiographic differentiation between inflammatory and neoplastic lesions is not possible.
- Positive-contrast vaginography – this is required prior to surgery to assess the extent and location of the abnormality. A vaginogram is a useful technique for diagnosis of double-vaginas, vaginal septae, and circumferential abnormalities. Vaginal septae are visible as dark bands within the contrast material. Circumferential strictures are visible as stenotic areas cranial to the urethral papilla. Procedure should be performed under heavy sedation or general anesthesia to help eliminate normal constriction of normal vestibular muscles which may mimic strictures. Patients should be fasted for 24 hours and given an enema 2 hours before the procedure. Iodinated contrast media (1 ml/kg) is passed through a Foley catheter, avoiding overdistension of the vagina. Vaginography is indicated when examining animals with vulvar hypoplasia as insertion of digits and instruments can be painful. It can also be useful to identify polyps, tumors, and rectovaginal fistulas.

 ## THERAPEUTICS

Appropriate Healthcare

- No treatment is required for congenital malformations or os clitorides in a bitch without clinical signs.

Non-Surgical

- Manual dilation, either digitally or with a smooth rigid object, can be attempted in patients that have an imperforate hymen or mild vestibulovaginal stenosis. This technique can be performed either in a sedated patient over several treatments, or with a single application of pressure in an anesthetized patient to achieve maximal dilation. This technique has variable success rates reported, and may only result in a reduction in clinical signs. It is unlikely to resolve moderate or severe stenosis. Some vaginal septae can be broken down by digital palpation.

Surgery

- Surgical correction of vertical vaginal bands or stenotic defects is indicated when urogenital signs persist or the intended use of the bitch is breeding. Larger vaginal septae (not possible to break down by digital manipulation) can be surgically removed via increased surgical access through an episiotomy (extending from the dorsal vulvar commissure towards the anus, along the median raphe), and can give increased access to 2 cm of the cranial vagina. Broad-based or elongated septae may have significant vascularization and require ligation. Circumferential strictures can be removed by resection of the stenotic area, vaginoplasty and vaginectomy. In mild cases, the ventral 180° of the stricture (3 to 9 o'clock) can be removed to allow adequate drainage. For short segmental hypoplastic areas (<1.5 cm) a vaginovestibuloplasty can be performed, with the dorsal incision extended through the stenotic area. The vaginal wall is subsequently closed in a T-pattern to increase the diameter of the vaginal lumen. Post-surgical dilatation of the vaginal vault may be required to prevent recurrence of vaginal strictures. An episioplasty can be performed to exteriorize the vulva in diagnosed cases of retracted or infantile vulva from under perineal skin folds (see Chapter 17).
- The surgical treatment of vaginal tumors consists of vaginal ablation to the external urethral orifice, and it is recommended that a concurrent ovariohysterectomy be performed to remove the source of steroid hormones that may have an underlying influence. Complete ablation may be difficult due to the intrapelvic location of the vagina. It should also be considered for cranial vaginal strictures and the unsuccessful removal vestibulovaginal abnormalities via episiotomy.
- Ovariohysterectomy or ovariectomy should be considered for bitches of no breeding value with clinical signs that are only apparent during estrus. It should also be considered as there may be a hereditary component associated with congenital conditions.

Client Education

- Depending on the degree of vaginal obstruction, a bitch can be bred naturally or by artificial insemination. A bitch with a diagnosed vulvovaginal abnormality requiring artificial insemination should be watched closely for dystocia; evaluation the week before the end of gestation is advised. Elective cesarean section, based on prior ovulation timing, tocodynamometry (uterine monitoring) or a drop in serum progesterone level to <2.0 ng/ml, should be considered for affected bitches. Normal parturition may be possible if there is sufficient relaxation of the vaginal walls at term gestation. It is unknown whether congenital malformations are hereditary.

Medication

Drug(s) of Choice

- Treatment with antibiotics alone should only be used if a vaginal culture result has a heavy growth of one or two organisms and there is cytological evidence of inflammation. Antibiotic selection should be based on sensitivity results.

Contraindications/Precautions

- As there is a possibility of a hereditary component to congenital anomalies, an accurate familial history should be collected and ovariohysterectomy should be considered.

Alternative Therapy

- Repeated manual dilation and application of corticosteroid creams may prevent reoccurrence of stenotic lesions and caudal dorsoventral bands and adhesions.

Patient Monitoring

- After treatment the bitch should be monitored for signs of vaginal discharge and urinary incontinence.

Prevention/Avoidance

- Unknown hereditary component.

Possible Complications

- Postoperative complications include adhesion formation, urinary tract infections and vaginitis. Treated patients that are used for breeding should be monitored closely for dystocia.

Expected Course and Prognosis

- Depends on the severity of disease. Prognosis is good for short dorsoventral bands and caudal strictures and adhesions. Prognosis is guarded for vaginal hypoplasia and segmental aplasia, or cranially located strictures and adhesions.

 COMMENTS

Associated Conditions

- Urinary tract infections.
- Vaginitis.
- Urinary incontinence.

Age-Related Factors

▪ Congenital conditions more frequently reported in young females. Neoplastic vaginal conditions have a mean age at presentation of 10.8 to 11.2 years.

See Also

Episioplasty/Vulvaplasty in the Bitch

Suggested Reading

Root, M.V., Johnston, S.D., Johnston, G.R. (1995) Vaginal septa in dogs: 15 cases (1983–1992). *J. Am. Vet. Med. Assoc.*, **206**, 56–58.

Crawford, J.T., Adams, W.M. (2002) Influence of vestibulovaginal stenosis, pelvic bladder, and recessed vulva on response to treatment for clinical signs of lower urinary tract diseases in dogs: 38 cases (1990–1999). *J. Am. Vet. Med. Assoc.*, **221**, 995.

Burk, R.L., Feeney, D.A. (eds) (2003) The abdomen, in *Small Animal Radiology and Ultrasonography*. Saunders, Philadelphia, pp. 427–432.

Kutzler, M., Keller, G.G., Smith, F. (2012) Os clitoridis incidence on radiographs submitted for coxofemoral dysplasia evaluations. Proceedings of the 7th International Symposium on Canine and Feline Reproduction, Whistler, Canada.

Feldman, E.C., Nelson, R.W. (eds) (2004) Vaginal Defects, Vaginitis and Vaginal Infections, in *Canine and Feline Endocrinology and Reproduction*. Saunders, Philadelphia, pp. 901–918.

Wykes, P.M., Olson, P.N. (2002) Vagina, Vestibule, and Vulva, in *Textbook of Small Animal Surgery* (ed. D. Slatter), Saunders, Philadelphia, pp. 1502–1510.

Purswell, B.J. (2010) Vaginal disorders, in *Textbook of Veterinary Internal Medicine* (eds S.J. Ettinger, E.C. Feldman), Saunders, Philadelphia, pp. 1929–1933.

Authors: David Beehan MVB MS DACT, Sarah K. Lyle DVM, PhD, DACT

Index

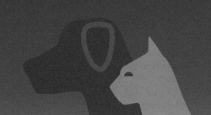